LABORATORY AND DIAGNOSTIC TESTING IN AMBULATORY CARE

A Guide for Health Care Professionals

4E

MARTI GARRELS, MSA, MT (ASCP), CMA (AAMA)

Medical Assisting Program Consultant
Retired Medical Assisting Program Director,
Lake Washington Institute of Technology
Kirkland, Washington

T0332102

ELSEVIER

ELSEVIER

3251 Riverport Lane
St. Louis, Missouri 63043

LABORATORY AND DIAGNOSTIC TESTING IN AMBULATORY CARE: ISBN: 978-0-323-53223-5
A GUIDE FOR HEALTH CARE PROFESSIONALS

Notices

Practitioners and researchers must always rely on their own experience and knowledge in evaluating and using any information, methods, compounds or experiments described herein. Because of rapid advances in the medical sciences, in particular, independent verification of diagnoses and drug dosages should be made. To the fullest extent of the law, no responsibility is assumed by Elsevier, authors, editors or contributors for any injury and/or damage to persons or property as a matter of products liability, negligence or otherwise, or from any use or operation of any methods, products, instructions, or ideas contained in the material herein.

Previous editions copyrighted 2015, 2011, and 2006.

Library of Congress Control Number: 2018949818

Director, Private Sector Education Content: Kristin Wilhelm
Content Development Manager: Lisa Newton
Content Development Specialist: Laura Klein and Erin Garner
Publishing Services Manager: Julie Eddy
Project Manager: Abigail Bradberry
Design Direction: Amy Buxton

Printed in India

Last digit is the print number: 9   8   7   6   5

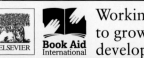

Bryan Edmonds, MBA, RMA(AMT), EMT
Medical Assisting Instructor/Program Coordinator
Milwaukee Area Technical College
Milwaukee, Wisconsin

Pamela Harvey MSN, RN
Instructor
North Florida Technical College
Starke, Florida
Adjunct Instructor for Health Science
Santa Fe College
Gainesville, Florida

Starra Herring, BSAH, BSHA, CMA (AAMA)-MA, AHI
Medical Assisting Program Director & Practicum Coordinator
MOA Program Director
Medical Billing and Coding Program Director
Stanly Community College
Locust, North Carolina

Judith Kline
Instructor of Medical Assisting
Miami Lakes Educational Center and Technical College
Miami Gardens, Florida

Jillian McDonald, BS, RMA (AMT) EMT, CPT (NHA)
Medical Assisting Program Director
Goodwin College
East Hartford, Connecticut

Pamela B. Primrose, PhD, MLS (ASCP)
Medical Laboratory Program Chair
Ivy Tech Community College
South Bend, Indiana

Samantha Saint-Onge, BBA, CMA
Program Director
Finlandia University
Hancock, Michigan

Bobbi Steelman, MAE, CPhT
Director of Education
Daymar Colleges Group
Bowling Green, Kentucky

Jessica Weinoldt, RT(R)(M)(CMA)
Medical Assistant Instructor
Lancaster County Career and Technology Center
Willow Street, Pennsylvania

PREFACE

This text is designed to provide students with a thorough understanding of the most common procedures and techniques of the current CLIA-waived tests and the cardiopulmonary diagnostic tests as they apply to the ambulatory care setting. The first two chapters provide an introduction to the clinical laboratory and the government regulations for setting up a CLIA-waived laboratory. Chapters 3 through 11, then present a consistent "triad" organization by first focusing on the *fundamental concepts* related to the laboratory procedures presented in each chapter, followed by the *application of the procedures,* and then concluding with *advanced concepts* to stimulate critical thinking. Color coded procedure boxes are integrated throughout with step-by-step instructions that are reinforced with numerous full-color photographs or illustrations. Throughout the text there is also a strong emphasis placed on proper patient interactions, specimen collections, safety, and government compliance. Measurable outcome-based procedure sheets and evaluation forms are provided in the workbook to measure psychomotor and affective (behavioral) competencies. Written exams are provided to measure cognitive (conceptual) competencies.

When writing the workbook and instructor materials, our intention was to provide instructors and health care practitioners with many customizable tools that will help them produce well-trained, qualified allied health professionals who are able to effectively work in the CLIA-waived laboratory setting, and in ambulatory settings where cardiopulmonary tests are performed.

OUTSTANDING FEATURES

An abundant supply of full-color photographs, illustrations, and tables provide powerful visual learning tools that are reinforced in the workbook.

Each of the procedural testing chapters is organized into three sections to bring the reader through progressive levels of learning:

- **Fundamental Concepts:** allows students to "see and understand" the basic human body structures and functions related to each chapter's testing procedures.
- **Procedures:** provides the scientific background of the tests being performed followed by visual step by step procedural figures that coordinate with the student's procedure sheets in the text and in the workbook.
- **Advanced Concepts:** generally involves problem solving and more difficult concepts. This section allows instructors the flexibility to determine the level of additional information the students will need to learn

Laboratory and diagnostic terms are presented at the beginning of each chapter and are boldfaced in blue text throughout the chapter. The terms are also reinforced via the workbook's terminology exercises.

ON-LINE RESOURCES:

Included with the purchase of this book is access to interactive web resources, located at **http://evolve.elsevier.com/Garrels/laboratory**. This on-line resource provides the following:

- Student Handouts, PowerPoint lectures on printable note sheets that are referenced to corresponding text images.
- *Animations and Clinical skills videos* that complement the content in the textbook and give students a chance to interactively engage in learning the material. Topics of the videos range from asepsis, infection control, and sterilization; to collecting and testing urine, blood, and microbiologic specimens; to performing hematology, blood chemistry, immunology, toxicology, and cardiopulmonary tests. The videos provide students the opportunity to visualize the skills being performed prior to performing them in the classroom laboratory.
- *Printable Workbook Log sheets and forms,* taken from the appendix in the workbook. These forms include laboratory maintenance forms, record-keeping logs, procedure check sheets for each test, and generic procedure sheets (if a student's program or a facility uses a method other than what is presented in the textbook), a sample health assessment form, and two student professionalism evaluation forms (for measuring behavioral competencies), and much more.

New to This Edition

Each chapter incorporates new information and updated figures to assist in the learning process. Important additions include the following:

- More than 80 updated pictures and drawings throughout the text.
- New Affective (Behavioral) check-off sheets used when dealing directly with patients.
- Updated butterfly needles used in venipuncture.
- DNA-Probe added to microbiology collection procedures.
- Updated History of Infection Control, and Emerging Infectious Disease in the Microbiology Chapter.
- Electrocardiography and Spirometry each have their own Chapters 10 & 11 (in the triad format: Fundamental Concepts, Procedures, Advanced Concepts).

Workbook for Laboratory and Diagnostic Testing in Ambulatory Care (ISBN 9780323532242)

This valuable learning tool contains measurable outcomes for all the conceptual and competency-based objectives in each chapter in order to fulfill national accreditation standards.

It contains *Affective-Behavioral Skill Competency Check Sheets* for specimen collections and patient instructions, and *Specific Procedure Check Sheets* for each of the laboratory and diagnostic test performed. The testing procedures are organized into *preanalytical*, *analytical*, and *postanalytical* testing phases.

These sheets can be used in the classroom and in clinical laboratory settings to verify individual competency that meets the "Good Laboratory Practice" criteria for quality assurance. In this new edition, the *workbook appendix* includes useful quality control log sheets, lab maintenance log sheets, report forms, a sample health screening assessment form, and two sample student/employee professional evaluation forms. These forms provide all the necessary documentation needed to prove laboratory quality assurance, safety compliance, and proper charting of test results.

TEACH Instructor's Resources for *Laboratory and Diagnostic Testing in Ambulatory Care,* located on the Evolve site at http://evolve.elsevier.com/Garrels/laboratory

The *TEACH Instructor's Resource Manual* was created to provide instructors or CLIA-waived lab supervisors with a wealth of material needed to run a successful class and/or clinical laboratory. All the materials have been "field-tested" to help ensure the accuracy and quality of material. This valuable tool is available on-line in Word document format, so that instructors have the ability to edit and update the files to suit their own needs.

The *TEACH Instructor's Resource Manual* on Evolve contains:

- TEACH lesson plans to help you prepare for class and make full use of the rich array of ancillaries and resources that come with your textbook. They are organized into easily understandable sections—Instructor Preparation, Student Preparation, the 50-Minute Lesson Plan, an Assessment Plan, and a Laboratory Activities Plan.
- In TEACH, the content covered in each textbook chapter is divided across several lesson plans, each designed to occupy 50 minutes of class time. The consistent time for each lesson plan allows you to re-sequence them in any order to fit your class calendar. And if you are using TEACH lesson plans from multiple Elsevier textbooks, their "building block" timing and design make it especially easy to combine them, even within the same class period.
- Information on how to set up course schedules, grading, record keeping, and so forth.
- Field-tested tips and supplies needed for each chapter.
- Comprehensive PowerPoint lecture slides that include the procedures covered in each chapter. (NOTE: The PowerPoint lectures in note-taking format are also available in the student resources.)
- An image library of all the images found in the text organized by chapter. (NOTE: The procedure images are located at the end of all the text pictures in each chapter.)
- Answer keys to student workbook exercises.
- Interactive electronic skill check-off sheets that will provide a numerical outcome result.
- Test Bank in ExamView format.

ONLINE LEARNING

The wealth of materials provided with this product suite (textbook, Workbook, and Evolve resources for both the student and instructor) also lends itself to being used in an online learning environment. In an online atmosphere, students can read the textbook, fill in their student notes from the PowerPoint printouts on Evolve, and complete their workbook exercises, all at home (and all at their own pace) prior to arriving on campus for their hands-on lab session. Using this method, the face-to-face student-instructor time could be fully devoted to reinforcing the text material, demonstrating the lab skills, and checking out the students in the lab.

ACKNOWLEDGMENTS

I would like to acknowledge the valuable input of all the reviewers, medical assisting educators, and students who have helped to make this fourth edition even better than the previous editions.

I am grateful to all the Elsevier publishers, editors, reviewers, and staff who have personally supported and guided me through this exciting adventure toward this fourth edition: Adrianne Rippinger, Rae Robertson, Katherine Judge, Elizabeth Tinsley, Michael Ledbetter, Susan Cole, Jennifer Bertucci, Jennifer Hermes, David Stein, Jeanne Genz, Kristen Mandava, Jayashree Balasubramaniam, Laura Klein, Abigail Bradberry, and Erin Garner.

It has been a pleasure to see the wonderful talents of my son-in-law and daughter, Zack and Gala Bent, who have graciously provided us with over 200 high-quality, up-to-date procedure photos and drawings during all four editions (with over 80 new figures in this fourth edition). I have also been blessed by the unwavering support from my husband, Mike. Thanks for seeing me through this arduous process!

Marti Garrels, MSA, MT (ASCP), CMA (AAMA)

CONTENTS

PROCEDURES

CHAPTER 1

Introduction to the Laboratory and Safety Training

OBJECTIVES

After completing this chapter, you should be able to do the following:

1. Define and match key terms and abbreviations in this chapter.
2. List the reasons why laboratory tests are ordered and describe how specimens are analyzed.
3. Demonstrate understanding of the types of medical laboratories and their personnel:
   - Describe the organization and function of medical laboratories.
   - Compare the advantages of performing laboratory tests in a physician's office laboratory versus an outside reference laboratory.
   - Identify the educational credentials of various personnel who work in laboratories.
   - Describe the necessary attributes required of the laboratory professional.
4. Identify and use laboratory requisitions and reports with proper documentation and confidentiality.
5. Interpret common metric system values used in laboratory test reporting.
6. Explain the categories of hazards found in medical laboratories.
7. Demonstrate understanding of the Centers for Disease Control and Prevention's (CDC's) Standard Precautions for infection control:
   - Explain the steps involved in the "chain of infection."
- Identify and apply the CDC's latest Standard Precautions for infection control and its recommendations regarding proper hand hygiene.
- Perform a medical hand wash followed by application of personal protective equipment (PPE) and proper removal of PPE.
- Locate Internet sources for updates on CDC and Occupational Safety and Health Administration (OSHA) recommendations regarding laboratory safety.
8. Demonstrate understanding of OSHA regulations and training:
   - Explain the latest OSHA regulations regarding the Bloodborne Pathogens Standard and the Hazard Communication Standard.
   - Identify waste classified as biohazardous and select appropriate containers for disposal.
   - Describe the proper actions that should be taken after exposure to bloodborne pathogens.
   - Complete a mock exposure incident report in the workbook appendix.
   - List and explain the safety rules that must be observed in the laboratory.
   - Identify and note the location of safety equipment, apparel, and safety manuals in the classroom laboratory.
   - Successfully complete a posttest on safety training.
   - Locate Internet sources for updates on OSHA regulations regarding laboratory safety.

KEY TERMS

ambulatory setting: outpatient facility versus hospital or bedridden setting

analyte: the substance being tested, such as glucose or cholesterol in a blood specimen

biohazards: dangers related to exposure to biological substances such as infectious and bloodborne pathogens

bloodborne pathogens: infectious microorganisms that are transmitted by blood or bloody body fluids from an infected host into the blood of a susceptible host via needlesticks or other sharps related injuries, mucous membranes, or open wounds

Bloodborne Pathogens Standard (BBPS): rigorous standard of policies and procedures developed by OSHA to protect employees who work in occupations where they are at risk of exposure to blood or other potentially infectious

materials (OPIMs) (i.e., other body fluids that may contain blood)

CD4 cells: T-lymphocytic white blood cells that fight infections

chemical hazards: dangers related to exposure to toxic, unstable, explosive, or flammable substances

chronic disorders: long-lasting, debilitating conditions

CLIA-waived tests: tests that provide simple, virtually erroneous-free results and no harm to the patient if incorrectly performed and require a minimum amount of judgment and interpretation

clinical laboratory: a facility or an area within a medical setting in which materials or specimens from the human body are examined or analyzed for diagnosis, treatment, and monitoring of disease and disease prevention

coagulation: clotting ability of blood

contaminated: an area that has been in contact with infectious materials or surfaces where infectious organisms may reside

C-reactive protein (CRP): biomarker for inflammation and is useful as a predictor of cardiovascular risk

critical value: a test result far from the reference range (low or high) indicating a threat to a patient's health (also referred to as "panic value")

cross-contamination: transmitting a pathogen from one individual to another

diabetes mellitus: disease caused by the lack of insulin or the inability to regulate blood sugar (glucose) levels

doffing: to take off

donning: putting on

Ebola: a bloodborne virus capable of causing a rare and deadly hemorrhagic disease

engineering controls: methods to protect workers by isolating or removing bloodborne pathogens from the workplace (i.e., biohazard disposal containers, safety devices on needles, and sharps containers)

ergonomic practices: proper movements and conditions that make a worker less prone to work-related injuries

exposure control plan: documented plan provided by a facility to eliminate or minimize occupational exposure to bloodborne pathogens in accordance with OSHA standards

glucose: simple sugar circulating in the blood

Hazard Communication Standard: federal law protecting employees' "right to know" about the dangers of all the hazardous chemicals to which they may be exposed under normal working conditions

health care–associated infections (HACIs or HAIs): disease spread within a health care facility (formerly referred to as nosocomial infections)

hepatitis A virus (HAV): highly contagious virus that enters the body through the gastrointestinal tract and attacks the liver

hepatitis B virus (HBV): most prevalent bloodborne virus that enters body via parental exposure or high-risk sexual activity that attacks the liver: an individual can build a protective resistance against this virus by prior immunization or vaccination

hepatitis C virus (HCV): bloodborne virus that attacks the liver and is very likely to reach the chronic stage later in life

homeostasis: steady state of internal chemical and physical balance

human immunodeficiency virus (HIV): retrovirus that attacks the immune system by destroying the white blood cells known as CD4+ or helper T lymphocytes

laboratory reports: results of laboratory tests that have been ordered

laboratory requisitions: written laboratory orders indicating the tests that should be performed

medical assistants: multiskilled professionals dedicated to assisting in patient care management in medical offices, clinics, and ambulatory care centers

occupational exposure: occurs when blood or other potentially infectious material comes in contact with open skin, eyes, or mucous membranes or by parenteral exposure (through the skin) in the workplace

opportunistic infections: infections that occur because of the body's weakened immune system and thus inability to repel pathogens normally found in the environment

panels or profiles: a series of tests associated with a particular organ or disease

parenteral contact: when blood enters the body through the skin or mucous membrane by means of a needle stick, bite, cut, or abrasion

pathogens: disease-causing microorganisms

patient compliance: a patient's willingness to follow a treatment plan and take an active role in his or her health care

percutaneous: through the skin

physical hazards: dangers related to electricity, fire, weather emergencies, bomb threats, and accidental injuries

polydipsia: excessive thirst

polyphagia: excessive hunger

polyuria: excessive urination

portal of entry: a body opening or break in the skin through which an infectious agent enters the body

portal of exit: the route by which an infectious agent leaves the host's body, such as through the mouth, broken skin, rectum, or body fluids

reference range: the numerical range of analyte values with which the general population will consistently show similar results 95% of the time

reservoir host: an infected person who is carrying an infectious agent (pathogen)

Standard Precautions: CDC recommendations for infection control within health care facilities to prevent transmission of disease through contact with blood, body fluids, or OPIMs

susceptible host: an individual who is unable to defend herself or himself against a pathogen

thrombosis: the formation of internal clots

transient microorganisms: organisms from contaminated objects or infectious patients that adhere to the skin and can be transmitted to others

transmission: the means by which an infectious agent or pathogen is transported from an infected individual to another person by indirect or direct contact

Universal Precautions: assumption that blood or other potentially infectious material from any patient or test kit could be infectious for HIV, HBV, or other bloodborne pathogens

venipuncture: removal of blood from a vein

work practice controls: policies that are recorded, monitored, and evaluated to protect employees from exposure to the pathogens in blood or body fluids

ABBREVIATIONS

CDC: Centers for Disease Control and Prevention
CLIA: Clinical Laboratory Improvement Act
HCAIs or HAIs: health care–associated infections
HHS: Health and Human Services
HMIS: Hazardous Materials Information System
NFPA: National Fire Protective Association
OPIMs: other potentially infectious materials, such as bloody body fluids

OSHA: Occupational Safety and Health Administration
PEP: postexposure prophylaxis; preventive treatment after exposure to blood or OPIMs
POCT: point-of-care testing
POL: physician's office laboratory
PPE: personal protective equipment
SDS: safety data sheets (formerly known as material safety data sheets [MSDS])

To enter the investigative world of medical laboratories, a general understanding of laboratory testing and the various laboratories that perform medical tests on specimens is needed. Then a solid foundation in laboratory safety issues is required before laboratory procedures can be performed in the ambulatory setting (outpatient facility versus hospital or bedridden setting).

❖ INTRODUCTION TO THE CLINICAL LABORATORY

The medical laboratory plays a critical role in patient care. This section provides information on the following:
- Why and how laboratory tests are performed
- Where the tests are performed
- How various medical laboratories are organized
- The people involved in the testing process
- The basic terminology and paperwork used in the laboratory

Purpose of Medical Laboratories

A medical or clinical laboratory is defined as a facility or an area within a medical setting in which materials, or specimens, from the human body are examined or analyzed for the purpose of diagnosis, treatment, and monitoring of disease and disease prevention. The results of the various laboratory tests performed on the specimens give the physician a wealth of information regarding the status of the patient or client.

Why Laboratory Tests Are Ordered

Physicians order laboratory tests for one or more of the three following reasons:

To screen patients for possible disorders. Screening test results are used to determine if a disease or medical condition exists in patients who may not have signs or symptoms of an underlying disease process. These tests are becoming increasingly popular because they can detect potential chronic disorders (long-lasting, debilitating conditions) such as coronary heart disease and diabetes well before irreversible damage occurs. Primary care physician offices and community health centers are encouraged by the latest Medicare policies to participate in screening programs. NOTE: The workbook appendix has a health screening report form that includes the various

screening tests that will be presented throughout the text and in the laboratory sessions.

To establish a diagnosis. Diagnostic test results help the physician identify or confirm a disease or medical condition. These results can significantly affect the medical care and treatment of the patient. Diagnostic tests should be conducted by well-trained individuals and must correlate with other clinical findings (e.g., the patient's medical history and physical examination).

To monitor the patient's condition or treatment. Monitoring test results helps the physician keep track of the patient's specific medical condition or response to treatment on a periodic basis. The following three medical conditions commonly require routine testing to monitor the effects of medication treatments:
- *Patients at risk of heart disease* who are taking cholesterol-lowering medications are checked periodically for levels of cholesterol and liver enzymes. The medication goal is to bring cholesterol levels to less than 200 mg/dL and to determine whether the medication is harming the liver, which would raise the levels of the blood enzymes alanine aminotransferase (ALT) and aspartate aminotransferase (AST) (this is covered in Chapter 6). They may also be tested for C-reactive protein (CRP), which is associated with the risk of a future myocardial infarction (heart attack) and indicates the health status of the patient's cardiovascular system.
- *Patients at risk of forming internal clots* (thrombosis) who are taking anticoagulant medications are checked to see if their blood coagulation (clotting) time is too fast or too slow.
- *Patients with diabetes* have their blood glucose (sugar) levels checked periodically at the office. They also may have their self-monitored blood glucose results interpreted by a physician. In both cases, the physician needs to determine if these patients are maintaining blood glucose levels within the recommended reference range (the numerical range of analyte values with which the general population will consistently show similar results 95% of the time).

Advances in medical instrumentation have allowed the monitoring of all these patients to take place in an ambulatory setting rather than in a hospital or reference laboratory. This allows the physician to see the results immediately while the patient waits and then advise the patient accordingly.

Three General Ways to Analyze Specimens

Medical laboratories analyze specimens in the following three basic ways:

Measuring the levels of analytes compared with reference values. The human body is a remarkable organism, capable of maintaining homeostasis (a steady state of internal chemical and physical balance). This universal ability is seen when a healthy population is tested for the presence of a particular analyte (a substance being tested, such as the level of glucose or cholesterol in a blood specimen). Most of the population tests within a range of similar results. This is referred to as the reference range for that analyte. When disease strikes, a person's homeostatic balance is disrupted, causing the analyte results to fall outside the reference range.

Figure 1.1 is an example of a reference laboratory's comprehensive report for blood tests. Note that the reference range for each analyte tested is listed above the patient's test value. If a test result is far from the reference range, it may be referred to as a critical value or *panic value* (indicating a threat to a patient's health). The laboratory report must mark or highlight the critical result requiring immediate attention. In the figure, Judith Johnson does not have any critical values. But she does have a few values outside of the reference range as indicated with an asterisk (*). A variety of laboratory reports are shown and discussed throughout this text.

Here is an example of a critical value that may be obtained by monitoring the level of a patient's glucose (sugar) analyte and comparing it with its established population's reference range. A physician obtained a variety of abnormal clinical signs and symptoms when examining a female patient—rapid weight loss, lack of energy, polyphagia (excessive hunger), polydipsia (excessive thirst), and polyuria (excessive urination). These symptoms caused the physician to suspect the disease diabetes mellitus (a disease caused by the lack of insulin or the inability to regulate blood sugar levels). The physician then ordered a blood glucose test and received a result of 300 mg/dL (milligrams per deciliter). The population's reference range for blood glucose levels was 70 to 110 mg/dL. The patient's extremely high (critical) glucose result, along with all the other signs and symptoms, indicated that her pancreas was unable to produce the insulin necessary to regulate glucose levels in a homeostatic way. Several tests can be performed to confirm the diagnosis of diabetes such as a second fasting blood glucose, hemoglobin A1C, or a 2-hour postprandial glucose. The physician would then prescribe a course of treatment and continue to monitor the blood glucose levels until the patient's test results returned to the proper reference range.

Observing and detecting abnormal cells under the microscope. Another way to analyze a specimen is to search for abnormal cells or pathogens (disease-causing microorganisms) under the microscope. In the ambulatory setting, this form of testing is generally limited to basic identification of abnormal cells and microorganisms found in urine, blood, or samples taken from infected tissues. Figure 1.2 shows numerous white blood cells and two red blood cells (see arrows) in a urine specimen.

This book discusses some of the normal and abnormal microscopic findings in urine, blood, and microbiology specimens

to highlight their significance. Additional training beyond this text is required to identify and report microscopic findings.

Detecting the presence or absence of an infection. The third way to analyze specimens is to test for the presence of pathogens causing an infection. In the ambulatory setting, increasing numbers of rapid screening tests are available to help the physician identify the presence of common pathogens. Figure 1.3 shows three Rapid Strep test strips: the first strip #1 is before testing, strip #2 shows a positive blue line result and a red control line, and strip #3 shows a no blue line (negative for strep) and a red control line. The red lines on both strips prove the strips are functioning correctly. The test result shown in the middle is positive for streptococcus A, and the test on the right is negative for streptococcus A. *Test kits* (all components of a test packaged together) are available that can detect the presence of bacteria that cause strep throat, peptic ulcers, and Lyme disease as well as the viruses that cause influenza, mononucleosis, and acquired immunodeficiency syndrome (AIDS). NOTE: These are simple screening tests and usually require further complex testing to confirm the diagnosis.

All negative and positive strep screens are sent to the microbiology laboratory for further analysis that includes culture, biochemical, and antibiotic sensitivity testing.

Types of Medical Laboratories and Personnel

The types of medical laboratories range from large, departmentalized institutions to small designated laboratory counters within an ambulatory setting. Personnel in the ambulatory setting interact with staff from all the other types of laboratories and need a basic understanding of how the various laboratories are organized and what types of health care professionals work in each setting.

Reference (or Referral) Laboratories

Reference, or referral, laboratories tend to be the largest laboratories, with specialized departments and extensive state-of-the-art equipment. Figure 1.4 is a sample organizational chart showing the departments typically found in a reference laboratory facility: Specimen Collection and Processing, Urinalysis, Hematology, Chemistry, Immunology/Immunohematology, Microbiology, Pathology, Cytology, Histology, Molecular Diagnostics, and Toxicology.

Reference laboratory professionals
- Pathologists are physicians with medical degrees who have specialized in test methodology and the diagnosis of diseases.
- Medical laboratory scientists and medical technologists have bachelor's degrees or may have a master's degree, are specialists in laboratory testing, and have received one of the following nationally recognized credentials after successfully passing a certification exam: MLS (ASCP) or MT (AMT).
- Medical laboratory technicians have 2-year associate degrees in laboratory training and have received one of the following nationally recognized credentials after successfully passing a certification exam: MLT (ASCP) or MLT (AMT).

LABORATORY REPORT
Biomedical Laboratories, Inc
100 Main Street
Athens, Georgia 30601

DATE REPORTED	DATE RECEIVED	PATIENT NAME—I.D.		PHONE	AGE	SEX
4/12/10	4/11/10	Judith Johnson	08575	(614) 592-1100	26	F

DATE COLLECTED	TIME COLLECTED	HOSPITAL I.D.	REQUISITION NO.	ACCESSION NO.
4/11/10	8:30 AM		91449	1235-G8

CLIENT NAME/ADDRESS	TEST REQUIRED
Woodside Medical Clinic 400 Main Street Athens, Ohio 45701	Comprehensive Metabolic Profile Lipid Profile CBC with Differential

PHYSICIAN	VOLUME	FASTING	PATIENT SS #	COMMENTS
J. Camerson, M.D.		X	248-71-2669	

CHEMISTRY   RENAL   ELECTROLYTES

GLUCOSE 70–110 mg/dL	B.U.N. 7–25 mg/dL	CREATININE 0.6–1.5 mg/dL	BUN/CREAT RATIO 6–20	CALCIUM 8.5–10.8 mg/dL	MAGNESIUM 0.6–1.0 mmol/L	PHOSPHORUS 2.5–4.5 mg/dL	SODIUM 135–147 mmol/L	POTASSIUM 3.5–5.3 mmol/L	CHLORIDE 96–109 mmol/L	CARBON DIOXIDE 21–28 mmol/L	FERRITIN M 20–450 F 8–350 ng/mL
91	24	1.3	18.5	9.8		3.3	140.6	4.45	105	24	

PROTEIN   LIVER

URIC ACID M 3.9–9.0 F 2.7–7.7 mg/dL	TOTAL PROTEIN 6.0–8.5 g/dL	ALBUMIN 3.5–5.5 g/dL	GLOBULIN 2.0–3.5 g/dL	ALB/GLB RATIO 1.0–2.4	TOTAL BILIRUBIN 0.2–1.3 mg/dL	DIRECT BILIRUBIN 0–0.4 mg/dL	ALK. PHOS 25–140 U/L	LD £ 240 U/L	AST (SGOT) £ 40 U/L	ALT (SGPT) £ 45 U/L	GGT M 0–65 F 0–45 U/L
	6.8	4.1	2.8	1.5	0.3		82		29	38	

THYROID   LIPIDS

T_3 UPTAKE 25–35 %	T_4 TOTAL 4.5–12 mg/dL	FTI $(T_3U¥T_4)$ 1.2–4.2	TSH 0.4–6.0 mIU/mL	T_4 FREE 0.70–1.53 ng/dL	T_3 TOTAL 85–205 ng/mL	TOTAL CHOL < 200 mg/dL	HDL CHOL > 40 mg/dL	LDL CHOL < 130 mg/dL	VLDL CHOL 5–40 mg/dL	TRIGLYCERIDES < 150	TOTAL CHOL/ HDL RATIO < 4.5
						158	43	83	32	*160	3.7

HEMATOLOGY

WBC 4.5–11 ¥10^3/mL	RBC M 4.5–6.2 F 4–5.5 ¥10^6/mL	HGB M 14–18 F 12–16 g/dL	HCT M 40–54 F 37–47 %	MCV 80–100 fL	MCH 27–34 pg	MCHC 31–36 %	RDW 11.5–14.5 %	PLATELET COUNT 150–400 ¥10^3/mL	RETICULOCYTE COUNT 0.5–2.5 %	ESR M 0–15 F 0–20 mm/Hr	PROTHROMBIN TIME 9–12 seconds
*12.3	4.27	13.4	39	91	31.3	34.5	13.7	258			

DIFFERENTIAL   SEROLOGY

NEUT 50–70 %	LYMPH 20–35 %	MONO 3–8 %	EOSIN 1–4 %	BASO 0–1 %	SYPHILLIS SCREEN NON- REACTIVE	MONO TEST NEG	RHEUMATOID FACTOR < 1:10	CRP < 0.8 mg/dL	ANTINUCLEAR ANTIBODY < 1:140	BLOOD GROUP	RH_e(D)
*83	*12	3	2	0							

URINALYSIS

APPEARANCE CLEAR	COLOR YELLOW	SP. GRAVITY 1.003–1.030	pH 5.0–8.0	PROTEIN NEG	GLUCOSE NEG	KETONES NEG	BILIRUBIN NEG	BLOOD NEG	NITRATE NEG	UROBILINOGEN < 2	LEUKOCYTE TEST NEG

FIG. 1.1 Blood test report showing the levels of a comprehensive panel of analytes. Compare the patient's results with the reference range found above each of the patient's values. Note the four results that fall outside of their reference ranges. In this report, the triglycerides, white blood cells (WBCs), and neutrophils (neut) are high, and the lymphocytes (lymph) are low. (From Bonewit-West K: *Clinical procedures for medical assistants*, ed 10, St. Louis, 2018, Elsevier.)

• Phlebotomists have undergone training on the job or by completing a phlebotomy training program and have received one of the following nationally recognized credentials after successfully passing a certification exam: PBT (ASCP), RPT (AMT), CPT (ASPT), CPT (NHA), and others.

NOTE: Continuing education is required to maintain certification for many of the certifying agencies.

These teams of laboratory professionals collect, process, and evaluate volumes of tests daily and are heavily regulated by the government to ensure that they produce accurate and reliable test results. It is interesting to note that 80% of final definitive

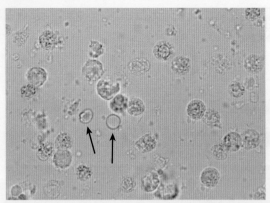

FIG. 1.2 Microscopic analysis of a urine specimen showing numerous granular white blood cells (WBCs) and two red blood cells (just left of center). The abundant WBCs show possible evidence of urinary tract infection. (From Brunzel NA: *Fundamentals of urine & body fluid analysis,* ed 4, St. Louis, 2018, Elsevier.)

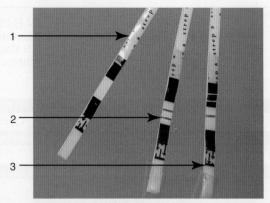

FIG. 1.3 Analyzing the presence of group A streptococcus infection. *Strip #1* is before testing, *strip #2* shows a positive blue line (indicating group A strep was present) and a red control line, *strip #3* shows a no blue line (negative for strep) and a red control line. (Photo by Zack Bent.)

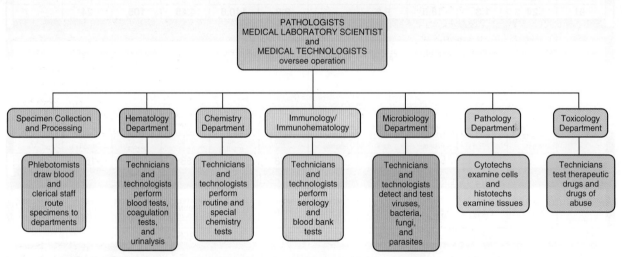

FIG. 1.4 Organizational chart for reference and hospital laboratories showing the departments and individuals involved in testing.

diagnoses come from the results of laboratory tests. The testing methods in each department require extensive training in instrument maintenance, problem solving, test interpretation, and statistical monitoring of test reliability.

Medical offices, health clinics, and hospitals send either their clients or their clients' specimens along with **laboratory requisitions** (laboratory orders indicating the tests that should be performed) to the reference lab. Some insurance companies require a specific reference laboratory for their clients. The client's specimen and requisition must go to the correct reference laboratory for proper insurance reimbursement.

Hospital Laboratories

Hospital laboratories are organized into departments and staffed similarly to reference laboratories. They are involved in diagnostic testing and monitoring the testing of inpatients as well as specimen collection and testing of outpatient specimens from ambulatory settings.

New technology has provided a new approach to patient testing in hospitals called point-of-care testing (**POCT**). Rather than sending specimens to the laboratory, a testing device can be brought directly to the patient's bedside, and accurate results can be immediately obtained. These user-friendly portable tests are administered by nurses and other health care professionals (e.g., critical care technicians) when a patient's medical condition, location, or treatment requires immediate results to determine proper medical care. Figure 1.5 shows a patient's blood hemoglobin numerical readout on a point-of-care hemoglobinometer.

Another popular point-of-care instrument is the i-STAT portable clinical analyzer (PCA) seen in Chapter 6. It uses disposable cartridges to determine a variety of analytes in whole blood. The analyzer stores up to 50 patient records and permits on-screen viewing of test results. It is capable of transmitting the results to a data management system by using infrared signals. Nonlaboratory hospital personnel must be trained to perform POCT properly.

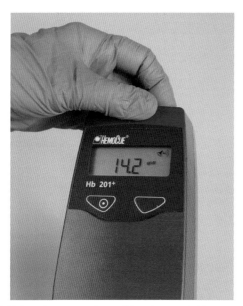

FIG. 1.5 Point-of-care testing with a hemoglobinometer to determine the patient's hemoglobin level. The specimen, taken from the patient's finger, registers the numerical result of 14.2 g/dL, a normal hemoglobin result (see lab report in Figure 1.1). (Photo by Zack Bent.)

The laboratory professionals that work in reference laboratories also work in hospital laboratories.

Ambulatory Care Settings

Unlike the extensive reference laboratories and hospital laboratories, an ambulatory laboratory generally consists of a small, limited space located within a designated area of the physician's office. Ambulatory care settings generally perform tests that have been designated by the government's Clinical Laboratory Improvement Act as CLIA-waived tests (tests that provide simple, unvarying results and require a minimal amount of judgment and interpretation). These government-approved tests provide rapid POCT for screening and monitoring patients in a variety of laboratory areas. The CLIA-waived user-friendly tests most frequently performed in the ambulatory setting that will be presented in this text are the following:
- Routine urinalysis and pregnancy testing
- Basic hematology tests—hemoglobin, hematocrit, sedimentation rate
- Coagulation—prothrombin time and its computed international normalized ratio result
- Chemistry—glucose, hemoglobin A_{1c}, lipid panel, alanine aminotransferase (ALT) and aspartate aminotransferase (AST), electrolytes, blood urea nitrogen (BUN), creatinine, and carbon dioxide (CO_2)
- Immunology/serology—mononucleosis test, *Helicobacter pylori* test, OraQuick test for HIV
- Microbiology—rapid tests for streptococcus A, influenza A/B, rapid urine culture
- Fecal occult blood

The physician's office laboratory (**POL**) has greatly benefited and will continue to benefit from the technical advancements

that have improved and simplified so many medical testing methods.

Advantages of physician's office laboratory testing. Ambulatory patients can now obtain their screening and monitoring test results immediately rather than needing to drive to an external laboratory. Also, the physician's interpretation and therapeutic recommendations can now be given during the same office visit. This has led to better patient care and patient compliance (a patient's willingness to follow a treatment plan and take an active role in his or her own health care).

Advantages of reference and hospital laboratories. Advantages are to provide physicians with the results of the more complex tests. Patient specimens must be sent to these laboratories for the critical test results that provide the physician with sufficient information to make definitive diagnoses. Because of the complexity of these diagnostic tests, they must be performed by individuals with extensive laboratory training, education, and credentialing. A complete description of such knowledge and training is beyond the scope of this book. See laboratory professional list in the Reference Laboratory and Hospital Laboratory sections.

Physician office laboratory personnel. Physician office laboratory personnel include physicians, physician assistants, nurse practitioners, medical assistants, and phlebotomists. Medical assistants are multiskilled professionals who assist in patient care management in medical offices, clinics, and ambulatory care centers. They perform administrative duties and clinical procedures, including performing phlebotomies and the basic CLIA-waived laboratory tests, and diagnostic cardiopulmonary tests. Medical assistants attend a 1- or 2-year program and are nationally credentialed as CMA (AAMA), RMA (AMT), NCMA (NCCT), or CCMA (NHA). There may also be medical laboratory technicians and medical laboratory scientists working in the larger POLs that service multiple physicians.

Table 1.1 lists all the health care professionals involved in medical laboratory and diagnostic testing. They are organized by educational credentials, from medical degrees to associate degrees and technical certificates. (NOTE: Nurses are not listed because laboratory training is not part of their education. They are often trained while working in physicians' offices.)

Attributes of a Laboratory Professional

Everyone performing laboratory tests, regardless of educational background and credentials or place of work, must possess the following personal characteristics to guarantee proper patient care:
- Professional attitude and appearance—discreet, respectful, proper attire, and personal hygiene
- Strong interpersonal communication skills with patients, coworkers, and supervisors
- Motivation, efficiency, commitment, and dedication to serving others in need
- Good organizational skills when setting up a series of tests—ability to manage time and multitask
- Focus, good power of observation, and the ability to pay attention to details during entire process
- Ability to solve problems if test results are unexpected

TABLE 1.1   Personnel Involved in Laboratory Testing

Title	Credential	Years of College Training and Degree	Laboratory Setting
Board-certified pathologists and specialists	MD or DO	8 or more years: medical degree	Reference and hospital laboratories
Primary care physicians and specialists	MD, DO, or ND (naturopathic doctor)	6 or more years: medical degree	Physician's office laboratory and health clinics
Physician Assistant and Nurse Practitioner	PA and NP	6 or more years: master's degree or doctorate degree	Physician's office laboratory and health clinics
Medical Laboratory Scientist, Medical Technologist, Clinical Laboratory Technologist	MLT (ASCP) and MT (AMT)	4 or more years: bachelor's or master's degrees	Reference and hospital laboratories
Medical Laboratory Technician, Clinical Laboratory Technician, Registered Laboratory Technician	MLT (ASCP)* MLT (AMT)	2 years: associate	Reference and hospital laboratories, and physician's office laboratories
Certified or Registered Medical Assistant	CMA (AAMA),* RMA (AMT),* NCMA (NCCT),* and CCMA (NHA)*	1–2 years: technical certificate or associate degree	Physician's office laboratory and ambulatory setting laboratories
Certified and Registered Phlebotomist	PBT (ASCP),* RPT (AMT),* CPT (ASPT),* CPT (NHA),* and others*	1 or less years: technical certificate	All laboratories needing blood specimen collection

*This book is designed to provide these professionals with the necessary information to perform specimen collection and CLIA-waived tests in ambulatory settings with confidence, accuracy, and precision.

- Honesty, integrity, and the ability to admit when unsure of procedure or results
- Manual dexterity, using both hands to accomplish the task
- Ability to perform precise calculations and measurements and neatly document all findings
- Good eyesight and normal color vision for reading color changes on test strips

Laboratory Documentation

Everyone involved in medical laboratory testing and specimen processing must understand and complete the paperwork and the electronic data accurately and completely. The documentation begins with the physician's laboratory test order being entered onto a requisition form and ends with the laboratory report being evaluated and filed in the patient's chart.

Laboratory Requisitions

When ordering tests from outside reference and hospital labs, laboratory professionals must understand all forms of written and electronic communication between their office and the laboratory. Communication begins when the physician orders a particular test or series of tests. The laboratory order is recorded on a requisition form that must be entirely completed. Different laboratories have different requisition forms, but most require all the following areas to be completed, as seen in Figure 1.6.

1. Demographics on the patient: name, zip code, date of birth, and gender. These are used to identify the patient when collecting specimens.

2. Insurance and billing information for the patient
3. Specimen collection information: date, time, and if the patient is fasting; medications taken
4. Priority status of specimen and where and how to send the reported results
5. Additional physicians needing the results
6. A listing of laboratory tests to be ordered. NOTE: Each test ordered has a procedure code on the left-hand side. (These codes are found in the latest CPT coding reference book.) Each test must also have a diagnostic code written on the requisition for insurance purposes. Figure 1.6 has a line to the right of each test to add the ICD-10 diagnostic codes. NOTE: The ICD-9 diagnostic reference code has been replaced by an updated alpha-numeric coding system known as ICD-10.
7. Also notice in Figure 1.6 that the *(a)* bar code in the top left and its corresponding *(b)* labels on the left are removed and placed on the specimen before sending it to the laboratory.

Electronic bar codes on requisitions are becoming more common, along with adhesive labels for the specimens, in an effort to eliminate specimen identification errors and maintain confidentiality. When these convenient labels are used, confirmation of the patient's identity with at least three identifiers is crucial (e.g., patient's name spelled out, birth date, phone number, or picture identification). As an additional safeguard, the patient should write his or her name or initials on the bar code label placed on the requisition and on the specimen labels.

a. G2349768

CLINICAL REQUISITION

① PATIENT INFORMATION - Please PRINT

Name_____
Last   First   M.I.

ZIP CODE_____

DOB_____ SEX _____
MO / DAY / YEAR

② BILLING

☐ PHYSICIAN/ACCOUNT

☐ PATIENT
(SEE REVERSE)

IF NO BILLING INFORMATION IS
PROVIDED, AND NO BOX IS CHECKED,
YOUR ACCOUNT WILL BE BILLED

③ SPECIMEN COLLECTION

DATE:_____
MO / DAY / YEAR

☐ AM
TIME:_____
☐ PM

Fasting   ☐ Yes   ☐ No

④ PRIORITY

☐ Routine   ☐ Phone

☐ Fax to DR._____

☐ at (   ) _____—_____

☐

⑤ PHYSICIANS

Ordering Physician if not
marked above
Report copy to:_____

_____

_____

SEE REVERSE SIDE FOR ASSIGNMENT OF
BENEFITS AND FINANCIAL AGREEMENT

ONLY CHECK (✓)ONE BOX IN THIS AREA

b.

G2349768

Name

G2349768

Name

G2349768

Name

G2349768

Name

TEST PANELS	ICD-10 DX CODE	TEST PANELS	ICD-10 DX CODE	TEST PANELS	ICD-10 DX CODE
☐ 29526 Metabolic Panel Basic		☐ 29525 Hepatic Function Panel		☐ 35839 Obstetric Panel	
☐ 29527 Metabolic Panel Comprehensive		☐ 29528 Renal Function Panel		☐ 29048 Lipid Panel	
☐ 23058 Electrolyte Panel		☐ 35285 General Health Panel		☐ 28192 Acute Hepatitis Panel	

TEST PANELS	ICD-10 DX CODE	TEST PANELS	ICD-10 DX CODE	TEST PANELS	ICD-10 DX CODE
☐ 25039 Activated Partial Thromboplastin (APTT)*		☐ 30055 Ferritin*		☐ 29127 Potassium	
☐ 29109 Amylase		☐ 29242 GGTP*		☐ 25045 Prothrombin Time*	
☐ 29921 BUN		☐ 29129 Glucose*		☐ 30178 PSA (Diagnostic)*	
☐ 30225 CA 125*		☐ 30089 hCG, Qualitative		☐ 30078 PSA (Screening)*	
☐ 30150 CA 27.29*		☐ 23409 Hemoglobin A1c*		☐ 25230 Sedimentation Rate	
☐ 28028 Calcium, localized		☐ 25316 Hgb & Hct*		☐ 29255 SGOT (AST)	
☐ 25015 CBC w/Differential*		☐ 28120 HIV-1/2 AB		☐ 30111 T3 Uptake*	
☐ 25014 CBC w/o Differential*		☐ 28121 HIV-1/2 AB w/WIB (if Ind)*		☐ 30113 T4. Free*	
☐ 30181 CEA*		☐ 29100 Iron (incl IBC)*		☐ 30213 T4 Total*	
☐ 29241 Cholesterol, Total*		☐ 23084 Magnesium		☐ 30017 TSH*	
☐ 29131 Creatinine		☐ 25437 Occult Blood (Diagnostic)*		☐ 25074 UA w/Micro C&S if indicated*	
☐ 31042 Digoxia*		☐ 25438 Occult Blood (Screening)*		☐ 25076 Urinalysis w/o Microscopic	
☐ 23857 Electrophoresis, Protein		☐ 29158 Phosphorus		☐ 25075 Urinalysis w/Microscopic	

REMINDER: IF YOU HAVE REQUESTED ANY TEST INDICATED IN RED OR NOTED WITH AN ASTERISK, THE PATIENT MAY NEED TO SIGN THE ADVANCE BENEFICIARY NOTICE (434) REFER TO SBMF MEDICAL NECESSITY GUIDE BOOK

FIG. 1.6 Bar code requisition form and labels for matching specimens with their laboratory order. Note the bar code and its number at the top *(a)* as well as its corresponding peel-off labels with the same requisition number and space for the patient's name *(b)*. The reference laboratory may also have the patient initial the requisition and the labels to confirm identity.

Figure 1.7 is another example of a laboratory requisition with a detailed organization of laboratory tests divided into the following categories:
- Panels or profiles—a series of tests associated with a particular organ or disease
- Hematology/coagulation tests—focus on the quantity and types of blood cells and coagulation times
- Chemistry tests—measure the levels of various chemicals, enzymes, and hormones
- Serology/immunology tests—analyze blood serum for evidence of infection or disease by evaluating antigen-antibody reactions in the laboratory
- Microbiology tests—identify the pathogen that is causing the disease

- Toxicology tests—measure the therapeutic levels and abuse of toxic drugs
- Urinalysis tests—indicate the prerenal, renal, and postrenal health status of the urinary system (i.e., the liver issues and the presence of diabetes, kidney stones, and cystitis respectively)

Notice how each test item has its five-digit procedure code on the left that is used for insurance billing. Each test item also has a collection container abbreviation on the right that tells the office which color-coded blood collection tube to use or which type of microbiology or urine specimen container to use. The codes are explained at the bottom of the requisition.

When the requisition is entirely completed, it goes to the laboratory with the patient or with the patient's specimen (e.g., blood, urine).

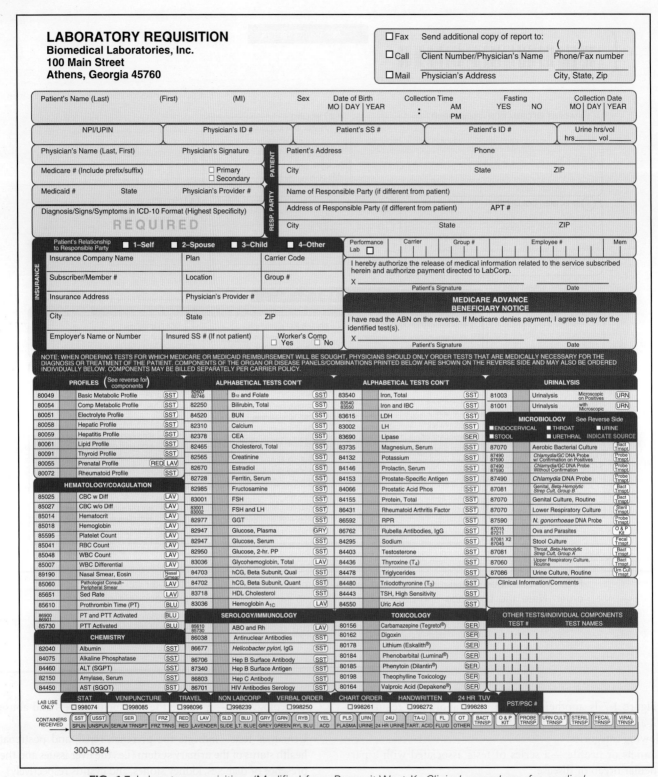

FIG. 1.7 Laboratory requisition. (Modified from Bonewit-West K: *Clinical procedures for medical assistants,* ed 10, St. Louis, 2018, Elsevier.)

Laboratory Reports

After the specimen has been tested, the laboratory calls in or sends the results on a laboratory report (refer to the results of laboratory tests as was seen in Figure 1.1). Another type of report is a computer printout, which shows the results of a chemistry panel of tests (Figure 1.8). Clinical laboratory test results

are now being incorporated into the electronic health record (EHR) as well.

New health care laws also allow laboratory results to be sent to patients if they request.

All laboratory reports must be reviewed by the physician as soon as possible. The physician must sign and date the report.

DATE AND TIME RECEIVED	ACCESSION NUMBER
10/20/2014 20:45	
LOCATION	DATE REPORTED
	10/21/2014

PHYSICIAN	PATIENT'S INFORMATION

TEST		RESULTS	REFERENCE RANGE	UNITS
Chemistry 23 - panel B				
Calcium, total, serum	LO	7.4	8.5-10.5	MG/DL
Phosphorus	LO	2.8	3.0-4.6	MG/DL
Uric acid	LO	3.2	3.5-7.2	MG/DL
Cholesterol	LO	123	151-240	MG/DL
Triglyceride		121	58-258	MG/DL
LDH		217	118-242	IU/L
SGOT (AST)	HI	41	10-37	IU/L
SGPT (ALT)	HI	45	10-40	IU/L
GGTP	LO	8	11-51	IU/L
Alkaline phosphatase		63	39-117	IU/L
Bilirubin, total		0.3	0.1-1.5	MG/DL
Albumin	LO	2.4	3.7-5.2	G/DL
Total protein	LO	3.6	6.0-8.5	G/DL
Albumin/globulin ratio		2.0	1.0-2.2	RATIO

Final report	(Summary)	Page 2 of 2

FIG. 1.8 Blood chemistry laboratory report. Note the patient's results compared with the reference range and the additional column indicating if the result is "HI" or "LO" compared with the reference range. (From Zakus SM: *Mosby's clinical skills for medical assistants,* ed 4, St. Louis, 2001, Mosby.)

TABLE 1.2 Metric Units of Measurement

Measurement	Metric Unit	Abbreviation	Relative Comparison to American Units
Weight	Gram	G, g, or gm	1 g is approximately the weight of a raisin and is used in place of ounces. 1 kg (the weight of 1000 g) is used in place of pounds.
Volume	Liter	L or l	1 L is a little more than a quart (used in place of the liquid measurements cup, quart, and gallon). 1 mL (1/1000 of a liter) is used in place of a liquid ounce or teaspoon.
Length	Meter	M or m	A **meter** is a little longer than a yard. **Centimeters** (1/100 of a meter) are used in place of inches. **Kilometers** (1000 meters) are used in place of miles.
Temperature	Centigrade (Celsius)	°C	0°C = freezing; 100°C = boiling (Fahrenheit: 32°F = freezing; 212°F = boiling) 4°–8°C = refrigerator temperature storage 15°–30°C = room temperature storage 37°C = body temperature

TABLE 1.3 Common Metric System Prefixes Used in Laboratory Reports

Metric Prefix	Abbreviation	Value to Unit	Examples in Laboratory Reports
Deci-	d	1/10 or 0.1	**dL or dl** = deciliter (one 10th of a liter)
Centi-	c	1/100 or 0.01	**cm** = centimeter, **cc** = cubic centimeter (which is the same volume as a milliliter = mL, one thousandth of a liter)
Milli-	m	1/1000 or 0.001	**ml or mL** = milliliter (one thousandth of a liter, which is the same as a cubic centimeter = cc); **mg** = milligram (one thousandth of a gram)
Micro-	mc	1/1,000,000	**mcg** = microgram (one millionth of a gram) (Note: When handwriting, use "mc" for micro, not the Greek letter μ.)

Depending on the results of the test, the physician may need to see or contact the patient. Each office has a specific protocol regarding how the patient is notified. Be sure to follow the protocol and then file the report in the patient's file folder after charting any additional information. Understanding the process and making sure all parties are informed in a timely manner are crucial.

Laboratory Measurements

Medical laboratories must communicate their test results in a universal way. Therefore, all laboratories report their results with international metric units for weight, volume, and length. Tables 1.2 to 1.4 show the most common metric units and time reporting used in medical laboratory reports.

Analytes measured in a liquid such as blood or urine are frequently expressed on laboratory reports in milligrams per deciliter (mg/dL). This is an expression of concentration, which is the *weight* of the analyte per *volume* of the specimen. If the analyte is very small, it is expressed in micrograms (mcg), where 1 mcg is 1/1,000,000 of a gram. Note: Use of "mcg" is preferred over the lower case Greek letter "μ" because of possible lab errors caused by misinterpretation. The Institute for Safe Medication Practices (ISMP, 2004) has published a list of error-prone abbreviations and strongly recommends that the use of "μg" be discontinued.

Many tests are temperature sensitive and must either be stored at room temperature or be refrigerated. The Centigrade temperature for refrigeration is usually 4° to 8°C (Figure 1.9), and room temperature is 15° to 30°C. (The workbook appendix for this chapter contains a daily temperature monitoring chart that must be filled out daily if test kits or supplies are refrigerated or stored at room temperature.)

When a *liquid* is measured in the laboratory, the most common volume is milliliter (mL or ml), which may also be referred

TABLE 1.4 Greenwich Time and International Military Time

Greenwich Time	Military Hours	Greenwich Time	Military Hours
12 midnight	0000 hours	12 noon	1200 hours
1:00 AM	0100 hours	1:00 PM	1300 hours
2:00 AM	0200 hours	2:00 PM	1400 hours
3:00 AM	0300 hours	3:00 PM	1500 hours
4:00 AM	0400 hours	4:00 PM	1600 hours
5:00 AM	0500 hours	5:00 PM	1700 hours
6:00 AM	0600 hours	6:00 PM	1800 hours
7:00 AM	0700 hours	7:00 PM	1900 hours
8:00 AM	0800 hours	8:00 PM	2000 hours
9:00 AM	0900 hours	9:00 PM	2100 hours
10:00 AM	1000 hours	10:00 PM	2200 hours
11:00 AM	1100 hours	11:00 PM	2300 hours

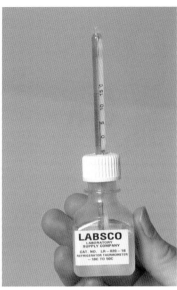

FIG. **1.9** Thermometer used to monitor refrigerator temperature. The reading of 6°C, an acceptable refrigerator temperature, would be logged.

to as a cubic centimeter (cc; the use of cc is discouraged, however, because it is often mistaken as "u," meaning units [ISMP, 2004]).

When the *length* of a test tube or a specimen within a capillary tube is measured, millimeters (mm) are used. There are approximately 25 mm in 1 inch, so 100 mm is approximately 4 inches.

NOTE: When recording whole numbers, *do not place a zero after the decimal* (e.g., the whole number 2 should be written 2, *not* 2.0). When recording a fraction, *a zero must be placed in front of the decimal* (e.g., one half should be written as 0.5, *not* .5).

SAFETY TRAINING IN THE LABORATORY

Potential hazards are present in the medical laboratory setting. Various government agencies have evaluated the most common laboratory dangers and created regulations and guidelines to help protect and to prevent harm to laboratory employees. These agencies continually monitor potential hazards and periodically update their regulations. Checking their websites and staying current with the latest changes and required dates of implementation are wise practices.

The hazards found in medical laboratories are divided into the following categories:

- Biohazards—dangers related to exposure to infectious or bloodborne pathogens (infectious microorganisms that are transmitted by the blood, body fluid, or OPIMs from an infected host into the blood of another)
- Chemical hazards—dangers related to exposure to toxic, unstable, explosive, or flammable materials
- Physical hazards—dangers related to electricity, fire, weather emergencies, bomb threats, and accidental injuries

Biohazard Training

Laboratory personnel must also learn how to prevent the spread of disease to themselves and others according to the regulations of two federal agencies: the Centers for Disease Control and Prevention (**CDC**) and the Occupational Safety and Health Administration (**OSHA**).

CDC and Infection Control

The basic means by which diseases are spread must be understood before beginning laboratory work.

Transmission and the chain of infection. For a disease to spread, the following conditions must exist as seen in Figure 1.10. A pathogen must be present in a reservoir host (an infected person who is carrying an infectious agent). The pathogen must then find a portal of exit (a means of leaving the infected host's body, e.g., through the mouth, broken skin, rectum, or body fluids). Next, each pathogen has a particular transportation mode or transmission (a means of transporting itself from the infected individual to another person, by direct or indirect contact, e.g., by air, food, hand-to-hand contact, insects, or body fluids). The pathogen must then find a portal of entry (a body opening or break in the skin) in another person. When inside the new person, the pathogen will not cause disease unless the person is a susceptible host (an individual who is unable to protect himself or herself against the infectious agent). A susceptible person who becomes infected becomes a reservoir host, and the cycle begins again.

Health care workers must understand the chain of infection and endeavor to break the chain whenever possible to stop the spread of disease. If a disease is spread within a health care facility, it is referred to as a health care–associated infection (HCAI or HAI) (also referred to as a nosocomial infection).

Standard precautions. The CDC has issued a list of Standard Precautions for infection control within health care facilities (Figure 1.11). The most important way to stop the transmission of infectious disease, and first on the list, is hand washing. Next on the list is wearing various barriers referred to as personal protective equipment (**PPE**), which is "specialized clothing or equipment worn by an employee for protection against infectious material." Examples of PPE are gloves, goggles, fluid-impermeable gowns, face shields, and masks. The remainder of the Standard Precautions list consists of recommendations for equipment disinfection, environmental control, linen disposal, bloodborne pathogen guidelines, and patient placement (e.g., isolation within a hospital setting). The serious occupational hazard of bloodborne pathogens has been further defined and regulated by OSHA and is discussed later in this chapter.

Hand hygiene. The most common mode of transmission of pathogens is by the hands. The major cause of HCAIs is the transmission of pathogens from health care workers' hands. These infections can also spread bacteria that may become resistant to antibiotics, which makes the treatment and eradication of infections more difficult.

Proper hand hygiene has proved to be the primary factor in infection control. Research has shown, however, that many

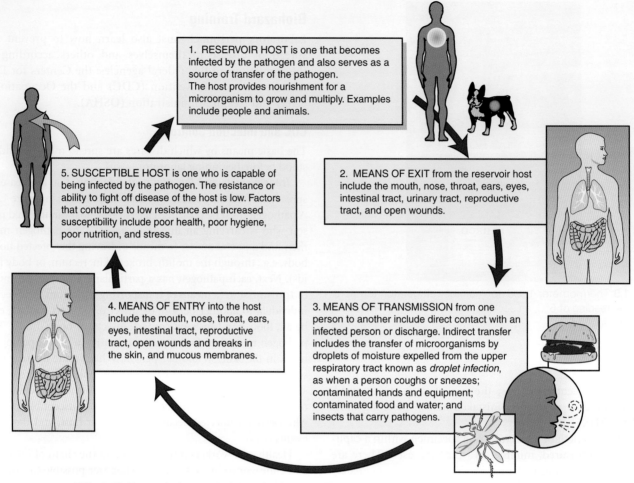

1. RESERVOIR HOST is one that becomes infected by the pathogen and also serves as a source of transfer of the pathogen. The host provides nourishment for a microorganism to grow and multiply. Examples include people and animals.

2. MEANS OF EXIT from the reservoir host include the mouth, nose, throat, ears, eyes, intestinal tract, urinary tract, reproductive tract, and open wounds.

3. MEANS OF TRANSMISSION from one person to another include direct contact with an infected person or discharge. Indirect transfer includes the transfer of microorganisms by droplets of moisture expelled from the upper respiratory tract known as *droplet infection*, as when a person coughs or sneezes; contaminated hands and equipment; contaminated food and water; and insects that carry pathogens.

4. MEANS OF ENTRY into the host include the mouth, nose, throat, ears, eyes, intestinal tract, reproductive tract, open wounds and breaks in the skin, and mucous membranes.

5. SUSCEPTIBLE HOST is one who is capable of being infected by the pathogen. The resistance or ability to fight off disease of the host is low. Factors that contribute to low resistance and increased susceptibility include poor health, poor hygiene, poor nutrition, and stress.

FIG. 1.10 Transmission and chain of infection. (From Bonewit-West K, Hunt S, Applegate E: *Today's medical assistant,* ed 3, St. Louis, 2016, Elsevier.)

health care workers do not practice routine hand washing. Their reasons have been as follows:
- Irritation and dryness caused by hand washing agents
- Inconvenient location of sinks
- Lack of soap and paper towels
- Too busy or insufficient time
- Understaffing or overcrowding
- Priority of patient needs
- Misinformation about risk of acquiring infection from patients

In response, new guidelines developed by the CDC and infection-control organizations now recommend that health care workers use an alcohol-based hand rub (gel, rinse, or foam) to routinely clean their hands between patient contacts as long as their hands are not visibly soiled. Alcohol-based hand rubs require less time, are more effective than soap for routine hand washing, are more accessible than sinks, reduce bacterial counts on hands, and improve skin condition. The following three ways to clean the hands are now recommended (Figure 1.12):
1. Washing with plain soap—good for removing microorganisms and dirt
2. Washing with antimicrobial detergent soap—better for removing and killing microorganisms
3. Using an alcohol-based hand rub—best for destroying transient microorganisms obtained from patients, specimens, and objects that are contaminated, that is, likely to have been in contact with materials or environmental surfaces where infectious organisms may reside

Antimicrobial soap hand wash. Laboratory employees' hands should be washed with antimicrobial soap (Figure 1.13) at the beginning and end of work, before eating, after using the rest room, and whenever hands have visible dirt or are visibly contaminated with blood or body fluids. Hand washing with soap and water involves the following process:
1. Remove all hand jewelry.
2. Use a paper towel to turn on water to avoid contamination of faucet and wet the hands with warm water (avoid hot water).
3. Apply 3 to 5 mL of liquid antiseptic soap to the hands. Use a towel on the pump dispenser to avoid contaminating the dispenser with soiled hands.
4. Rub the hands together for at least 15 seconds, covering all surfaces of the hands and fingers with soap. Intertwine the fingers and scrub the backs and fronts of both hands.
5. Clean the fingernails with a brush if necessary or by scraping the nails in a circular motion on the palm of the opposing hand.

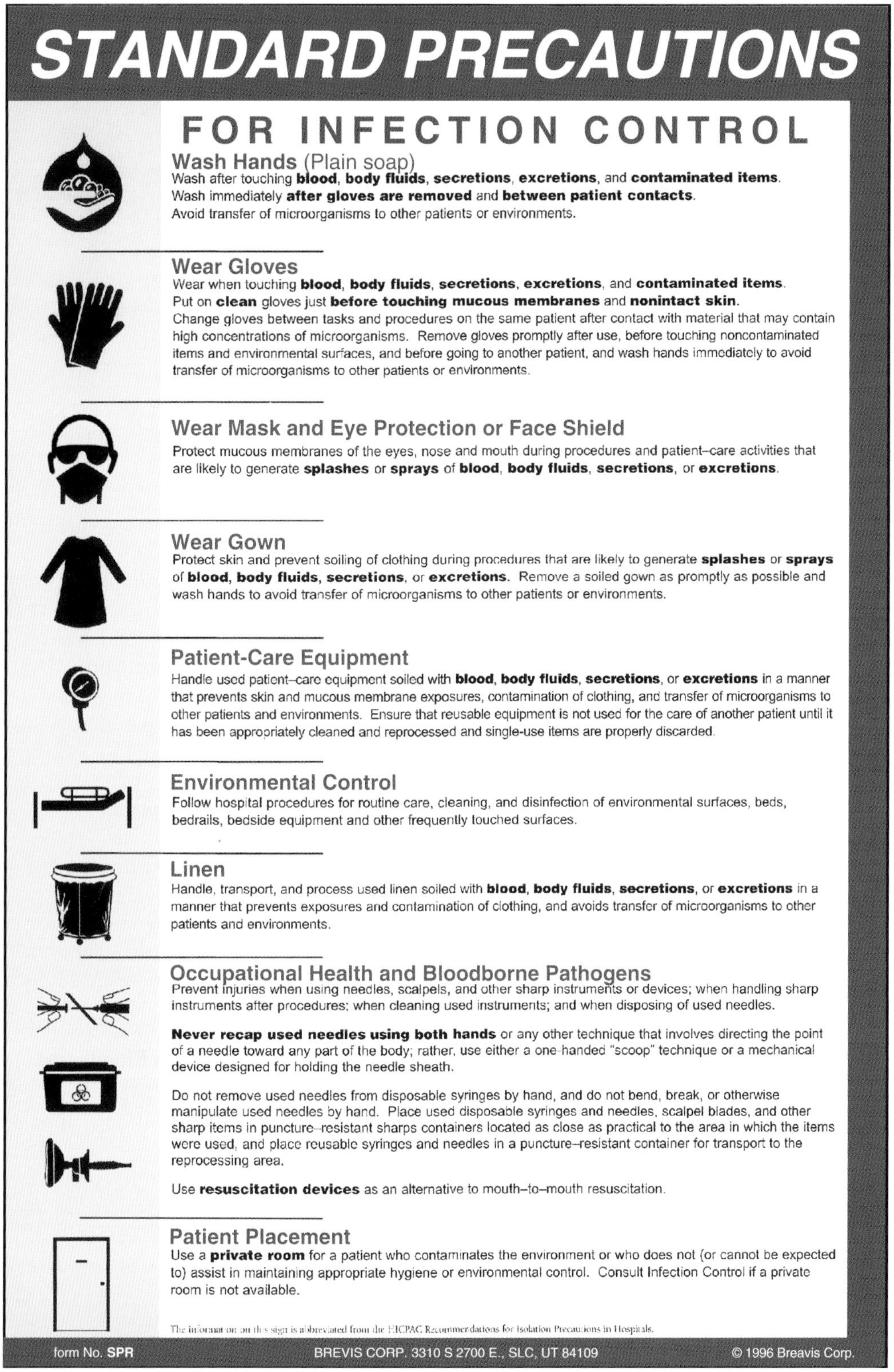

STANDARD PRECAUTIONS

FOR INFECTION CONTROL

Wash Hands (Plain soap)
Wash after touching **blood**, **body fluids**, **secretions**, **excretions**, and **contaminated items**. Wash immediately **after gloves are removed** and **between patient contacts**. Avoid transfer of microorganisms to other patients or environments.

Wear Gloves
Wear when touching **blood**, **body fluids**, **secretions**, **excretions**, and **contaminated items**. Put on **clean** gloves just **before touching mucous membranes** and **nonintact skin**. Change gloves between tasks and procedures on the same patient after contact with material that may contain high concentrations of microorganisms. Remove gloves promptly after use, before touching noncontaminated items and environmental surfaces, and before going to another patient, and wash hands immediately to avoid transfer of microorganisms to other patients or environments.

Wear Mask and Eye Protection or Face Shield
Protect mucous membranes of the eyes, nose and mouth during procedures and patient–care activities that are likely to generate **splashes** or **sprays** of **blood**, **body fluids**, **secretions**, or **excretions**.

Wear Gown
Protect skin and prevent soiling of clothing during procedures that are likely to generate **splashes** or **sprays** of **blood**, **body fluids**, **secretions**, or **excretions**. Remove a soiled gown as promptly as possible and wash hands to avoid transfer of microorganisms to other patients or environments.

Patient-Care Equipment
Handle used patient–care equipment soiled with **blood**, **body fluids**, **secretions**, or **excretions** in a manner that prevents skin and mucous membrane exposures, contamination of clothing, and transfer of microorganisms to other patients and environments. Ensure that reusable equipment is not used for the care of another patient until it has been appropriately cleaned and reprocessed and single-use items are properly discarded.

Environmental Control
Follow hospital procedures for routine care, cleaning, and disinfection of environmental surfaces, beds, bedrails, bedside equipment and other frequently touched surfaces.

Linen
Handle, transport, and process used linen soiled with **blood**, **body fluids**, **secretions**, or **excretions** in a manner that prevents exposures and contamination of clothing, and avoids transfer of microorganisms to other patients and environments.

Occupational Health and Bloodborne Pathogens
Prevent injuries when using needles, scalpels, and other sharp instruments or devices; when handling sharp instruments after procedures; when cleaning used instruments; and when disposing of used needles.

Never recap used needles using both hands or any other technique that involves directing the point of a needle toward any part of the body; rather, use either a one-handed "scoop" technique or a mechanical device designed for holding the needle sheath.

Do not remove used needles from disposable syringes by hand, and do not bend, break, or otherwise manipulate used needles by hand. Place used disposable syringes and needles, scalpel blades, and other sharp items in puncture–resistant sharps containers located as close as practical to the area in which the items were used, and place reusable syringes and needles in a puncture–resistant container for transport to the reprocessing area.

Use **resuscitation devices** as an alternative to mouth–to–mouth resuscitation.

Patient Placement
Use a **private room** for a patient who contaminates the environment or who does not (or cannot be expected to) assist in maintaining appropriate hygiene or environmental control. Consult Infection Control if a private room is not available.

The information on this sign is abbreviated from the HICPAC Recommendations for Isolation Precautions in Hospitals.

form No. **SPR** | BREVIS CORP. 3310 S 2700 E., SLC, UT 84109 | © 1996 Brevis Corp.

FIG. 1.11 Centers for Disease Control and Prevention's Standard Precautions for infection control. (Copyright © Breavis Corp.)

6. Rinse the hands with water flowing down from the wrists to the fingers and dry thoroughly.
7. Use a clean, dry paper towel to turn off the water faucet.
8. Apply appropriate hand lotion or cream provided by employer.

Healthy, intact skin acts as a barrier against cross-contamination (transmitting a pathogen from one individual to another) and harbors fewer pathogens. When the skin is damaged, transient microorganisms (organisms from contaminated objects or from infectious patients that adhere to the skin

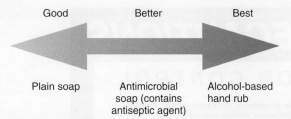

FIG. 1.12 Effectiveness of hand hygiene preparations in killing bacteria.

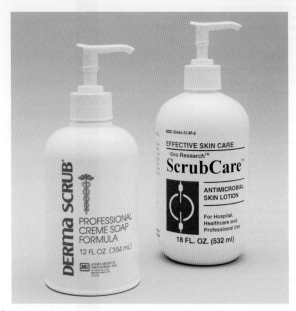

FIG. 1.13 Hand washing with antimicrobial soap should be used at the beginning and end of work, after using the rest room, and before eating. Also, antimicrobial hand lotion should be applied to prevent the skin from drying and cracking. (Photo by Zack Bent.)

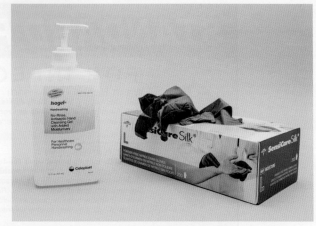

FIG. 1.14 Sanitize hands with alcohol-based hand rub before and after using disposable gloves. (Photo by Zack Bent.)

3. Continue rubbing the hands together until the alcohol dries (15 to 25 seconds).
4. Make sure the hands are completely dry before putting on gloves.
5. Wash the hands with soap and water when a buildup of emollients can be felt on the hands.

Fingernail hygiene consists of maintaining natural nail tips at ¼ inch in length and refraining from using nail polish. Artificial nails should not be worn by employees who have contact with any patients.

Personal protective equipment. Along with hand hygiene recommendations, the CDC also recommends when and how to use PPE. OSHA also specifies and regulates the circumstances in which PPE must be used. (It also requires the employer to provide employees with their needed PPE along with training on how to use it.) These OSHA requirements are discussed next and in Procedure 1.1 located at the end of this chapter.

OSHA Biohazard Training in Bloodborne Pathogens Standard

The federal Department of Labor has appointed OSHA to find ways of promoting worker safety and health in every workplace in the United States. On the basis of the history of hazards to health care workers, OSHA has developed a rigorous standard of policies and procedures called the **Bloodborne Pathogens Standard (BBPS)** to protect employees who work in occupations where they are at risk of exposure to blood or other potentially infectious materials (**OPIMs**). **Occupational exposure** is defined as skin, eye, mucous membrane, or parenteral contact with blood or OPIMs in the workplace. **Parenteral contact** means the blood entered the body through the skin or mucous membrane by means of a needle, bite, cut, splash, or abrasion. Those who work in a medical laboratory or perform **venipuncture** (removal of blood from a vein) are at an increased risk for occupational exposure to bloodborne pathogens.

OSHA regulations require that an **exposure control plan** be provided by your facility to eliminate or minimize your

and can be transmitted to others) are harder to remove. Therefore, gloves and alcohol-based hand rubs are also required.

Alcohol-based hand rub. Hand sanitizing with alcohol-based hand rubs should be routinely used between patients and after having direct hand contact with patients, their wounds, broken skin, or body fluids (specimen containers) or after touching equipment used on the patient. Some patients may harbor "colonies" of infectious microorganisms on their skin with no sign of infection. Therefore, the Standard Precautions pertaining to the use of gloves and proper hand hygiene apply to *all* patients. Use an alcohol-based hand rub routinely before putting on gloves and after removing gloves.

The following are tips on how to use an alcohol-based hand rub:

1. Apply 1.5 to 3 mL (or manufacturer's recommended amount) of an alcohol gel or foam to the palm of one hand and then rub the hands together (Figure 1.14).
2. Cover all surfaces of the hands and fingers, including the areas around and under the fingernails as described in the washing with soap and water procedure above.

occupational exposure to bloodborne pathogens. It is a key document developed to assist the employer in implementing and ensuring compliance with the BBPS, thereby protecting employees. It consists of the following elements:

- Determination of employee risk of exposure
- Implementation of methods of exposure control when dealing with all patients. It demands Universal Precautions (the assumption that the blood or body fluid containing blood from *any* patient or test kit could be infectious) by providing engineering and work practice controls to improve safety of employees, PPE for employees, and safe housekeeping practices
- Hepatitis B vaccination for employees at risk of bloodborne pathogen exposure
- Postexposure evaluation of patient and employee immediately after an exposure incident
- Evaluation of circumstances surrounding exposure incidents
- Communication of hazards by annual training of employees
- Documentation showing compliance to all the aforementioned elements

New employees of a laboratory receive initial training in the BBPS and subsequent annual training to learn of any changes in the standard. The following OSHA training session is divided into three sections:

1. Education on the causes, symptoms, and transmission of bloodborne pathogen diseases
2. Instruction on preventive measures to minimize exposure
3. Actions and procedures to follow when exposed to blood or OPIMs

Diseases caused by bloodborne pathogens. Four main bloodborne pathogens pose a threat to health care workers: human immunodeficiency virus (HIV), hepatitis B, and hepatitis C, and Ebola. Note: Hepatitis A is not caused by a bloodborne virus but is similar to hepatitis B and hepatitis C in that it is a viral infection of the liver. Table 1.5 summarizes the comparative information on the four bloodborne viruses and a note at the bottom explaining infectious hepatitis A virus (HAV). An additional bloodborne virus has emerged that also requires universal precautions: the Zika virus that is transmitted via the bite of the Aedes species of mosquito.

The human immunodeficiency virus (HIV) is a retrovirus that attacks the immune system by destroying the white blood cells known as CD4+ helper T lymphocytes. An HIV infection has four stages:

1. An *acute stage* after exposure characterized by flulike symptoms with swollen glands
2. An *asymptomatic period* or clinical latency in which no symptoms are readily apparent but the person is still infectious
3. A *symptomatic stage* with the appearance of opportunistic infections (infections that occur because of the body's inability to repel pathogens normally found in the environment)
4. The *AIDS (acquired immunodeficiency syndrome) stage,* when the immune system is severely weakened and the following conditions start to appear: an extreme decrease in the number of CD4 cells (the T lymphocytic white blood cell

that fights infection); any combination of the following opportunistic infections that are known to occur when the CD4 cells are no longer defending the body—Kaposi sarcoma, *Pneumocystis* pneumonia, cytomegalovirus infection, herpes simplex 1 and 2 infection, mycobacterial infection (e.g., tuberculosis), candidiasis (yeast infection), cryptosporidiosis, toxoplasmosis, and cryptococcosis.

Currently, there is no preventive vaccination for HIV or any cure for the infection of CD4 cells. Management consists of early diagnosis of the HIV infection followed by treatment to reduce the growth rate of the retrovirus and its effect on the CD4 cells.

Hepatitis B virus (HBV) is the most prevalent bloodborne virus. It first infects the liver with acute flulike symptoms and possible jaundice. Most people recover and become immune to the virus, but approximately 2% enter the chronic stage and develop cirrhosis of the liver, cancer, or both. The good news is that a vaccine is available to produce immunity against the virus before an exposure incident. OSHA requires employers to provide the hepatitis B vaccine series free of charge to all health care employees who may be exposed to blood or OPIM. (Some health care employees who work only with medical records would not need the vaccination.)

Hepatitis C virus (HCV) is another bloodborne virus that attacks the liver. It is not as prevalent as HBV, but it is much more likely to reach the chronic stage. In fact, 75% to 85% of infected HCV individuals reach the chronic phase with cirrhosis of the liver, cancer, and death. Because no vaccine for HCV exists, health care workers cannot establish an immunity against the disease. Health care workers exposed to HCV are at risk.

Hepatitis A virus (HAV) is not a bloodborne virus; however, similar to HBC and HCV, it does attack the liver. It is highly contagious and is transmitted by direct or indirect contact through the gastrointestinal tract rather than blood. Patients with HAV are generally placed in isolation during their illness.

Additional facts regarding the bloodborne viruses

- The average health care professional is more likely to contract HBV or HCV than HIV.
- Although all these diseases have initial flulike symptoms, HIV attacks the immune system, causing swollen glands, but HBV and HCV attack the liver, causing jaundice (a yellowing of the skin caused by excess bilirubin levels).
- HCV is becoming a threat because many individuals are chronic carriers, and no vaccination is available.

Preventive measures to minimize exposure. Practicing Universal Precautions is the most important way to prevent exposure incidents. The most common exposure to bloodborne pathogens in health care is from accidental puncture wounds with contaminated needles, glass, or other sharp items. All sharp items should be treated with respect. Mucous membrane exposure through splashes or aerosols can also occur, so goggles and masks or face shields should be used when performing procedures or tasks in which potential splashes or aerosols may occur.

The HBV vaccine should be made available to all health care employees who have the potential of being exposed to blood and OPIMs. Employers must provide a three-vaccination series, and new employees should begin their series within the first 2 weeks of employment. Any employee who does not wish to be

TABLE 1.5	**Four Bloodborne Pathogens***			
	Human Immunodeficiency Virus (HIV)	**Hepatitis B Virus (HBV)**	**Hepatitis C Virus (HCV)**	**Ebola Virus**
Transmission	Contact with infected blood or blood products, semen, vaginal secretions; perinatal transmission. Must get into bloodstream by direct entry into a vein or break in skin or mucous linings	Found in body fluids; spread by blood transfusions, contaminated needles, and sexual contact. HBV is the most common bloodborne pathogen	Intravenous drug use, body piercing, organ and blood transfusions, contaminated needles. Contaminated needles carry a 10-fold greater chance of causing HCV than HIV	First human was infected through contact with an infected animal. Person-to-person transmission is when blood or body fluids enter through broken skin or via mucous membranes
Symptoms	Flulike symptoms, fever, diarrhea, swollen glands, and fatigue. HIV infection leads to AIDS and an inability to fight infections	Flulike symptoms generally do not appear until 6 months after viral infection; they can include jaundice, fatigue, and abdominal and joint pain	Milder than HBV; symptoms (if appearing) occur generally 1–2 months after exposure; they include jaundice, fatigue, dark urine, abdominal pain	Fever, severe headache, muscle pain, weakness, fatigue, diarrhea, vomiting abdominal (stomach) pain, unexplained hemorrhage (bleeding or bruising)
Effects	After infection, HIV is not curable; the majority of infected individuals do not develop AIDS until many years after infection	Most people recover and become immune; death can result in the 2% who become chronically infected	85% of infected individuals acquire chronic form; of those, cirrhosis of the liver develops in 1%–15%	Infection results are internal bleeding
Prevention	No vaccination available; self-testing is now available for early detection and early treatment to prevent the retrovirus from replicating itself	HBV vaccination	No vaccination available	Health care: PPE, infection control, sterilization, isolation
Treatment	Postexposure prophylaxis must start in 1–2 hours; antiretrovirals (AVRs) control the HIV infection, but it is never cured	Postexposure treatment with immunoglobulins should begin as soon as possible—within 24 hours and no later than 7 days	Treated with immunoglobulin, HepatoZYME (inhibits viral synthesis), and alpha interferon	No vaccine or medicine (no antiviral drug). Patient needs supportive care and strong immune system
Trends	Health care workers are more likely to contract HBV and HCV infections than HIV, although the incidence of HIV infection is rising	10- to 49-year-old people are most affected; approximately 1.25 million are chronically infected	2.7 million have chronic form; this number is expected to triple in the next 5–10 years; it is the leading cause of liver disease and liver cancer	2014–2016: largest outbreak, affecting thousands

*Hepatitis A virus is not bloodborne disease. It is usually spread by fecal contaminated food. The symptoms are jaundice, fatigue, abdominal pain, and flulike symptoms. The infection results in immunity; symptoms can last 6 to 9 months. Prevention is HVA vaccination and good hygiene. Treatment consists of immunoglobulins and isolated bed rest to prevent spread.

vaccinated must sign a Hepatitis B Vaccine Declination form. Health care students should also begin the series if they will be working with blood and blood products.

Many advances have also been made in HIV/AIDS prevention and treatment, including rapid self-testing and effective antiretroviral therapies that have reduced the development of HIV opportunistic diseases and early deaths. Early detection of HIV infection is now recognized as a critical component in controlling the spread of HIV infection. Figure 1.15 shows the OraQuick self-test kit.

Engineering controls are efforts and research aimed at isolating and removing bloodborne pathogens from the workplace. Some examples of engineering controls involve the use of the following:

• Biohazard bags for blood-contaminated paper and plastic products and biohazard sharps disposal containers made of puncture-resistant material that will safely receive contaminated needles, syringes, and other sharp implements immediately after use

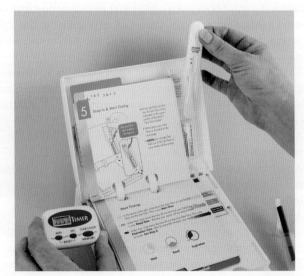

FIG. 1.15 The new OraQuick self-test kit for HIV. This test and the rapid blood test for HIV are presented in Chapter 7: Immunology. (Photo by Zack Bent.)

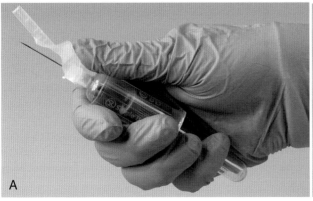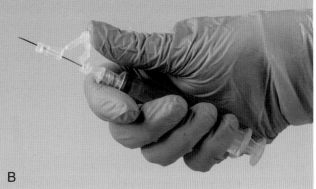

FIG. 1.16 Examples of needle safety devices being activated immediately after drawing blood. **A,** One-hand, thumb-activated device. **B,** One-hand, thumb-activated spring device. (Photo by Zack Bent.)

- Safer medical devices to cover contaminated needles immediately after use (Figure 1.16), self-sheathing needles, and needleless systems when performing intravenous (IV) therapy
- Plastic supplies and equipment to replace breakable glass supplies when collecting and processing blood

The OSHA standard requires that everyone in the workplace explore new procedures and products regularly to provide greater safety to the health care worker while affording comfort and quality of care to the patient.

Work practice controls are policies that are recorded, monitored, and evaluated to protect employees from exposure to the pathogens in blood or body fluids. Various individuals (both administrators and front-line workers) are assigned the task of identifying, evaluating, and implementing changes in work behavior to reduce the risk of exposure. The implementation and commitment to adhere to work practice controls is required of each individual.

Examples of safe practices in the medical laboratory include the following:
- Do not eat, drink, smoke, or apply makeup or contact lenses in areas with a reasonable likelihood of exposure.
- Sanitize the hands before donning and after doffing gloves.
- Bandage cuts and other lesions on the hands before gloving.
- Label all biohazard containers and appliances.
- Place all biohazard waste in appropriately labeled biohazard containers (e.g., sharps versus bag containers).
- If mucous membranes (eyes, mouth, nose) come in contact with blood, flush them with water as soon as possible.
- Do not store food or drink with biohazardous materials.
- Wear and use appropriate protective barriers and closed-toe shoes when working with blood or OPIMs.
- Use mechanical means to pick up broken contaminated glass.
- Double-package specimens with a biohazard label when sending them to another laboratory.

In the medical laboratory, gloves and fluid-impermeable gown barriers are routine requirements when dealing with blood or OPIMs. Each procedure should be evaluated to determine if face shields or goggles and masks are also necessary to protect the mucous membranes. This equipment should be used if the procedure is likely to generate splashes or sprays of blood, body fluids, secretions, or excretions.

Housekeeping guidelines in the laboratory consist of several measures:
- Disinfect counters at the beginning and end of each day with an OSHA-approved disinfectant such as freshly diluted 10% bleach solution. Figure 1.17 shows a double-bottle system that dilutes the bleach with water on demand and a CaviWipe container with tissues to thoroughly disinfect contaminated surfaces. NOTE: Always wear protective gloves when working with either of these products.
- When a waste receptacle contains biohazardous material, it must be red, contain the universal symbol for biohazard, or both (Figure 1.18). An understanding of the various waste receptacles and their functions is vital (Figure 1.19).
  1. Regular wastebaskets should be used for paper wrappers, paper towels, and other materials that do not have blood or body fluids on them.

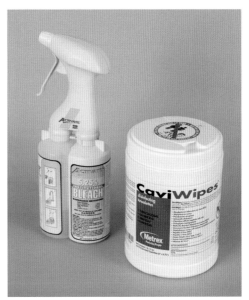

FIG. 1.17 A bleach and water dispenser automatically delivers a freshly diluted 10% bleach solution and CaviWipes for thorough disinfection of contaminated surfaces. (Photo by Zack Bent.)

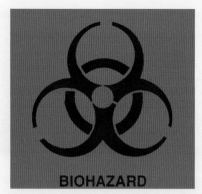

FIG. 1.18 Biohazard label.

2. Biohazard wastebaskets containing red plastic liners and bags with biohazard labels should be used for contaminated gloves, gowns, gauze, and soft plastic supplies.
3. Biohazard sharps containers with biohazard labels should receive only sharp items such as needles and glass that could cut or penetrate a soft biohazard bag. They should be snapped closed when they are approximately three-fourths full.
4. Biohazard-labeled bags and sharps containers are gathered into large cardboard boxes supplied by a regulated waste facility. The boxes are collected and incinerated twice at a cost based on the total weight of the waste. Do not throw unnecessary items in biohazard receptacles.

If a biohazard spill of blood or OPIMs occurs, it should be cleaned with a spill kit specifically designed to protect the person during the cleanup process (e.g., gloves and cleanup tools), the area should be decontaminated using the absorbent material and chemicals, and everything should be disposed of properly in a biohazard-labeled bag or box (Figure 1.20).

Procedure after exposure to blood. If exposed to blood by a percutaneous (through the skin) injury or a splash on the mucous membranes of the eyes or mouth, the following postexposure steps must be taken immediately:

1. Flush with water and wash the exposed area.
2. Report the incident immediately to your supervisor.
3. File an incident report that includes detailed information about how the exposure occurred. (See the Sample Blood and Body Fluid Exposure Report form in the workbook appendix for this chapter.)
4. Seek medical attention and permission to determine if the patient was infected with HIV, HBV, or HCV; then determine baseline blood defenses for each of the viral infections. If HIV is suspected, retest at 6, 12, 24, and 52 weeks after exposure to see if any change indicates infection.
5. Because a possibility always exists that the blood contained infectious viruses, postexposure prophylaxis (**PEP**) (preventive treatment after being exposed to blood or OPIMs) must

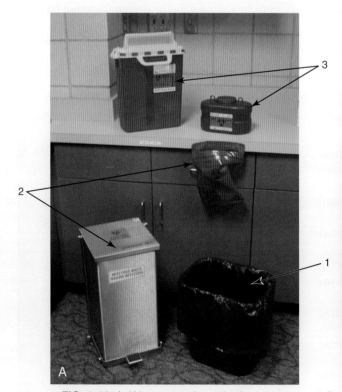

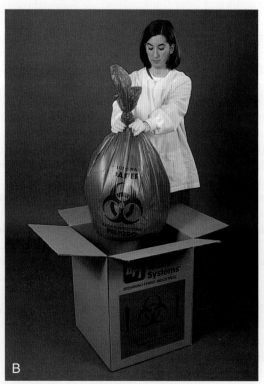

FIG. 1.19 A, Waste containers in the laboratory. *1,* Regular waste receptacle; *2,* nonsharps biohazard waste receptacles; and *3,* biohazard sharps containers. **B,** Biohazard waste is collected in boxes for managed-waste pickup. (**B,** from Bonewit-West K: *Clinical procedures for medical assistants,* ed 10, St. Louis, 2018, Elsevier.)

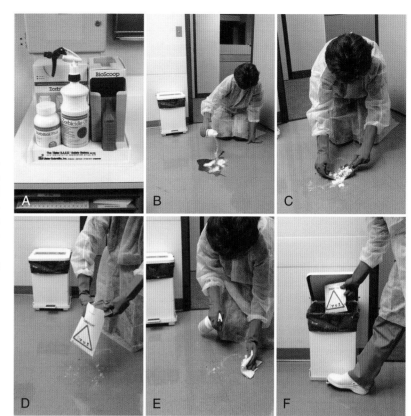

FIG. 1.20 Biohazard spill kit and cleaning procedure. **A,** Biohazard spill kit. **B,** Apply absorbent powder to spill. **C,** Scoop up powder into the supplied dust pan. **D,** Carefully place filled dust pan into biohazard envelope. **E,** Spray area thoroughly and wipe remaining residue. **F,** Deposit biohazard envelope into biohazard container. (From Proctor D, Adams A: *Kinn's the medical assistant: an applied learning approach,* ed 12, St. Louis, 2014, Saunders.)

begin as soon as possible. The PEP for each of the viral infections is based on the risk evaluation of a qualified health care professional and may consist of the following:

- Hepatitis B: Passive HBV immune globulin and active HBV vaccine should be administered within 72 hours.
- Hepatitis C: Immunoglobulin, HepatoZYME, and alpha interferon should be administered as soon as possible.
- HIV: Antiretrovirals (ARVs) are now proven to reduce HIV infection, although they do not eliminate it. Therefore, it is crucial to begin taking the daily pill as directed by the physician.

6. Counseling and confidentiality are also available and required by OSHA.

Documentation of BBPS compliance. Compliance with all the steps involved in OSHA's BBPS must be proven by each facility's documentation of its exposure control plan. The paperwork that must be presented during an OSHA inspection includes the following:

- Written job categories of employees at risk of exposure to blood
- HBV vaccination guidelines and records for each employee at risk
- Record of initial and annual Universal Standards training sessions for bloodborne pathogens and safety training for each employee
- Definition and listing of safe work practices
- Sharps injury log of all work-related needle sticks and cuts from sharp objects contaminated with blood, including date

and time of exposure, details of the procedure being performed, the exposure, the exposure source, the exposed person, and postexposure follow-up
- A written plan to maintain the privacy of employees
- Documentation showing the evaluation of new technology by employees and their selection of safety devices based on effectiveness in decreasing injuries, acceptance by users, and ability to not adversely affect patient care

Chemical Hazard Training

Hazardous chemicals in the workplace are also regulated by OSHA in a federal document referred to as the Hazard Communication Standard. The document states that employees have the right to know about the dangers of all the hazardous chemicals to which they may be exposed under normal working conditions. As with the BBPS, the employer must develop a program that consists of taking an inventory of hazardous chemicals in the workplace, labeling the chemical hazards, collecting and maintaining a safety data sheet (**SDS**) for each hazardous chemical, properly storing and disposing of hazardous chemicals, and providing employees with information and training. Examples of chemical hazards are dangerous acids, caustics, flammables, and inhalants.

In small medical laboratories, most of the chemicals used are fortunately in small, prepackaged quantities. The most common chemical hazard is the bleach used to disinfect counters. All labels on chemicals such as bleach should be read to understand their hazards. Figure 1.21 shows a bleach label with the

Product Label Example

1. **BRITE BLEACH** Contains No Phosphates

2. Active Ingredient: Sodium Hypochlorite 5%

3. 64 fl. oz (2 Quarts)

4. **Caution: Keep Out Of The Reach Of Children**

BRITE: Household Uses

5. Use *BRITE* to clean your bathroom and kitchen. *BRITE* is an excellent disinfectant and deodorizer. *BRITE* cleans by removing stubborn stains and eliminating odor-causing germs from surfaces all around the house.
• Toilet Bowls — Pour in 1/2 cup of *BRITE*. Brush entire bowl. Let stand 10 minutes. Do not use with toilet bowl cleaners. See caution statement.
• Kitchen Sinks — Cover stains with water. Pour 1/2 cup of *BRITE* directly into standing water.
• Floor — Clean with a solution of 1 cup of *BRITE* per gallon of sudsy water. Do not use on cork.
• Bathtubs and Showers — Clean with a solution of 1 cup of *BRITE* per gallon warm water.
Laundry
Direction for Use:
For best results, use the proper amount of *BRITE* in your wash water.
• Large top-loading automatic: 1-1/2 cups
• Regular top-loading automatic: 1 cup
• Front-loading automatic: 1/2 cup
• Heavy-soiled laundry: increase 1/2 cup
• Hand laundry: 2 gallons of sudsy water, 1/4 cup *BRITE*

6. WRITE for a free *BRITE* "Guide to Cleaner Laundry" booklet or other information on laundry and house cleaning to the BRITE Co., P.O. Box 12345, Braselton, WA 44150.
For Use On The Following Fabrics: Cotton, linen, synthetics, permanent press and all color-fast fabrics. Do not use *BRITE* on silk, wool, mohair, leather, spandex or non-color fast fabrics.

7./8. **Caution:** *BRITE* may be harmful if swallowed or may cause severe eye irritation if splashed in eyes. If swallowed, feed milk. If splashed in eyes, flood with water. Call Physician. **Skin irritant:** If contact with skin, wash off with water. Do not use *BRITE* with ammonia or products containing acids such as **toilet bowl cleaners, rust removers, or vinegar;** to do so will release **hazardous gases.** Prolonged contact with metal may cause pitting or discoloration. **Do not use this bottle for storage of any other liquid but** *BRITE.*

FIG. 1.21 Product label. Note the eight required elements for labeling a hazardous chemical.

following eight container label requirements provided by the manufacturer:
1. Brand name of the chemical
2. Common or chemical name
3. Amount of the contents
4. Signal words such as *danger* (if flammable, corrosive, or highly reactive with other substances), *poison* (if toxic when ingested or inhaled), *warning,* or *caution* (if any other hazardous condition is present)
5. Instructions for the safe use of the chemical (storage, usage, and disposal)
6. Manufacturer information
7. Description of possible hazards such as physical hazards (ability of material to explode, ignite, or react with other chemicals), health hazards (whether material can irritate tissue or cause cancer), toxicity (whether material is toxic if swallowed or inhaled), and safety precautions (whether material requires protective clothing, gloves, or eye protection)
8. First-aid instructions if necessary

Along with being properly labeled, each hazardous chemical must be listed on a chemical hazard inventory sheet and have its

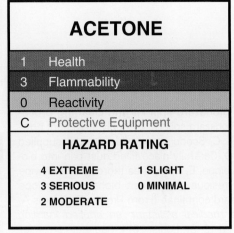

HMIS Label

ACETONE

1	Health
3	Flammability
0	Reactivity
C	Protective Equipment

HAZARD RATING

4 EXTREME	1 SLIGHT
3 SERIOUS	0 MINIMAL
2 MODERATE	

FIG. 1.22 Hazardous Materials Information System (HMIS) showing the labeling of acetone (used in staining procedures).

own SDS. The sheets are compiled in an inventory notebook available to all employees.

On the basis of the information in the SDS or the manufacturer's label, chemical hazard labels must be placed on all containers holding hazardous chemicals. The National Fire Protection Association (NFPA) and the Hazardous Materials Information System (**HMIS**) are two of the most popular systems for labeling hazardous chemicals. The systems use standard labels to communicate hazards through the use of colors, numbers, letters, and symbols (Figure 1.22).

The HMIS is a five-part rectangle that provides identification of the chemical using the information that appears on the SDS in four categories:
• Blue: health hazards (injuries that may occur if material is inhaled or ingested, skin irritants or carcinogens present in material)
• Red: flammability (volatility of material, ability of material to ignite)
• Yellow: reactivity (stability of the chemical, whether it reacts with other chemicals)
• White: the need for PPE (such as gloves, masks, and gowns)
The numerical ratings range from 0 for no hazard to 4 for extreme hazard. An alphabetical designation is used to denote recommended PPE.

Another way to label hazardous chemicals is the National Fire Protective Association (**NFPA**) label that uses the same four colors in a diamond pattern and a similar rating system of 0 to 4. Examples of typical NFPA-labeled solutions found in the laboratory are shown in Figure 1.23.

Each facility must use a labeling system that everyone understands. Another way of identifying extremely hazardous chemicals is to use icons representing each chemical hazard: flammable, explosive, corrosive, poisonous, radioactive, compressed gas, and carcinogenic as seen in Figure 1.24.

Physical Hazard Training

The third area requiring safety awareness involves potential physical hazards. This area relies on common sense and physical

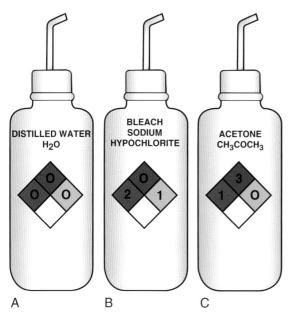

FIG. 1.23 A to C, Laboratory dispenser bottles with National Fire Protective Association labels indicating acetone and bleach hazards. Compare the label for acetone with the Hazardous Materials Information System label in Figure 1.22, and compare the bleach (sodium hypochlorite) label with the BRITE manufacturer label in Figure 1.21.

hazard orientation in areas such as lifting, weather alerts, bomb threats, and electrical dangers.
- Make sure electrical instruments are grounded and the wires are intact when working with electrical instruments. Never operate electrical equipment with wet hands. Note the electrical hazard icons in Figure 1.25.
- Run periodic drills for physical safety (e.g., fire drills, emergency weather protocol, terrorist attacks).
- Lift with the legs, not the back, and avoid twisting the back when carrying something heavy from one place to another.
- Keep hair shorter than shoulder length or tie it back to avoid contamination or getting it tangled in moving instruments.
- Never push waste down into a wastebasket with the hands or reach into a biohazard disposal container.
- Learn ergonomic practices (proper movements and conditions that make you less prone to work-related injuries) such as proper positioning of seats and computers to prevent carpal tunnel syndrome, leg cramping, and undue stress on back and neck.

Laboratory Safety Evaluation

Laboratory safety training is completed by performing the following:
1. Complete the Chapter 1 Review Questions at the end of this chapter (NOTE: answers are found in the back of the textbook) and all the Chapter 1 workbook questions.
2. Complete the following Evolve online interactive exercises for Chapter 1:
   - Exercise on ordering laboratory tests
   - Exercise on matching laboratory departments with their functions

 Flammable!

 Explosive!

 Corrosive!

 Poison!

 Radioactive!

 Compressed Gas!

 Carcinogenic Cancer-causing agent!

FIG. 1.24 Warning signs for extremely hazardous chemicals.

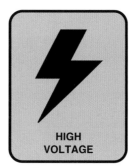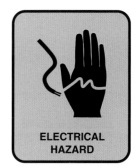

FIG. 1.25 Warning signs for electrical hazards.

3. Tour the laboratory using the Laboratory Safety Checklist at the end of Chapter 1 in the workbook. Be sure to locate or be familiar with how to use the biohazard spill kit (see Figure 1.20), the eye wash station (Figure 1.26), and the chemical spill kit (Figure 1.27).

4. Turn in the OSHA Bloodborne Pathogen Quiz at the end of Chapter 1 in the workbook and a mock exposure incident form in the appendix of the workbook.

5. Observe and perform Proper Use of Personal Protective Equipment found in Procedure 1.1.

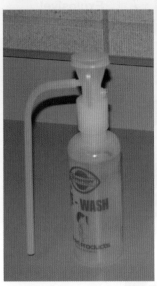

FIG. 1.26 Eye wash station.

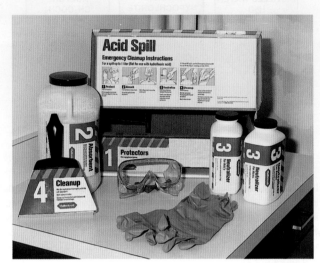

FIG. 1.27 Chemical spill kit. (From Stepp CA, Woods M: *Laboratory procedures for medical office personnel,* Philadelphia, 1998, Saunders.)

PROCEDURE 1.1   Proper Use of Personal Protective Equipment

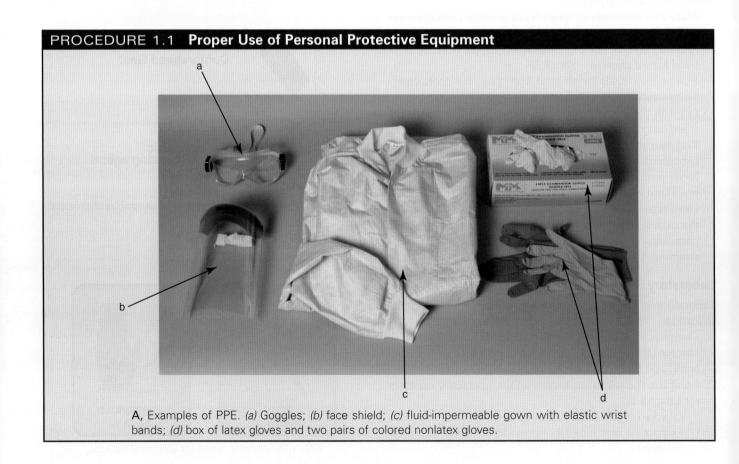

A, Examples of PPE. *(a)* Goggles; *(b)* face shield; *(c)* fluid-impermeable gown with elastic wrist bands; *(d)* box of latex gloves and two pairs of colored nonlatex gloves.

PROCEDURE 1.1   Proper Use of Personal Protective Equipment—cont'd

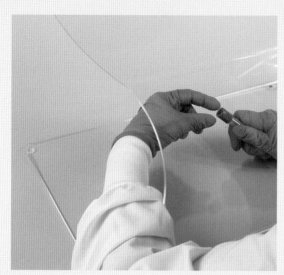

B, A Plexiglass shield provides splash protection in place of goggles and face mask when performing laboratory procedures.

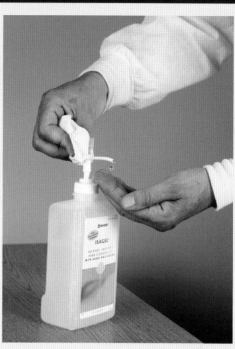

C, Sanitize the hands before donning personal protective equipment.

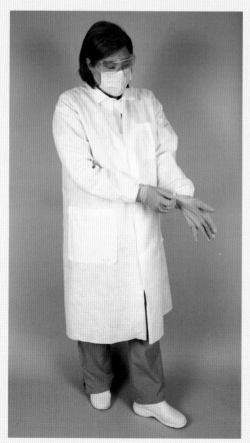

D, Order of donning PPE: (1) fluid-impermeable coat, (2) face protection, (3) gloves.

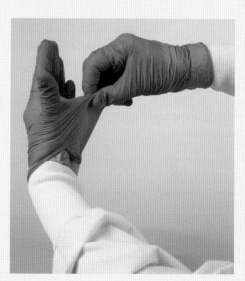

E, Removing gloves correctly. Pull off the glove on the non-dominant hand using the dominant hand.

Continued

PROCEDURE 1.1 Proper Use of Personal Protective Equipment—cont'd

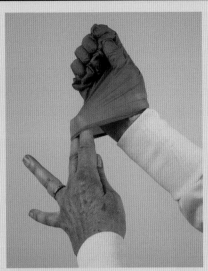

F, Hold the dirty glove in the dominant hand while slipping the nondominant fingers under the cuff.

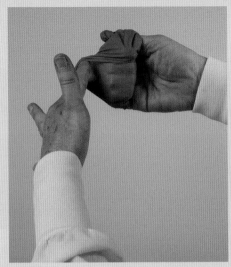

G, Flip the glove inside out while holding the other glove on the inside.

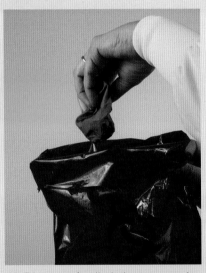

H, Dispose of soiled gloves properly.

PPE used in health care settings is displayed in Figure A. In the laboratory fluid-impenetrable gowns with cuffs at the wrists *(Ac)* and nonpowdered gloves *(Ad)* are typically worn to protect the clothes and hands from direct contact with specimens. Latex gloves are not recommended because of potential allergic reactions. Vinyl, nitrile, and other nonlatex gloves are now available in a variety of sizes and colors. A Plexiglass shield can also be placed between you and your work area (see Figure B).

Procedure

1. Before **donning** (putting on) PPE, remember to perform either the hand wash or the hand rub appropriately as described in the Hand Hygiene section of the text.

2. Also refer to the Chapter 1 videos on the Evolve website showing proper aseptic hand wash and alcohol-based hand rub methods (see Figure C).
3. If the procedure to be performed has the potential of splashing, eye goggles *(Aa)* or a face shield *(Ab)* or both will be required to protect the mucous membranes of the eyes, nose, and mouth.
4. Follow the proper sequence for donning PPE: (1) put on the gown, (2) put on any face protectors, and (3) don disposable nonsterile, nonpowdered, nonlatex, well-fitting gloves. Extend the gloves over the gown cuffs (see Figure D).
5. Keep gloved hands away from the face.
6. Remove gloves if they become torn. (Perform hand hygiene before donning new gloves.)
7. Avoid touching other surfaces and items not involved in the testing process.
8. The outside of the front of the gown is considered contaminated. The clean areas of the gown and gloves are on the inside and the back of the gown.
9. The sequence for removing PPE is to take off (1) the gloves, (2) then the face shield, and (3) then the gown.
10. The proper removal and disposal of gloves is as follows:
    a. Remove one glove by grasping the outside with the other gloved hand and pulling it off (see Figure E).
    b. Wad up the removed glove in the gloved hand. Slip an ungloved finger under the cuff and fold it over until you can grasp the inside area of the second glove (see Figure F).
    c. Pull off the second glove inside out with the first glove still inside (see Figure G).
    d. If the gloves have visible blood or body fluid on them, dispose of them in a biohazard waste receptacle (see Figure H).
11. Next, remove the goggles and then the gown.
12. Close the gown with the clean inside protected before hanging it up. The gown must not leave the lab area.
13. Perform hand hygiene (hand wash or hand rub) immediately after removing PPE.

▌ R E V I E W   Q U E S T I O N S *

1. The head of a hospital laboratory is usually a _____.

2. Phlebotomists perform _____.

3. Two nonhospital locations of medical laboratories are _____ and _____.

4. The educational degree of a pathologist is _____.

5. Five qualities important in a laboratory professional are:

   _____

   _____

   _____

   _____

   _____

6. Match the prefix on the left with the definition on the right.

   _____ milli-   **a.** one hundredth

   _____ centi-   **b.** one millionth

   _____ deci-   **c.** one tenth

   _____ micro-   **d.** one thousandth

7. Write the abbreviation for the following units:

   milliliter _____

   deciliter _____

   centimeter _____

   micrometer _____

   cubic centimeter _____

8. The three major types of hazards are _____, _____, and _____.

9. An example of a physical hazard is _____.

10. An example of a chemical hazard is _____.

11. What is an appropriate surface disinfectant for use in the laboratory?

12. Bloodborne pathogen precautions apply only to patients who are known to have infectious disease.

    True _____   False _____

13. Laboratory apparel includes fluid-impermeable laboratory coats and closed-toe shoes.

    True _____   False _____

*Answers to these Review Questions are located in the Appendix on p. 278.

WEBSITES

CDC information on Zika virus:
https://www.cdc.gov/zika/pdfs/zika-key-messages.pdf
Food and Drug Administration's website:
www.fda.gov; use the search function to find information on HIV
National Institutes of Health's website showing the latest research on the hepatitis viruses A to E:
www.niaid.nih.gov/topics/hepatitis/research/Pages/activities.aspx
Health and Human Services (**HHS**) information on disease control:

www.hhs.gov/diseases/index.html
OSHA's Bloodborne Pathogens Standard:
www.osha.gov/SLTC/bloodbornepathogens/index.html
OSHA's website showing standards for Ebola virus:
www.osha.gov/SLTC/ebola/standards.html
OSHA information on SDS:
https://www.osha.gov/Publications/HazComm_QuickCard_SafetyData.html

Regulations, Microscope Setup, and Quality Assurance

OBJECTIVES

After completing this chapter, you should be able to do the following:

1. Define and match key terms and abbreviations in this chapter.

Laboratory Regulations

2. Explain the purpose of CLIA 1988 and its benefit to the patient and demonstrate knowledge:
   - Cite the three levels of complexity listed in CLIA 1988.
   - Describe the process of obtaining certification to perform CLIA-waived laboratory tests and provider-performed microscopy.
   - Locate the latest information regarding CLIA-waived testing on the Internet.

Microscopic Procedure

3. Label the parts of a compound microscope and explain the functions of each.
4. Perform a microscopic procedure according to the stated task, conditions, and standards listed in Procedure 2.1 in the workbook, including focusing a slide under low, high

dry, and oil immersion and then cleaning and maintaining a microscope.

Quality Assurance, Quality Control, and Risk Management

5. Discuss the Centers for Disease Control and Prevention's latest tips for quality assurance: "Ready? Set? Test!"
6. List and describe the three analytical phases of laboratory testing requiring quality assessment.
7. Discuss quality control, including:
   - Explain the difference between quality assurance and quality control.
   - Define *accuracy, precision,* and *reliability* when observing the results of standard controls.
   - Identify trends, shifts, random error, out-of-control, and patient panic values.
8. Discuss current risk management and Health Insurance Portability and Accountability Act issues as they apply to the physician's office laboratory.
9. Understand the uses and benefits of electronic medical records and bar coding as they relate to medical laboratories.

KEY TERMS

accuracy (correctness): when controls consistently fall within 2 standard deviations of the mean

bar code: a pattern of narrow and wide bars and spaces that is encoded with its own particular meaning, just like words in a language are made up of letters and symbols (used for patient and specimen identification)

calibration: the process of setting an instrument to accurately respond to the test reagents or devices

Certificate of Waiver (CoW): CLIA document that allows a facility to perform only waived tests

CLIA-waived tests: tests that provide simple, virtually error-free results and require a minimum amount of judgment and interpretation and no patient injury if incorrect

control sample: a manufactured specimen that has a known value of the analyte being tested

external controls: manufactured liquid positive and negative controls with known values that are tested before the patient specimen to check the reliability of the instrument, the reagents, and the testing technique

internal control: built-in positive control used in qualitative tests to prove the device or test kit is working properly

invalid test: when the internal control area on a qualitative test shows no reaction during the testing process

kit: all components of a test packaged together

Levey-Jennings chart: a graph used to plot and visualize the results of control samples over time to ensure that test methods are consistently accurate

mean: the average test result of a series of control tests

medical office risk management: overseeing the physical and procedural risks that may bring about an injury or legal action against the practice

nonreactive or negative: a result indicating the absence of the substance that the test is designed to detect

optics check: confirming that the light source and light sensor in optical analyzers are working properly

precision (reproducibility): the ability to produce the same test result each time a test is performed

proficiency testing program: proving laboratory competency by testing a sample specimen from an outside accreditation agency and obtaining the correct result

protected health information (PHI): any health information in any form (written, electronic, or oral) that contains patient-identifiable information (e.g., name, Social Security number, telephone number) that must be kept confidential

qualitative test: test that simply looks for the presence or absence of a substance

quality assurance (QA): overall process to aid in improving the reliability, efficiency, and quality of laboratory testing in general; process oriented

quality control (QC): process in which known manufactured samples (controls) are routinely tested to establish the reliability, accuracy, and precision of a specific test system product

quantitative test: test that produces a numerical value indicating the amount of a substance present

reactive or positive: a visible result indicating the presence of a substance a test is designed to detect

reagents: substances or ingredients used in a laboratory test to detect, measure, examine, or produce a reaction

reliability: when both accuracy and precision are accomplished

semiquantitative test: test that determines the approximate quantity of an analyte (i.e., small, moderate, large)

standard deviation (SD): statistical term describing the amount of variation from the mean in a dataset

wet mount specimens: microscope slides that contain cells in water without a stain

ABBREVIATIONS

CDC: Centers for Disease Control and Prevention
CLIA: Clinical Laboratory Improvement Amendments
CMS: Centers for Medicare and Medicaid Services
FDA: Food and Drug Administration
HHS: Health and Human Services

HIPAA: Health Insurance Portability and Accountability Act
PPM: provider-performed microscopy
PPMP certification: provider-performed microscopic procedures certification

This chapter presents additional government regulations, microscope setup, and quality assurance (QA) procedures as they apply to the medical laboratory.

❖ CLIA: GOVERNMENT REGULATIONS

Whenever a specimen is removed from a human body and an analysis occurs that translates to a result, that activity is considered a medical laboratory test. As stated earlier, physicians use test results for the following reasons: (1) to *screen* and detect possible diseases, (2) to confirm a clinical *diagnosis* and make treatment decisions, and (3) to *monitor* the progress of diseases and treatments. If testing is not performed properly, the incorrect results can pose a threat to the patient's overall care and treatment. For example, if a clinical laboratory misreads or misreports a patient's blood sample as having a normal cholesterol level when in fact the patient's cholesterol level is abnormally high, that patient may not receive the necessary treatment to prevent a heart attack. In addition, if the report is misread as high when it is actually normal, the patient may receive unnecessary treatment that could potentially cause harm.

To protect patients from inaccurate test results, Congress passed the Clinical Laboratory Improvement Amendments (**CLIA**) in 1988. CLIA 1988 required that all laboratories examining materials derived from the human body for diagnosis, prevention, or treatment purposes be certified by the Secretary of Health and Human Services (**HHS**). The Centers for Medicare and Medicaid Services (**CMS**) administers the certification process by requiring all medical laboratories to register and pay a certification fee based on the level of complexity of the tests they perform.

CLIA Levels of Complexity and Their Certification Requirements

There are four complexity levels: high complexity, moderate complexity, provider-performed microscopy (**PPM**; a subset of moderate complexity), and waived testing. The Food and Drug Administration (**FDA**) is involved in determining the level of complexity for all commercial medical laboratory tests on the market.

CLIA Certificate of Waiver

The CLIA Certificate of Waiver (CoW) is used predominantly by physician's office laboratories (POLs), ambulatory settings, and institutions with point-of-care testing (POCT).

According to CLIA, CoW laboratories can perform only tests that are determined by the FDA to be so simple that there is little risk of error. Examples of CLIA-waived tests with their appropriate procedure codes are listed in Table 2.1.

The number and types of tests waived under CLIA have increased from the 8 originally approved tests in 1992 to now more than 100 tests. The number of waived laboratories has also grown exponentially, from 20% to more than 60% of the total laboratories enrolled in CLIA.

To become a CLIA-waived laboratory, the physician or facility simply needs to enroll in the CLIA-waived program through CMS, pay an applicable certification fee of $150 every 2 years, and follow the manufacturer's instructions for each FDA-approved waived test.

The following are some benefits of becoming a CLIA-waived lab in an ambulatory setting:
- Rapid availability of results while the patient is available for immediate follow-up
- Simple tests have minimal need for training
- Portability of many waived tests allows for easier testing in nontraditional settings

CLIA High and Moderately Complex Laboratories

Hospital and reference laboratories are staffed with highly educated laboratory professionals who have been trained to perform the complex tests in the various laboratory departments, such as

TABLE 2.1 Tests Granted Waived Status Under CLIA 1988

CPT Code	Test Name	Use
Original Eight Tests Approved in 1988		
Hematology		
83026	Hemoglobin by copper sulfate—nonautomated	Monitors hemoglobin level in blood
85013	Blood count; spun microhematocrit	Screens for anemia
85651	Erythrocyte sedimentation rate—nonautomated	Nonspecific screening test for inflammatory activity; increased in the majority of infections and most cases of carcinoma and leukemia
Chemistry		
82962	Blood glucose by glucose monitoring devices cleared by FDA for home use	Monitoring of blood glucose levels
Urine and Feces		
81003QW	Dipstick or tablet reagent urinalysis—nonautomated for bilirubin, glucose, hemoglobin, ketones, leukocytes, nitrites, pH, protein, specific gravity, and urobilinogen	Screening of urine to monitor or diagnose various diseases and conditions such as diabetes, the state of the kidney or urinary tract, and urinary tract infections
81025	Urine pregnancy tests by visual color comparison	Diagnosis of pregnancy
84830	Ovulation tests by visual color comparison for human luteinizing hormone	Detection of ovulation (optimal for conception)
82271	Fecal occult blood	Detection of hidden blood in feces from any cause, benign or malignant (colorectal cancer screening)
Examples of More Recently Approved Waived Tests		
Hematology (see Tests in Chapter 5)		
85014QW	STAT-CRIT/hematocrit	Screen for anemia
85018QW	HemoCue hemoglobin system	Measures hemoglobin level in whole blood
85610QW	ProTime test	Measures time it takes to clot blood and calculates patient's INR
Blood Chemistry (see Tests in Chapter 6)		
80061QW	Cholestech LDX	Measures total cholesterol, HDL cholesterol, triglycerides, and glucose levels in blood
82947QW	HemoCue B—glucose photometer	Measures glucose levels in whole blood
83036QW	Bayer A1CNOW+	Measures percent concentration of hemoglobin A_{1c} in blood, which is used in monitoring long-term care of people with diabetes
80047QW	i-STAT basic metabolic panel	Measures sodium (Na), potassium (K), chloride (Cl), ionized calcium (Ca), total carbon dioxide (TCO_2), creatinine (Crea), glucose (Glu), blood urea nitrogen (BUN), hematocrit (Hct), and hemoglobin (Hgb) in whole blood
82274QW	iFOB fecal occult blood	Immunologic detection of hidden blood in feces
Drug Screening (see Chapter 9)		
G0434QW	Multiple drug cup test	Screening test to detect presence of amphetamines, barbiturates, benzodiazepines, THC, cocaine metabolites, methadone, methamphetamines, opiates, oxycodone, and PCP in urine
K121247	Alcohol saliva test for ethanol	Measures amount of ethanol in saliva
Immunology and Serology (see Chapter 7)		
86308QW	Rapid whole blood mononucleosis tests	Qualitative screening test for presence of heterophile antibodies to aid in diagnosis of infectious mononucleosis
86318QW	Rapid whole blood test for *Helicobacter pylori* antibodies for determining possible cause of peptic ulcers	Immunoassay for rapid, qualitative detection of immunoglobulin G antibodies specific to *H. pylori*
86618QW	Rapid whole blood test for *Borrelia burgdorferi* (causative agent of Lyme disease)	Qualitative detection of immunoglobulin G and M antibodies to *B. burgdorferi*
86701QW	Rapid HIV-1 antibody test with whole blood	Qualitative immunoassay to detect antibodies to HIV-1 in fingerstick and venipuncture whole blood specimens
86703QW	OraQuick rapid HIV-1 and HIV-2 antibody test	Qualitative immunoassay to detect antibodies to HIV-1 in oral liquid specimen

TABLE 2.1	Tests Granted Waived Status Under CLIA 1988—cont'd	
CPT Code	**Test Name**	**Use**
Microbiology (see Chapter 8)		
87804QW	Quick influenza A and B test	Qualitative detection of influenza type A and B antigens in nasal wash and nasopharyngeal swab specimens
87889QW	Quick *Streptococcus* A test	Rapidly detects *Streptococcus* A antigen from throat swabs as an aid in diagnosis of strep throat, tonsillitis, and scarlet fever
Urinalysis (see Chapter 3)		
81003QW	Bayer Clinitek 50 urine chemistry analyzer—qualitative dipstick for glucose, bilirubin, ketones, specific gravity, blood, pH, protein, urobilinogen, nitrites, leukocytes (automated)	Screening of urine to monitor or diagnose various diseases and conditions such as diabetes, the state of kidney or urinary tract, and urinary tract infections
82044QW	Bayer Clinitek 50 urine chemistry analyzer—microalbumin, creatinine	Semiquantitative measurement of microalbumin and creatinine in urine for detection of patients at risk for developing kidney damage
84703QW	Bayer Clinitek 50 urine chemistry analyzer— pregnancy test using cartridge in analyzer	Qualitative test for hCG hormone in urine to detect pregnancy
Semen		
89321QW	Fertell male fertility test	Measures concentration of motile sperm
83900Q	SpermCheck vasectomy	Detects presence of sperm

CPT, Current Procedural Terminology; *FDA*, Food and Drug Administration; *hCG*, human chorionic gonadotropin; *HDL*, high-density lipoprotein; *INR*, international normalized ratio; *PCP*, phencyclidine; *THC*, tetrahydrocannabinol.

hematology, chemistry, microbiology, and blood bank. To be registered and certified by CLIA, professional laboratories must obtain a Certificate of Registration and then be surveyed to receive a Certificate of Compliance and then a Certificate of Accreditation. They must maintain their accreditation status by being surveyed periodically to validate that they are performing only tests within their level of complexity and that their personnel are qualified and sufficiently trained in the test procedures.

All testing procedures are continuously monitored by the following systems:

1. Quality assurance (QA)—the overall process to aid in improving the reliability, efficiency, and quality of all laboratory tests in general. QA has three major phases: preanalytical, analytical, and postanalytical. Each of these steps must be evaluated regarding the effectiveness of the laboratory's policies and procedures in producing and documenting the test results, the identification of any problems, and the correction of the problems. The policies must ensure the accurate and prompt performance and reporting of tests.
2. Quality control (QC)—a part of QA that takes place during the analytical phase. It uses manufactured samples with known values that are tested along with the patient samples to establish the reliability, accuracy, and precision of a specific test system.
3. Proficiency testing program—biannual confirmation of laboratory competency by testing specimens from an outside accreditation agency and obtaining the correct results (**proficiency testing**).

Further details concerning high and moderate complexity testing may be found at the government websites for HHS, CMS, **Centers for Disease Control and Prevention (CDC)**, and FDA. The purpose of this text, however, is to explore the lesser regulated CLIA certificates most commonly used in physicians' offices, ambulatory care, and point-of-care settings, specifically the CLIA-waived tests and the PPM tests.

CLIA: Provider-Performed Microscopy Procedures Certificate

The PPM procedures (PPMP) certificate allows qualified health care providers to conduct waived testing and basic microscopic examinations during the patient's visit. The microscopic tests are performed on specimens that are not easily transportable. To receive **PPMP certification**, the physician or medical facility must enroll in the CMS program for PPMP certification, pay applicable certificate fees of $200 every 2 years, and maintain certain QA and administrative requirements such as the following:

- Proficiency testing by an outside agency to evaluate microscopic accuracy twice a year
- Documentation of microscope and centrifuge maintenance
- Confirmation that competent personnel are interpreting the microscopic findings

Some of the microscopic tests that require proper preparation are presented in this text. The preparations for these microscopic tests include the following:

- Urine sediment preparation as part of a complete urinalysis
- Direct wet mount preparations for the identification of bacteria, fungi, parasites, and abnormal human cellular elements
- Potassium hydroxide preparations for identifying fungi
- Cellulose tape preparations for identifying pinworms

The actual reading and reporting of the microscopic findings must be done by the physician or a laboratory professional trained and certified to interpret the particular test. Table 2.2 lists the approved PPM tests and their numerical Current Procedural Terminology (CPT) codes.

TABLE 2.2	CLIA-Approved Provider-Performed Microscopy Tests
CPT Code	**Microscopic Test**
Q0111	Wet mounts, including preparations of vaginal, cervical, or skin specimens to view organisms in living state
Q0112	All potassium hydroxide preparations to detect fungal infections
Q0113	Pinworm examinations to detect *Enterobius vermicularis*
Q0114	Fern test (to detect leakage of amniotic fluid caused by ruptured membranes)
Q0115	Postcoital direct, qualitative examinations of vaginal or cervical mucus to detect presence and motility of sperm after sex regarding infertility
81015	Urinalysis, microscopic only to examine, count, and categorize solid structures in urine
81000	Urinalysis, by dipstick or tablet reagent for bilirubin, glucose, hemoglobin, ketones, leukocytes, nitrite, pH, protein, specific gravity, urobilinogen, and any number of these constituents; nonautomated, with microscopy
81001	Urinalysis, by dipstick or tablet reagent for bilirubin, glucose, hemoglobin, ketones, leukocytes, nitrite, pH, protein, specific gravity, urobilinogen, and any number of these constituents; automated, with microscopy (Note: This may be used only when the laboratory is using an automated dipstick urinalysis instrument approved as waived.)
81020	Urinalysis; two- or three-glass test: to determine the location of an infection in the male urinary system
89055	Fecal leukocyte examination to count and categorize white blood cells in a fecal specimen
G0027	Semen analysis; presence and motility of sperm, excluding Huhner test to detect the presence and motility of sperm
89190	Nasal smears for eosinophils to identify and count eosinophils to assess allergic reactions

MICROSCOPE PROCEDURE

If the physician chooses to register and perform basic microscopic examinations of specimens, his or her employees will need to learn how to set up a microscope slide for observation. They will also need to focus and maintain the microscope for optimal performance. The microscopic structures and procedure for using a clinical microscope are described in the following section. Procedure 2.1: Using a Microscope skill checklist is found at the end of Chapter 2 in the workbook.

Identifying the Parts and Functions of a Microscope

The microscope can be divided into the following three basic functional areas:

1. *The foundational structures*—consisting of the base, arm, stage, and mechanical slide holder and its controls
2. *The illuminating structures*—consisting of the light source and condenser, with the condenser containing both a control knob and an iris diaphragm lever to open and close the diaphragm
3. *The magnifying structures*—consisting of the objectives lenses that are attached to the revolving nosepiece, the ocular lenses, and the coarse and fine focus adjustment knobs

As you look at the picture of the microscope in Figure 2.1, note the name of each lettered structure in the text as it is described in the three subsequent categories.

Foundational Structures and Their Functions

First, always carry the microscope with two hands—one under the *(a) base* and the other holding the *(b) arm*. The slide with the specimen is placed on the *(c) stage* and clipped into place with the *(d) mechanical holder,* which can then precisely move the slide back and forth and side to side when the operator turns the *(e) mechanical controls* located under the stage.

Illuminating Structures and Their Functions

The slide is illuminated by the *(f) light source* in the base of the microscope. The light flows up into the *(g) condenser,* where it becomes highly concentrated. The condenser can be raised or lowered to a position just under the slide by using the *(h) condenser adjustment* when viewing densely stained specimens. The condenser can be lowered for more transparent wet mount specimens (slides that contain cells in water without a stain). The condenser also contains the *(i) iris diaphragm lever,* which opens the iris for dense slides and closes the iris, thus reducing the amount of light, for more transparent slides (similar to the way the iris of the eye opens and closes the pupil).

Magnifying Structures and Their Functions

After the light flows up through the condenser and through the slide on the stage, it enters one of three or four *(j) objectives lenses*. These lenses are usually color coded, with tubes of different lengths marked with the magnification power. The shortest tubes are the low power objectives and are usually marked with 4× or 10× magnification, meaning they make the image 4 or 10 times larger, respectively. The middle-length tube contains the high power objective and usually magnifies 40×. The longest tube objective usually magnifies 100×. This extremely high power objective contains the only lens that requires oil to be placed between it and the slide to prevent air from bending (refracting) the light out of focus. Thus, it is called the *oil immersion objective.* The *(k) revolving nosepiece* is used to move from one objective to another. (Note: Do not turn the objectives by pushing on the objective tubes.)

After passing through the objectives, the lighted image strikes a mirror that sends the image through the *(l) ocular lenses* (eyepieces), where the operator can see the result. The ocular lenses enlarge the image an additional 10 times, which is

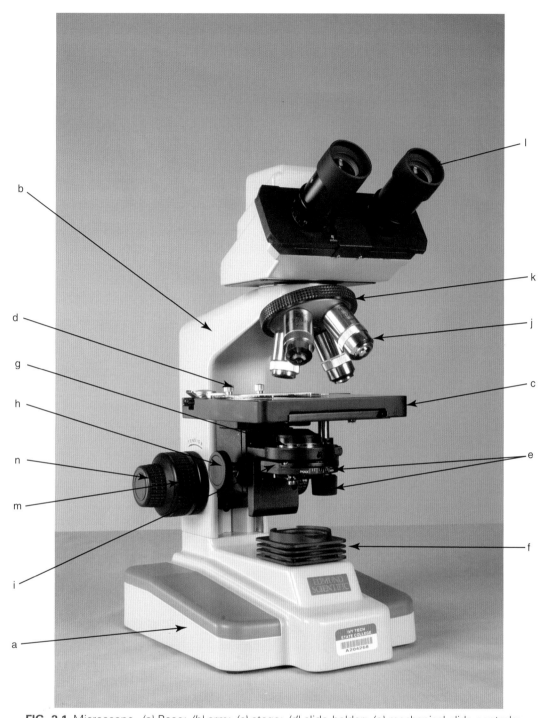

FIG. 2.1 Microscope. *(a)* Base; *(b)* arm; *(c)* stage; *(d)* slide holder; *(e)* mechanical slide controls; *(f)* light source; *(g)* condenser; *(h)* condenser adjustment; *(i)* iris diaphragm lever; *(j)* low power objective; *(k)* nosepiece; *(l)* ocular lens; *(m)* coarse focus adjustment; *(n)* fine focus adjustment.

multiplied by the objective magnification to determine total magnification.

Objective Magnification (×) Times	Ocular Magnification (×) =	Total Magnification
Low power 4×	10×	40×
Low power 10×	10×	100×
High power 40×	10×	400×
Oil immersion 100×	10×	1000×

The ocular lenses can also be adjusted to focus each eye individually and can move closer together or apart to become aligned with the operator's eye span. The specimen is brought into focus by starting with the low power objective and then turning the *(m) coarse adjustment* knob followed by moving the hand to the *(n) fine adjustment* knob to focus the objects more clearly.

After all the names and locations of the parts of the microscope have been mastered, the first microscope laboratory procedure can be undertaken as seen in Procedure 2.1 and in the workbook.

PROCEDURE 2.1 Using a Microscope

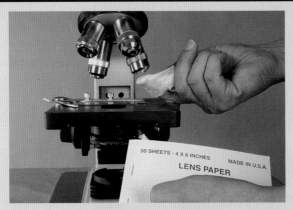

A, Clean with lens paper.

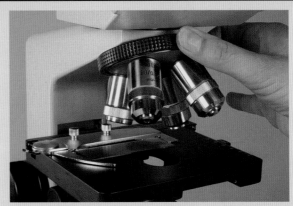

B, Move the objectives by rotating the nosepiece to where the low power objective is pointing down toward the slide.

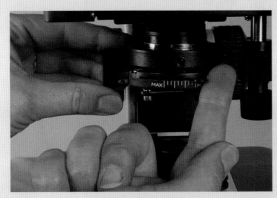

C, Adjust the condenser height control on the left and the diaphragm control on the right.

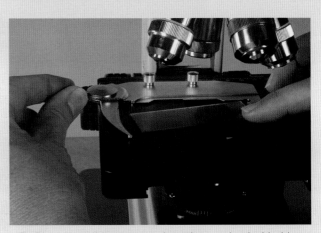

D, Place the slide on stage into the mechanical holder.

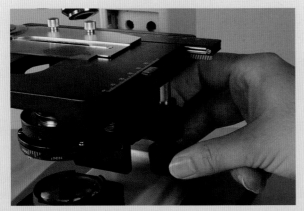

E, Use the mechanical stage controls to move the slide sideways or forward and back to place the slide above the light source.

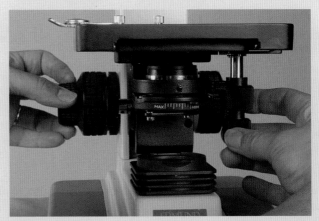

F, After finding the image with the large coarse knob, use the small fine focus knob with one hand while moving the slide slightly using the mechanical stage control with the other hand.

PROCEDURE 2.1 Using a Microscope—cont'd

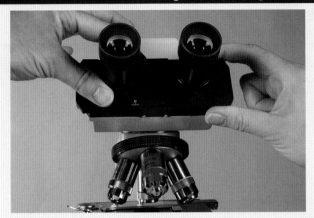

G, Adjust the oculars to the width of your two eyes and then adjust each of the oculars to your eyes' vision.

Equipment and Supplies
Microscope; lens paper; a stained slide; immersion oil; soft, lint-free tissue

Set Up the Microscope and Slide (see Figure 2.1)
1. Always carry the microscope with one hand under the base *(a)* and the other grasping the arm *(b)* of the scope.
2. Clean the ocular *(l)* and objective *(j)* lenses with lens paper (clean the oil immersion lens last). Note that in Figure A the soft part of the finger is used to clean the lens. Use a different part of the lens paper for each lens and always clean the oil immersion lens last to keep from spreading the oil to the other lenses.
3. Turn the nosepiece *(k)* until the low power objective is directly above the stage (Figure B). Do not push the objective tubes.
4. Turn the coarse adjustment *(m)* until the stage *(c)* and the low power objective *(j)* are farthest apart.
5. Turn on the light source *(f)* and turn the condenser adjustment *(h)* until the condenser *(g)* is at its highest level for viewing stained slides. With the other hand, completely open the iris with the diaphragm lever *(i)* to adjust for the maximum amount of light (Figure C).
6. Place the slide in the slide holder *(d)* (Figure D) and use the mechanical controls *(e)* to move the stained portion of the slide directly above the light source (Figure E).
7. Adjust the ocular lens *(l)* to align with your eyes.

Low Power Focus
8. Always start with the low power objective in place and initially focus using the coarse adjustment. While looking through the oculars, turn the coarse adjustment *(m)* until color starts to appear and then turn very slowly, bringing the image into coarse focus (Figure F). *Tip:* Moving the mechanical slide knob slightly back and forth with your right hand while finding the focus position with your left hand helps realize movement for ease in focusing.
9. Next, move the focusing hand to the fine focus adjustment *(n)* and turn it one way and then the other until the image becomes clear. Both eyes should see a clear image. If not, adjust the oculars by turning their individual focus controls. In Figure G, the left hand is adjusting the ocular focus while the right hand is pulling the ocular lenses apart to align with the operator's eyes.
10. When the image is in focus, move the slide so that the object of interest is in the center of the visual field. Then turn the nosepiece to high power.

High Power Focus
11. Refocus the image by turning the fine adjustment one way and then the other until you see color and then the clear image. (NOTE: Do not use the coarse adjustment because it will make too drastic a change and possibly

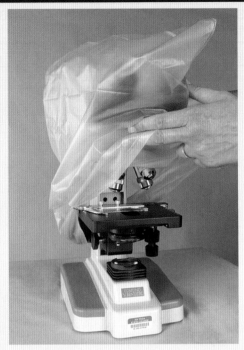

H, After cleaning the lenses and stage, always store the microscope with its protective cover.

break the slide or damage the objective. If you are unable to focus with the fine adjustment, go back to low power and start again with the coarse and fine focus adjustments.) Move the slide so that the desired object is again in the middle of the visual field.

Oil Immersion Preparation and Focus
12. You are now ready to use the oil immersion lens for maximum magnification. Turn the nosepiece halfway between high power and the oil immersion objective.
13. Place a drop of oil directly on the slide where the condenser light is shining through the slide.
14. Carefully turn the nosepiece until the oil immersion lens dips into the oil and snaps into place.
15. Now, while looking into the oculars, move the small fine focus adjustment back and forth until the image pops into view. The slide can be moved and refocused by using the mechanical stage controls with one hand, while the other hand is turning the fine focus to continuously make adjustments while moving to different areas of the slide. The instructor or supervisor will verify the successful focused result.

Cleanup and Microscope Maintenance
16. When you are finished observing the slide, turn off the light and turn the nosepiece back to the low power objective. By using the large coarse focus knob, maximize the distance between the lens and the stage. Remove the slide, and clean the stage with soft, lint-free tissue. Clean the oil off the slide with tissue or xylene.
17. With a new piece of lens paper, clean the ocular lenses and then the objective lenses. Always clean the oil immersion lens last. Do not forget to remove any residual oil from the stage.
18. Cover the microscope with a dust-proof cover (Figure H) and store it in a clean, protected area.

Continued

PROCEDURE 2.1   Using a Microscope—cont'd

KEYS TO PROPER CONDENSER AND OBJECTIVE LENS SETTINGS BASED ON THREE COMMON SLIDES

	Liquid Urine	Stained Blood Slide	Stained Microbiology
Condenser setting	Down with diaphragm almost closed	All the way up against the bottom of the slide with the diaphragm open	All the way up against the bottom of the slide with the diaphragm open
Objective lens setting	Low and then high "dry" lenses only—no oil immersion (10× and 40×)	Start on low, then high, and then oil immersion for identification	Start on low, then high, and then oil immersion for identification

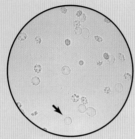

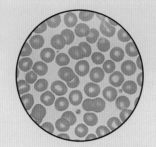

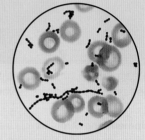

A (From Stepp CA, Woods M: *Laboratory procedures for medical office personnel*, Philadelphia, 1998, Saunders; Zakus SM: *Mosby's clinical skills for medical assistants*, ed 4, St. Louis, 2001, Mosby.)

B (From Rodak BF: *Hematology: clinical principles and applications*, ed 4, St. Louis, 2012, Saunders.)

C (From Proctor D, Adams A: *Kinn's the medical assistant: an applied learning approach*, ed 12, St. Louis, 2014, Saunders.)

GOOD LABORATORY PRACTICES

The CLIA CoW is the least regulated category of laboratory testing. Waived tests can be performed by individuals with little or no previous experience in laboratory testing, and they do not require the rigorous QC or QA documentation, periodic surveys, and proficiency testing of the other CLIA categories. These facts, along with the ever-increasing number of approved waived tests, have raised the following question: Are the waived test results accurate and reliable? The HHS, CMS, FDA, CDC, laboratory professionals, and test manufacturers are all looking for ways to better educate the personnel performing waived tests. Anyone performing a test on a specimen must know how to achieve accurate and reliable results to ultimately improve the quality of health care.

Quality Assurance

How can the patient be assured that the results were obtained in a reliable, efficient, and well-monitored way? This is where QA becomes a factor. Remember, QA is an overall process to aid in improving the reliability, efficiency, and quality of the laboratory as a whole. Also remember that QA has three major phases: preanalytical, analytical, and postanalytical.

Table 2.3 describes the QA that must be assessed and documented during the three phases of laboratory testing. Table 2.4 lists the problems or variables that may occur within each phase causing inaccurate results. These tables are a good review of the concepts presented in this chapter. Everyone involved in the laboratory process must take personal responsibility for his or her part in providing safe, high-quality patient care.

Eight quality assurance questions should always be asked when testing specimens:

1. Are the patients and specimens properly identified?
2. Are the patients' charts up to date, with the proper patient test information?
3. Was the QC performed and documented?
4. Did the laboratory get the right answers for the QC?
5. Do the waived test results correlate with the patient's history or symptoms?
6. Are there any complaints about the laboratory testing?
7. Are the testing personnel trained before performing laboratory testing?
8. Are there periodic discussions about laboratory concerns?

Quality Control

A major concern facing all medical laboratories is how to ensure that the test **kit** or test instrument is producing the correct results consistently. As mentioned earlier, if the patient's test result is *not* right, it can have a harmful effect on the patient's future course of diagnosis and treatment. The answer to the problem during the analytical phase is to implement QC for each test. This is done by testing a **control sample** (a manufactured specimen that already has a known value) before testing the patient specimen. If the control sample's test result is within

TABLE 2.3 Quality Assurance and the Three Stages of Laboratory Testing

Preanalytical Phase	Analytical Phase	Postanalytical Phase

1. Physician examines the patient and **orders the tests** that need to be performed to:
  a. Screen for possible disorders
  b. Confirm tentative diagnosis
  c. Monitor existing disorder
2. A **requisition** is completed, and the patient is instructed in any preparatory procedure, such as fasting (no eating) medications taken or not taken before some blood tests, or first morning urine specimen (for some urine tests).
3. An appropriate **specimen is collected** in the proper container:
  a. Urine
  b. Blood in proper tubes
  c. Specimen from infected site
  d. Fecal specimen
4. The specimen is processed:
  a. Labeled in the presence of the patient
  b. Stored at proper temperature
  c. Preservatives or additives are added if needed
5. The specimen is transported to:
  a. A laboratory area in the office
  b. A reference laboratory
  c. A hospital laboratory
	6. If tested in the physician's office laboratory, **quality control** is run and logged before patient testing:
	  a. The instrument is calibrated daily, and results are logged.
	  b. Controls provided by the manufacturer are run, and results are logged.
	  c. A proficiency test is successfully run on the sample from an outside source twice annually, and results are logged.
	7. If all the preceding are verified, the **patient specimen is tested.**
	8. A **laboratory report** is produced showing the results of the tests:
	  a. In-office results are recorded directly on the patient's chart with reference ranges and on a patient log.
	  b. Reference laboratory reports are sent to the office by mail, phone, fax, or electronically. They are logged when received.
		9. The specimen is **properly disposed** of in biohazard container and sent to a managed waste company.
		10. **Quality control results are analyzed** to determine if the test method is "in control" based on precision, accuracy, reliability, shifts, trends, and random errors.
		11. Patient reports are interpreted and signed by:
		  a. The ordering physician
		  b. Laboratory pathologists
		  c. Additional consulting physicians
		12. **The patient is notified** in the proper confidential manner. Communication is documented in the patient record.
		13. The **final signed report is filed** in the patient record.

TABLE 2.4 Variables That Can Negatively Affect the Quality of Laboratory Results

Preanalytical Phase	Analytical Phase	Postanalytical Phase

• Improper patient identification
• Improper patient instruction or compliance (e.g., did not fast, did not collect first morning urine specimen)
• Improper collection of specimen (e.g., wrong time, wrong container, wrong volume, wrong site)
• Improper labeling of specimen
• Improper processing of specimen (e.g., spun versus unspun blood)
• Improper storage of specimen (e.g., refrigerator or room temperature)
• Improper transportation of specimen (e.g., timing, temperature, light exposure)
• Contamination
	• Instrument not functioning correctly
	• Instrument not calibrated
	• Not running and observing controls before patient test
	• Reagents or test kit expired
	• Reagents or test kit not stored at proper temperature
	• Reagents from one kit used with another kit
	• Poor testing technique of operator
	• Not following manufacturer's instructions regarding
	  1. Amount of specimen
	  2. Amount of reagents
	  3. Steps involving time
	  4. Proper temperature for testing (e.g., refrigerated test kit must first come to room temperature before testing)
		• Incorrectly recording in-office results on patient log or patient record
		• Not identifying when controls are out of their range and problem-solve reasons for this
		• Not providing physician with reference range along with patient's results to aid in interpretation
		• Not notifying physician when results have arrived from outside reference laboratory
		• Not notifying patient in proper confidential manner regarding results of test
		• Results lost in mail or fax machine
		• Report filed in wrong patient chart

the acceptable range of its known value, then the values from patients' specimens are surmised to also be reliable. When all the QC sample results are recorded on a dated log sheet, the overall performance of the test system can also be monitored over time.

In CLIA-waived laboratories, two different types of tests require QC: qualitative and quantitative.

Quality Control Monitoring of Qualitative Waived Tests

The method of simply testing for the presence or absence of an analyte (the substance being tested in the specimen) is considered a qualitative test. Most qualitative test kits are designed to show three possible test results expressed as the following:

- Reactive or positive—a result that indicates the presence of the substance a test is designed to detect
- Nonreactive or negative—a result that indicates the absence of the substance a test is designed to detect
- Invalid test—when the internal control area on a qualitative test shows no reaction during the testing process

Figure 2.2 shows three qualitative pregnancy test kits. These individual testing devices usually have a built-in positive control ("C") that produces a colored band to prove the device is

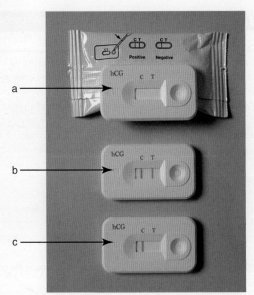

FIG. 2.2 Qualitative pregnancy tests. *a)* Test kit before adding urine specimen; *b)* a positive reaction in the test area *(T)* indicates that the pregnancy hormone human chorionic gonadotropin (HCG) is present; *c)* a negative reaction (nonreaction) in the test area indicates that no pregnancy HCG is present. NOTE: In both tests *(b* and *c)* the internal control area *(C)* indicates the results are valid.

operational. If the built-in internal control does not show a color reaction, the test would need to be repeated. If the repeated test also fails, the test system would be considered invalid, and corrective action must be taken by checking for the following possible causes:

1. Were the directions followed?
2. Were the reagents (substances used in a test to detect, measure, examine, or produce a reaction) added in the correct order and at the correct time?
3. Were the reagents outdated or stored at the wrong temperature (e.g., room temperature, in the refrigerator)?
4. If everything seems accurate and problems still exist, contact the manufacturer and use a new kit.

Many manufacturers also supply and recommend external controls (liquid positive and negative controls that are tested the same way as the patient's liquid specimen to check the reliability of the instrument and the testing). These manufactured external controls must be run daily, weekly, or monthly as recommended by the manufacturer to further check the reliability of the test system. The dated results of these external controls must also be logged and evaluated. You will be using the qualitative log sheets in your workbook when testing for occult blood, immunology tests, and microbiology tests.

Quality Control Monitoring of Semiquantitative Waived Tests

It is also possible to semiquantify the amount of an analyte by its color reaction with a particular reagent, as seen when testing urine specimens (see Chapter 3). A urine test strip contains reagent pads that react specifically with each analyte, causing a variety of color changes. The more a particular analyte is present in urine, the darker the color will be on the reagent pad. This is referred to as a semiquantitative test. Whereas a *qualitative* test indicates if a particular analyte is present, *semiquantitative* testing determines the approximate quantity of an analyte. Urine reagent strips provide both qualitative and semiquantitative measurements, with results recorded as negative and/or positive or in ranges such as trace, 1+, 2+, or 3+ or small, moderate, or large.

Quality control monitoring consists of running two manufactured liquid controls, one with normal results and a second with abnormal results. The manufacturer will provide the semiquantitative predicted results of its control to be compared with the results obtained when running the liquid control. If the results do not match, the same four questions listed in the preceding section should be addressed and the necessary corrections made.

Quality Control Monitoring of Quantitative Waived Tests

Quantitative test results have a numerical value indicating the amount of a substance present. (e.g., See the Laboratory Report with all its numerical readouts in Chapter 1, Figure 1.1.) The quantitative result for each test is compared with a population's reference range. The typical reference range for fasting glucose level in the general population shows 70 to 110 mg/dL. If the patient's results are drastically less than or greater than the reference range, it may be clinically significant. For example, if the glucose level in a patient with diabetes is drastically low, the patient could transition into insulin shock. If the glucose level is drastically high, the patient could present with a diabetic coma.

Optics. Monitors that measure the quantity of a substance often send a light through the specimen or reflect off the specimen to determine how much of the analyte is present. With this method of testing, an optics check (process of confirming that the light source and light sensor in optical analyzers are working properly) must be performed daily with the results documented on a log sheet. The manufacturer may refer to this process as *calibrating the instrument.* Calibration is the process of setting the instrument's optics to the test reagents or test devices that will be used. See the step B showing the calibration step performed on the Cholestech in Chapter 6, Procedure 6.3. **Coding** the instrument to the manufacturer's new test strip number may also be necessary after receiving a new set of testing supplies to reset the instrument's optics. Be sure to read the manufacturer's directions to determine if and when optic checks and/or coding are necessary.

External controls. Quantitative tests produce numerical results that indicate whether the analyte value is high, normal, or low compared with its reference range. Therefore, it is often necessary to run two or three levels of manufactured control samples on the instrument to ensure that all levels are being accurately detected (i.e., high, low, and normal controls). These QC samples are generally manufactured liquids that are tested in the same way as the patient's specimen. They, too, must be documented on log sheets at specific intervals (daily, weekly, or monthly), dated, and evaluated over time.

External controls can be further evaluated by statistical means. For example, if a control specimen was tested 10 times, the results could be added and then divided by 10 to determine a mean (average test result). Each result could then be compared with the mean, and a mathematical calculation could be made to determine how much each control result varied from the mean. Another mathematical calculation could then be made to determine the standard deviation (SD) (a statistical term describing the amount of variation from the mean in a dataset). After these figures are determined, a graph can be created showing the value of the mean and the value of one and two SDs above and below the mean (abbreviated as +1 SD, +2 SD, −1 SD, and −2 SD). When manufactured controls are being run, the goal is to make sure the results fall within ±2 SDs of the manufacturer's mean (referred to as the control's range). In Figure 2.3, the mean for a glucose normal standard control is 100 mg/dL. If 1 SD is calculated to be 5 mg/dL, then ±1 SD would be 105 and 95 mg/dL. Two SDs would be equal to 10 mg/dL, and their values above and below the mean would be 110 and 90 mg/dL, respectively. In this example, 6 days of control results have been plotted and all the results fall within ±2 SDs. This indicates the test method is "in control." (NOTE: CLIA-waived test controls have been statistically measured by the manufacturers and will be packaged with the control "range" already determined.)

The graph in Figure 2.3 is called a Levey-Jennings chart, which is used to plot the ongoing results of test control samples. If a control test result falls higher or lower than 2 SDs or outside the manufacturer's given range, it is considered "out of control," and corrective action must be taken before testing and reporting patient samples.

By plotting quantitative results on a Levey-Jennings chart over time, the laboratory professional can identify possible problems and correct them before running patient samples. Examine each of the graphs in Figures 2.4 to 2.6 and note the possible causes for each of the patterns. In all these cases, the control may be within 2 SDs, but reason for concern still exists.

The following are some patterns seen in weekly control graphs and examples of ways they may be corrected:

Excessive scatter (see Figure 2.4): Values scatter widely above and below the mean. Possible cause: operator variability (e.g., days 2 and 5 were logged by technician A, and days 1, 3, 4, and 6 by technician B). Correction: Observe each technician's technique to see how he or she is performing the test and interpreting the results.

Trends (see Figure 2.5): Values move up or down incrementally in the same direction on each subsequent day. Possible cause: Reagents are outdated or the instrument is losing its calibration. Correction: Use a new set of reagents and run a calibration check.

Shift (see Figure 2.6): Values shift from a consistent set of results to another set of results. Possible cause: new reagents, new person testing, or sudden deterioration of reagents. Check lot numbers and expiration dates on reagents and observe new technician's performance.

Additional statistical terms must be understood when analyzing control results. Accuracy (correctness) occurs when control results consistently fall within 1 SD of the mean. Precision (reproducibility) is the ability to produce the same test result each time a test is performed. Reliability is the result when both accuracy and precision are accomplished. Reliability is the goal that must be achieved before testing patient specimens.

A way to visualize these three terms is to take the mean of a control and place it in the middle, or bull's eye, of a target (Figure 2.7). The two circles around the mean represent 1 SD and 2 SDs. The arrows in *A* are inaccurate because they all incorrectly miss the center of the target, and they are not precise because they are scattered around the central area. The arrows in *B* are precise because they are clustered together (reproducible), but none of them are accurate because they all incorrectly miss the inner circle. The goal for a *reliable* test system is seen as the arrows in *C* that show all the values *accurate* (in the center of the target) and *precise* (all showing a similar value). NOTE: These same terms apply when observing CLIA-waived control results. The controls should fall close to the manufacturer's stated mean (the bull's eye), and they should also be within the manufacturer's stated range (the circle around the bull's eye).

See Figure 2.8 for an example of the manufacturer's liquid control ranges for a glucose meter.

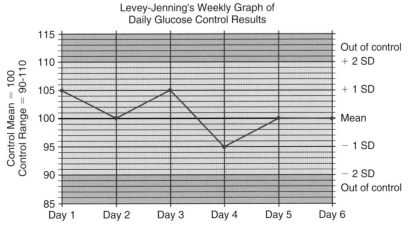

FIG. 2.3 Weekly glucose control results that are in control. *SD,* Standard deviation.

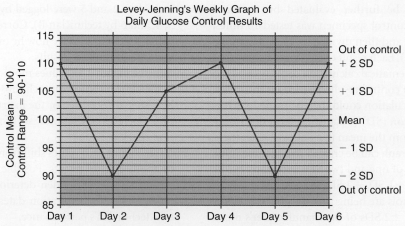

FIG. 2.4 Weekly glucose control results showing excessive scatter. *SD,* Standard deviation.

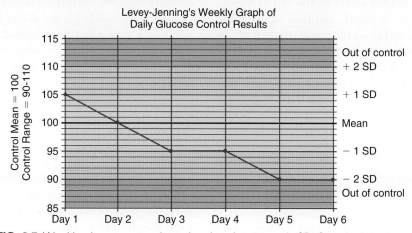

FIG. 2.5 Weekly glucose control results showing a trend. *SD,* Standard deviation.

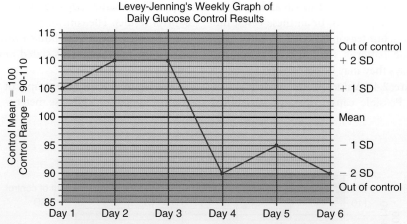

FIG. 2.6 Weekly glucose control results showing a shift. *SD,* Standard deviation.

A proficiency testing program requires a lab to enroll in an accreditation organization that sends the lab unknown samples to test twice a year. The received samples must be run in exactly the same manner as patient specimens. The results are then sent back to the accreditation agency so it can confirm that the results agree with their known values. This method of QC is *required* for CLIA complex tests (including physician-provided microscopy) and is *recommended* for CLIA-waived testing.

Quality Assurance and Quality Control Checklists

This text is designed to follow the latest booklet and its check sheet provided by the CDC titled "Ready? Set? Test!" (Figure 2.9). You will also find a helpful 10 step outline in Chapter 2 of your

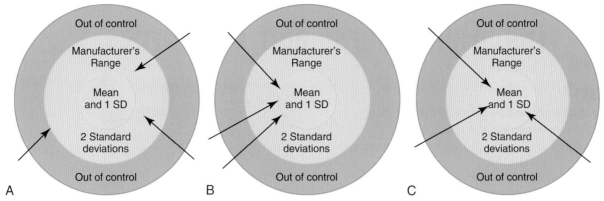

FIG. 2.7 Visual examples of quality control test results using a target to facilitate understanding of terms. **A,** Results are not *accurate* (not within required standard deviations, or the bull's eye) and are not *precise* (not consistently reproducible or hitting the same area). **B,** Results are precise but not accurate. **C,** Results are both precise and accurate and are therefore *reliable. SD,* Standard deviation.

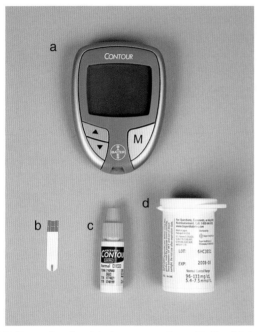

FIG. 2.8 Example of a *(a)* glucose *meter* with its *(b) test strip* that calibrates the instrument when inserted and "draws in" the specimen or liquid control. *(c) External liquid control* used to check whether its results fall in the normal range and *(d)* the test strip container with the *lot number, expiration date,* and *manufacturer's normal control range of 96 to 133 mg/dL (the mean would be 114 mg/dL).*

workbook Appendix titled "Quality Assurance Recommendations for Certificate of Waiver (CoW) Laboratories."

HIPAA Privacy Rule

Another area of concern that has generated governmental intervention in the medical community is that of patient confidentiality. On April 14, 2003, the Health Insurance Portability and Accountability Act (**HIPAA**) Privacy Rule went into effect. HIPAA is a federal law consisting of several components, one of which contains provisions to protect a patient's privacy. The

privacy rule provides patients with more control over the use and disclosure of their health information. During the three phases of laboratory testing, many individuals handle what is referred to as protected health information (PHI), which is any health information in any form (written, electronic, or oral) that contains patient-identifiable information, such as name, Social Security number, and telephone number. This information must be kept confidential. Because of this new approach to medical records and medical information, employees are trained regarding how their specific office uses, stores, maintains, and transmits laboratory testing information. No test result should be given to a patient or family member without the physician's permission. If a patient asks for his or her results or those of another person, you should explain that you are not authorized to disclose that information and that the physician will interpret and explain the results to the patient or family member based on the full medical findings and knowledge of the patient. It is also important to guard the patient's test results from being seen or heard by others.

Risk Management

Medical office risk management is a term that refers to both the physical and the procedural risks that may bring about an injury or legal action against a practice. In the laboratory and office, the best defense against legal accusations is proper documentation. The following documentation recommendations contribute to sound risk management practices in the laboratory:

- Provide written office procedures that inform patients how to prepare for tests (e.g., how to collect home specimens, fasting requirements, or special diets) and document in the patient's record when this occurred.
- Be accurate and consistent when charting and documenting test and control results on the lab logs.
- Use appropriate abbreviations and legible writing on the patient chart and logs.
- Chart corrections made in the legally required manner (line through error; correction, date, and initials of person correcting error).

Tips, Reminders, and Resources

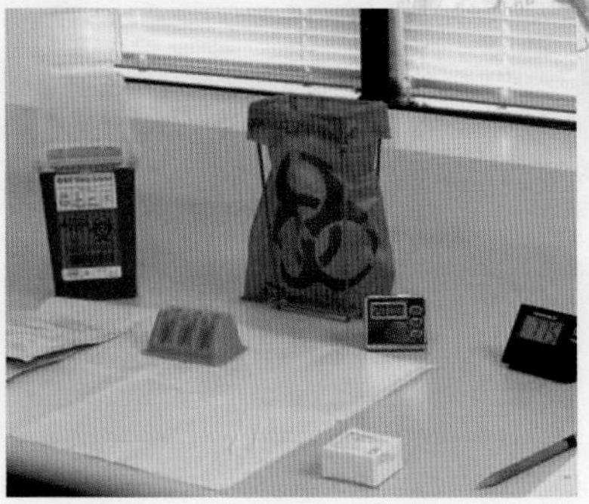

Ready?

☐ Clean work surfaces before and after testing.

☐ Perform testing in a well lit area.

☐ Check and record temperatures of the testing and reagent storage areas.

☐ Check inventory regularly to ensure you will have enough reagents and supplies on hand for testing.

☐ Check and record expiration dates of reagents/kits, and discard any reagents or tests that have expired.

☐ Check that all kit reagents came from the same kit lot. Do not mix reagents.

☐ Inspect reagents for damage, discoloration, or contamination, and discard if found.

☐ Prepare reagents according to manufacturer's instructions.

☐ Allow time for refrigerated reagents/samples to come to room temperature prior to testing.

☐ Inspect equipment and electrical connections to be sure they are working.

☐ Perform calibration checks, as needed, following the manufacturer's instructions.

☐ File the old manufacturer's instructions and replace with the new copy if there are changes.

☐ Communicate all changes in the manufacturer's instructions to other testing personnel and to the person who directs or supervises testing.

☐ Treat and test quality control (QC) samples the same as patient samples.

☐ Perform QC as recommended in the manufacturer's instructions.

Set?

☐ Check patient identification and test orders.

☐ Discuss pretest instructions and counseling needs with the patient.

☐ Wear appropriate personal protective equipment (PPE) such as gloves.

☐ Collect and label a good sample for testing.

☐ Clean hands and change gloves between patients.

☐ Use the proper biohazard containers to dispose of waste and sharps.

Test!

☐ Do not test samples that are improperly collected or handled.

☐ Have the manufacturer's instructions or a quick reference guide at the work station.

☐ Follow the manufacturer's instructions in the exact order.

☐ Follow required timing for testing.

☐ Identify and correct problems before reporting test results.

☐ Identify and report critical values in a timely manner.

☐ Perform or refer confirmatory or additional testing, if needed.

☐ Make sure patient reports are legible and reported in a timely manner.

☐ Make sure reports are standardized and easily distinguishable from referral laboratory test reports.

☐ Report patient test results only to authorized persons.

☐ Document verbal reports, followed by a written test report.

☐ Report public health diseases.

☐ Dispose of biohazardous waste safely.

☐ Participate in proficiency testing (PT).

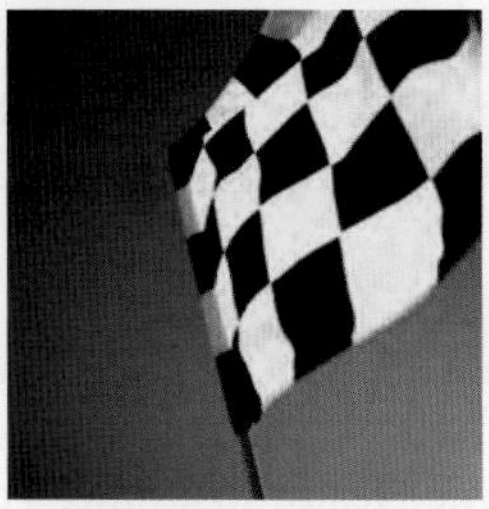

FIG. 2.9 "Ready? Set? Test!" (From Centers for Disease Control and Prevention, Division of Laboratory Science and Standards, *To Test or Not to Test?* Booklet. http://www.cdc.gov/dls/waivedtests/ReadySetTestBooklet.pdf.)

- Document immediately when diagnostic tests have been received, reviewed, filed, and communicated to the patient.

Electronic Medical Records and Bar Coding

As the demand for more laboratory and safety documentation increases, technological advancements in the area of electronic communications to ease this burden are increasing as well. These advancements will also make the process of test documentation more accurate. For example, electronic medical records are replacing patients' physical charts. These records will be accessible at each phase of the testing process by laptop computers or desktop computers located in the reception area, examination rooms, laboratory area, and reference laboratories. In most of the large reference laboratories and hospitals, the various departments are directly linked to a central computerized health information system. This system takes the test results directly from the laboratory's instruments to the patient's electronic medical record and then immediately alerts the physician about the results.

Another electronic aid to the laboratory is the use of bar code labels on all requisitions and specimens. Bar coding was introduced to the health care industry in the mid-1970s, when blood banks and blood collection centers began using the technology for error-free tracking, tracing, and positive patient identification (Figure 2.10). Today bar coding is used in virtually every hospital department to help improve accuracy and timely information management. Statistics show that the error rate for manual data entry is 1 in 300 characters compared with 1 in 3 million characters for bar code scanning.

So what exactly is a bar code? Without getting too technical, a bar code is a pattern of narrow and wide bars and spaces. Each pattern is encoded with its own particular meaning, just like words in a language are made up of letters and symbols. When a beam of light scans the bar code, the light reflects differences between the dark bar areas and the space areas. These differences are transformed into electrical impulses that are measured, decoded, and entered into a computer.

The single most important use of bar codes in the medical laboratory is for positive patient and specimen identification throughout the entire testing process. An understanding of an office's or reference laboratory's labeling system is important. A typical system consists of a specific bar code printer that prints the bar code labels on the basis of typed input from a computer. As the operator enters the patient's name and the test ordered, a series of bar code labels is generated and then attached to the laboratory requisition and the collected patient specimens. Before the labels can be applied to the specimens, patients must be identified by at least two of the following patient identifiers, depending on specific office protocol:

1. Always ask the patient to give his or her name. Do *not* say, "Are you Mrs. Smith?"
2. Have the patient state his or her Social Security number, *or*
3. Ask the patient's birth date, *or*
4. Ask the patient's telephone number.

After positive identification is made that agrees with the requisition and the bar code labels, have the patient print his or her name on the label that will be affixed to the requisition. The smaller bar code labels are then affixed to the tubes of blood after they have been filled.

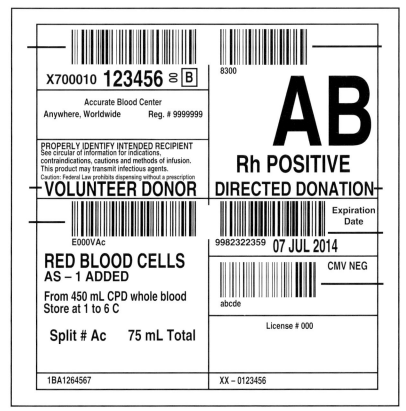

FIG. 2.10 Blood bank bar code label.

REVIEW QUESTIONS*

1. What is the purpose of CLIA 1988?
2. What is the purpose of proficiency testing?
3. A slide is initially brought into focus by using the _____ power objective.
4. Ocular lenses have a magnification of _____.
5. The _____ directs and concentrates light through the slide and into the objective lens.
6. The revolving _____ contains the objectives.
7. The _____ objective usually has a magnification of 100×.
8. The total magnification is calculated by multiplying the 10× ocular lens by the magnification of the _____ lens.
9. Match each quality control term on the left with its definition on the right.

_____ standard deviation	**a.** uninterrupted rise or decline from the mean
_____ trend	**b.** average value of a set of control tests
_____ mean	**c.** variability from the mean in a dataset

---

*Answers to these Review Questions are located in the Appendix on p. 278.

WEBSITES

CDC site with educational information on CLIA-waived testing, including an excellent brochure and online course: "Ready? Set? Test!":
wwwn.cdc.gov/dls/waivedtests/
CPT codes for CLIA-waived tests:
www.doh.wa.gov/portals/1/Documents/Pubs/681018.pdf

Tests granted waived status under CLIA with CPT codes:
www.cms.gov/Regulations-and-Guidance/Legislation/CLIA/Downloads/waivetbl.pdf
FDA listing of CLIA-waived tests since 2000:
www.accessdata.fda.gov/scripts/cdrh/cfdocs/cfClia/testswaived.cfm

CHAPTER 3

Urinalysis

OBJECTIVES

After completing this chapter, you should be able to do the following:

1. Define and match key terms in this chapter.
2. Demonstrate an understanding of the urinary system by:
   - Describing the structures and functions of the organs, the formation of urine, the significance of renal threshold, the flow of urine, and the composition of urine
   - Defining medical terms related to the urinary system and urinalysis
3. Instruct the patient in the proper method of urine collection for voided urine, clean-catch midstream urine for bacterial studies, and timed urine specimens.
4. Describe the three parts of urinalysis: physical, chemical, and microscopic.
5. State the tests involved in physical urinalysis and recognize the diseases that cause abnormal results.
6. State the 10 dipstick tests involved in manual chemical urinalysis, causes of false positive and false negative and recognize the diseases that cause abnormal results.
7. Describe the automated method for performing chemical urinalysis, including microalbumin testing.
8. Perform physical and chemical assessments of urine samples demonstrating the following criteria:
   - Perform the stated task, conditions, and standards listed in the Procedure Sheets in the student workbook.
   - Apply the correct quality control.
   - Follow the most current Occupational Safety and Health Administration (OSHA) safety guidelines.
9. Describe the standardized urine microscopic method (e.g., KOVA), and perform a microscopic urinalysis setup according to the conditions required while following the most current OSHA safety guidelines.
10. Recognize the pictures of various elements in normal and abnormal urine microscopic sediment.
11. Correlate abnormal microscopic results with certain pathologic conditions and correlate the results with the physical and chemical urinalysis results, identify discrepancies.

KEY TERMS

anuria: no flow of urine; complete absence of urine production

Bence Jones protein: protein found in the urine of patients with multiple myeloma

bilirubin: waste product from the breakdown of hemoglobin

casts: cylindrical structures excreted in the urine in the shape of the renal tubules and ducts caused by precipitation of Tamm-Horsfall mucoprotein, albumin, or both

diuresis: increase in the volume of urine output from the kidney

dysuria: painful urination

electrolytes: elements or compounds that form positively or negatively charged ions when dissolved and can conduct electricity

glomerular (Bowman) capsule: cup-shaped structure surrounding the glomerulus that collects the glomerular filtrate

glomerulus: structure in the renal corpuscle made up of tangled blood capillaries in which the hydrostatic pressure in the capillaries pushes substances through the capillary pores into the glomerular capsule

glycosuria: sugars (especially glucose) in the urine

hematuria: intact red blood cells in the urine

hemolysis: rupture of red cell membranes and release of hemoglobin

iatrogenic: adverse effect or complication caused by treatment or diagnostic procedures

ketonuria: ketones in the urine

lyse: rupture and disintegration of cells

micturition: expelling of urine from the body; also referred to as voiding and urination

nephron: functional unit of the kidney

nocturia: voluntarily getting up frequently during the night to urinate

oliguria: decrease in the flow and volume of urine (i.e., <500 mL/24 hr)

pH: scale from 0 to 14 that measures the level of acidity or alkalinity of a solution

polyuria: frequent urinary flow producing abnormally large amounts of urine (i.e., >2000 mL/24 hr)

porphyrin: intermediate substance in the formation of heme (part of hemoglobin)

proteinuria: proteins in the urine

pyuria: white blood cells in the urine

reducing substances: substances that easily lose electrons

renal corpuscle: part of the nephron that contains the glomerulus and glomerular capsule

renal threshold level: blood reabsorption limit of a substance and the point at which the substance is then excreted in the urine

renal tubules: parts of the nephron composed of proximal convoluted tubules, the nephron loop (loop of Henle), and distal convoluted tubules

retroperitoneal: located behind the peritoneal cavity

sediment: the solid material at the bottom of the centrifuged tube of urine

specific gravity: in urinalysis, the weight of urine compared with the weight of an equal volume of water; measures the amount of dissolved substances in urine

supernatant: the liquid portion of urine on top of the spun sediment

ureters: two slender, muscular tubes 10 to 12 inches long that carry the urine formed in the two kidneys to the urinary bladder

urethra: tube that carries urine to the outside of the body

urethral meatus: urethral opening through which urine is expelled from the body

urinary bladder: hollow muscular organ that holds urine until it is expelled

❖ FUNDAMENTAL CONCEPTS AND COLLECTION PROCEDURES

Anatomy and Physiology of the Urinary System

Before the results of urine testing can be interpreted, the overall anatomy and function of the urinary system must be understood.

Structures of the Urinary System

The urinary system consists of the two kidneys, two ureters, a urinary bladder, and a urethra (Figure 3.1).

Kidneys. Each person normally has two kidneys, which are reddish-brown, "kidney" bean-shaped organs. The kidneys are 4 to 5 inches long and are located in the **retroperitoneal** space (behind the peritoneal cavity) slightly above the waistline in the posterior wall of the abdominal cavity. Each kidney is composed of three main sections: the cortex, which is the outer part that contains the glomeruli and arterioles; the medulla, which is the middle light pink area; and the

renal pelvis, which is the light brown hollow inner area (Figure 3.2A).

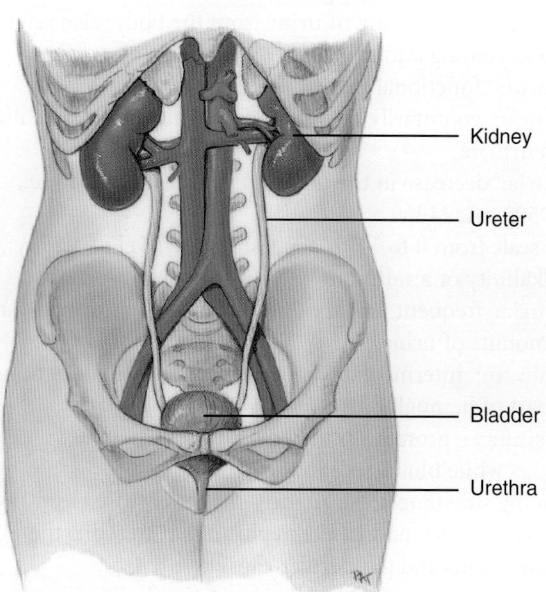

Ureters. The two **ureters** are slender, muscular tubes 10 to 12 inches long. They carry the urine formed in the kidneys to the urinary bladder.

Urinary bladder. The **urinary bladder** is a hollow muscular organ that holds the urine until it is expelled by a process called **micturition** (also referred to as *voiding* and *urination*).

Urethra. The **urethra** is a tube that carries urine to the outside of the body. The length of a woman's urethra is approximately 1.5 inches. A man's urethra is longer, approximately 8 inches. The opening at the end of the urethra, where the urine is expelled, is called the **urethral meatus**.

Function of the Urinary System

The urinary system has the following functions:
- It removes unwanted waste substances.
- It stabilizes blood volume, acidity, and electrolytes.
- It regulates extracellular fluids of the body and the absorption of calcium ions by activating vitamin D.
- It secretes the hormone erythropoietin, which controls the rate of red blood cell (RBC) formation, and the hormone renin, which regulates blood pressure.

The functional unit of the kidney is the microscopic **nephron** located within the cortex and medulla of the kidney. Approximately 1 million nephrons are in each kidney. The nephrons filter waste substances from the blood and simultaneously maintain the essential water and electrolyte balance of the body (Figure 3.2B). The structural components of the nephron are the renal corpuscle and renal tubules (Figure 3.3).

The **renal corpuscle** consists of two structures: the **glomerulus** and the **glomerular (Bowman) capsule**. The glomerulus is made up of tangled blood capillaries in which the hydrostatic pressure in the capillaries pushes substances through the capillary pores. The filtered substance is called the glomerular filtrate, and it is collected in the glomerular (Bowman) capsule, a cup-shaped structure surrounding the glomerulus.

Renal tubules are composed of proximal convoluted tubules, the nephron loop (loop of Henle), and distal convoluted tubules. The glomerular filtrate fluid flows through these tubules and undergoes changes in composition. Also in the medulla of the

FIG. 3.1 The urinary system. (From Applegate EJ: *The anatomy and physiology learning system*, ed 4, St. Louis, 2011, Saunders.)

Kidney

Ureter

Bladder

Urethra

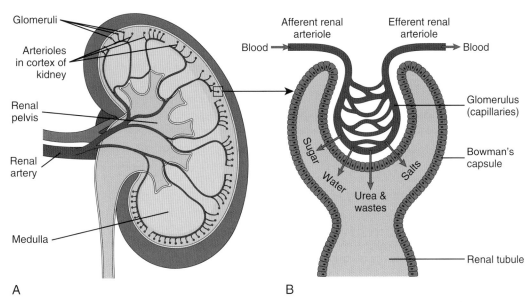

FIG. 3.2 A, Sections of the kidney. **B,** Enlarged view of renal corpuscle consisting of the glomerulus and glomerular (Bowman) capsule. (From Chabner D: *The language of medicine,* ed 10, St. Louis, 2014, Saunders.)

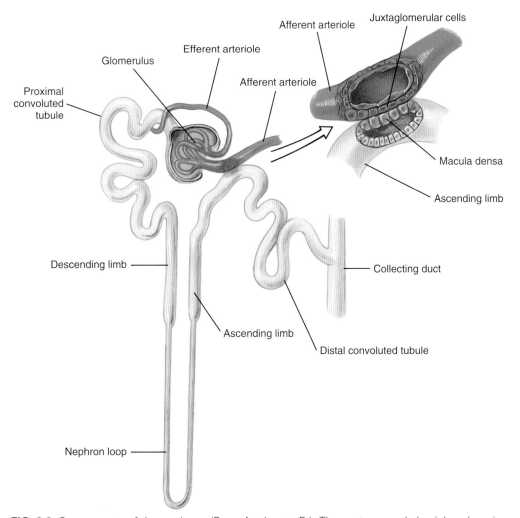

FIG. 3.3 Components of the nephron. (From Applegate EJ: *The anatomy and physiology learning system,* ed 4, St. Louis, 2011, Saunders.)

kidney are collecting tubules and ducts that empty into the renal pelvis.

Formation and Flow of Urine

Urine is formed in the nephron by three mechanisms: filtration, reabsorption, and secretion.

Filtration. Filtration is the process by which fluids and dissolved substances in the blood are forced through the pores of the glomerulus into the glomerular capsule by hydrostatic pressure. Substances such as water, salts, glucose, and nitrogen waste products (urea, creatinine, and uric acid) can pass through the pores. Substances such as RBCs and proteins are too large and therefore remain in the blood.

Reabsorption. In the process of reabsorption, some of the substances that flow through the renal tubules that are needed by the body cross back into the blood by the peritubular capillaries surrounding the tubules. Examples of reabsorbed substances are glucose, water, and **electrolytes** (elements or compounds that form positively or negatively charged ions that, when dissolved, can conduct electricity).

When blood levels of a substance such as glucose reach a point at which no more can be reabsorbed, the substance is excreted in the urine. This is the **renal threshold level** for that particular substance. For example, the renal threshold level for glucose is 160 to 180 mg/dL.

Secretion. The final process in the formation of urine is called *secretion,* in which substances are transported from the peritubular blood capillaries into the renal tubules. Metabolized drugs, uric acid, potassium, and hydrogen ions are examples of substances that are secreted into the urine.

Flow of blood and urine through the urinary system. Blood is carried into the kidney by the renal artery, which eventually branches into the afferent arterioles. The afferent arterioles carry blood into the capillaries of the glomerulus, and the efferent arterioles carry the blood out of the glomerulus. The glomerular filtrate is collected in the glomerular capsule (Bowman capsule) and flows through the proximal convoluted tubules to the nephron loop; then to the distal convoluted loop, the collecting tubule at which point the fluid is now referred to as urine, and the collection duct; and finally to the calyces of the renal pelvis. The urine then passes through the ureters to the urinary bladder, where it is stored until released by the process of urination—micturition—or voiding. The main structures involved in the formation and excretion of urine, in sequence, are the following:

1. Bloodstream—Blood enters the kidney via the renal afferent arterioles.
2. Glomerulus
3. Glomerular (Bowman) capsule
4. Renal tubules
5. Collecting ducts
6. Renal pelvis
7. Ureter
8. Urinary bladder
9. Urethra
10. Urinary meatus—Urine is expelled from the body.

NOTE: The Evolve site for this text has animated pictures showing the formation of urine as it is filtered from the arterioles and then processed through the nephron.

Composition of urine. Water makes up 95% of urine. Urine also contains nitrogen waste products such as urea, uric acid, ammonia, and creatinine. Urea, uric acid, and ammonia are derived from the breakdown of protein, and creatinine is a waste product of muscle metabolism. Other waste products found in urine include chloride, sodium, potassium, calcium, magnesium, phosphate, and sulfate.

Approximately 1200 mL of blood passes into the renal arteries per minute, with a daily output of 1200 to 1500 mL of urine per day. This amount varies depending on the amount of fluid intake and the amount of fluid lost from perspiration, feces, and water vapor from the lungs.

The following terms are related to urination:

1. **Diuresis**—increase in the volume of urine output from the kidney, which can be caused by the following:
   - Intake of excessive amounts of fluids, especially those that contain caffeine
   - Some drugs, such as diuretics
   - Some types of diseases, such as diabetes mellitus, diabetes insipidus, and renal diseases that prevent the kidney from concentrating the urine
2. **Anuria**—no flow of urine that can occur because of renal failure or severe obstruction (i.e., kidney stone or tumor)
3. **Dysuria**—painful urination caused by an inflamed urethra from a urinary tract infection (UTI), kidney stone, sexual activity
4. **Nocturia**—voluntarily getting up at night frequently to urinate caused by an enlarged prostate, prolapsed bladder, overactive bladder, diabetes, tumors, and so on
5. **Oliguria**—decrease in the flow and volume of urine (<500 mL/24 hr) that can occur in the following situations:
   - Decreased fluid intake
   - Vomiting
   - Profuse sweating
   - Diarrhea
   - Kidney disease
6. **Polyuria**—frequent urinary flow producing abnormally large amounts of urine (>2000 mL/24 hr)

Urine Specimen Collection

The urine sample is usually easily obtained, but all types of urine collection methods have the following general requirements:

- The volume needed is usually between 25 and 50 mL.
- The outside of the filled container should be cleaned with a disinfectant.
- The outside of the specimen container must be correctly labeled with the patient's name, the collection date and time, and the type of specimen (e.g., random specimen, first morning specimen, clean-catch midstream, or catheterized). Do not label the lid of the container because it may become separated from the specimen.

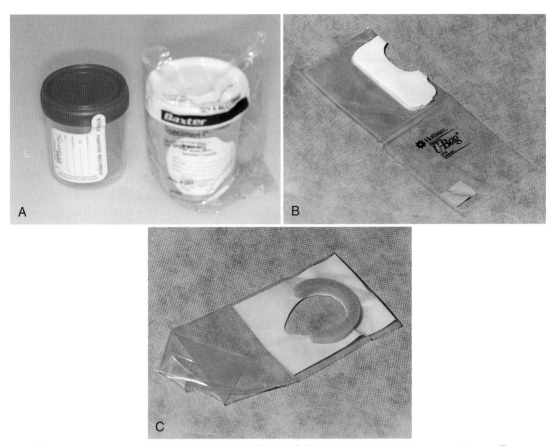

FIG. 3.4 A, Adult urine specimen container. **B** and **C,** Pediatric urine specimen containers. (From Stepp CA, Woods M: *Laboratory procedures for medical office personnel,* Philadelphia, 1998, Saunders.)

Use the correct urine containers (Figure 3.4). The physician's office should provide the patient with a urine container. Containers from the patient's home, such as glass jars, should not be used because their previous contents can affect the accuracy of the tests. The most common types of containers are disposable, nonsterile plastic cups with lids. For infants and children who are not toilet trained, special pliable polyethylene bags called pediatric urine containers (PUCs) are available that contain an adhesive section to adhere to the skin. If urine is being collected for microbiological studies, a sterile urine container must be used.

- If a woman is having a menstrual period, collection of a urine sample should be postponed. If this is not possible and a urine specimen must be collected immediately, the requisition must note that the patient is menstruating. This will indicate the cause of a false-positive result for blood.
- The urine should be tested as soon as possible after collection. If it is going to sit for more than 1 hour, it must be refrigerated, or preservatives must be added.

The method of collection for urine specimens is dictated by the type of test being ordered. For example, special collection procedures are performed if the urine will be cultured for bacteria or if a 24-hour test is ordered. Documentation of the method used to collect the specimen should be noted on the specimen container, the requisition form, and the patient's chart.

Random Specimen

A random specimen is usually collected in the medical office. This specimen is not regarded as the specimen of choice because of the potential for variation in urine concentration based on time of collection and consumption of fluids which can dilute the specimen if collected shortly thereafter. The patient should collect the midstream portion of urine when voiding but it is not required for a random collection. The patient is instructed to void a small amount of urine into the toilet to flush away the normal bacteria in the area around the urinary opening and to get a steady midstream flow. The second portion is collected in the container to a volume of at least 25 mL. After the specimen has been collected, the remaining urine in the bladder can be emptied into the toilet. A specimen collected this way is more representative of the contents of the bladder. The lid should be tightly placed on the container, and the outside of the container should be disinfected. The sample container (not the lid) should be appropriately labeled.

First Morning Specimen

The first morning specimen is usually the specimen of choice because it is the most concentrated and has the greatest amount of dissolved substances. Provided the patient has not voided during the night, the first morning urine specimen has formed over an approximately 8-hour period providing higher levels of cellular elements and analytes. Because this urine is more concentrated, the probability of detecting abnormalities increases and the microscopic elements remain intact for a longer period.

The patient must collect the first morning specimen soon after rising and preserve it by refrigeration until it is brought into the physician's office. The collection procedure is the same as that described for the random specimen.

Clean-Catch Midstream Urine Specimen

Clean-catch midstream specimens are strongly recommended for culture and antibiotic susceptibility testing when the physician suspects the patient has a UTI. The urethra and urinary meatus normally harbor many microorganisms. Therefore, when a urine specimen is collected, for culture to determine the source of a UTI, only the organisms causing the infection should be cultured. To avoid contamination, the midstream clean-catch method of collection is used. This method consists of having the patient clean the urinary opening first using antiseptic wipes, as seen in Figure 3.5. The patient then urinates into the sterile container by using the midstream method. See Procedure 3.1: Instructing Patients How to Collect a Clean-Catch Urine Specimen located at the end of this fundamental section.

Note: If the medical assistant does not know if the urine specimen will be needed for culture, collect a clean-catch midstream just in case.

When the urine requires further evaluation, it may be necessary to send it to an outside lab in a sterile tube with preservative to keep the organisms alive during transportation. This transferring of the clean-catch midstream urine specimen to a sterile vacuum tube is covered in the microbiology chapter (see Chapter 8).

Other options for collecting urine specimens for culturing are bladder catheterization and suprapubic aspiration. In catheterization, a sterile tube called a *catheter* is passed through the urethra into the bladder to remove urine. With suprapubic aspiration, urine is removed by passing a needle through the abdominal wall into the bladder.

Timed Urine Specimen

Some tests require that a urine specimen be collected at a certain time. One example is a 24-hour urine specimen. Collecting all the urine produced over a 24-hour period allows greater accuracy of measurement for urinary components. Substances produced in the urine are affected over time by body metabolism, exercise, and hydration. Substances measured in a 24-hour specimen include calcium, creatinine, cortisol, catecholamines, lead, potassium, protein, and urea nitrogen. In addition, this type of specimen is used the diagnosis of the cause, control, and prevention of kidney stones.

24-hour collection procedure. Urine containers for 24-hour collection (Figure 3.6) are quite large, holding approximately 3000 mL. They are dark in color to screen out ultraviolet light and avoid decomposition of substances.

The following guidelines should be given to the patient:

- Depending on the analyte being measured, the specimen should be kept refrigerated or a preservative should be added to the container before the start of urine collection.

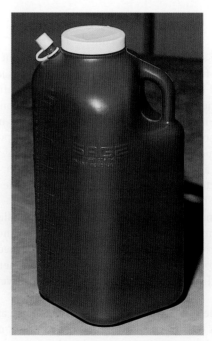

FIG. 3.6 A 24-hour urine container. (From Stepp CA, Woods M: *Laboratory procedures for medical office personnel,* Philadelphia, 1998, Saunders.)

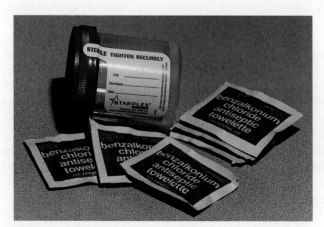

FIG. 3.5 Supplies for collecting a midstream clean-catch specimen. (From Stepp CA, Woods M: *Laboratory procedures for medical office personnel,* Philadelphia, 1998, Saunders.)

- Some containers may contain a preservative such as HCl, boric acid, thymol, or toluene. Patients should be instructed about the possible hazards associated with these preservatives. NOTE: The proper preservative must be selected to avoid interference with the analyte being tested.
- The patient should be provided with verbal and written directions.
- The patient should be instructed to moderately limit the intake of fluids during the collection process. Also, the patient should not consume alcohol 24 hours before and during the collection procedure.
- The physician should determine whether medication should be discontinued during the procedure because some medications, such as thiazides, phosphorus-binding antacids, allopurinol, and vitamin C, could alter the results. See Procedure 3.2: Instructing Patients How to Collect a 24-hour Urine Specimen at the end of this fundamental section.

Behavioral Criteria When Working with Patients

Before performing Procedures 3.1 and 3.2, it would be helpful to look over the proper way to show awareness of a patient's concerns related to the procedures that will be performed (Table 3.1).

NOTE: You will also find this table in your workbook along with the following two procedures.

TABLE 3.1 CAAHEP Affective Competency I.A.3

Competency	I.A.3. Show awareness of a patient's concerns related to a procedure being performed			
Objective(s)	Given the conditions, and provided the necessary supplies, the student will demonstrate awareness of patient concerns as he or she provides patient care in a role-play scenario for a student-partner.			
Time frame	15 minutes			
Grading	Pass = 100% accuracy; All steps must be completed as written for "pass." Students are permitted two graded attempts. Grading instructions: When step is performed as written, record a "✓" for "pass." When step is omitted or there is an error in written procedure, record instructor initials for "fail," and the procedure must be repeated.			

		GRADED ATTEMPT 1		GRADED ATTEMPT 2	
Step #	Procedure	Pass	Fail	Pass	Fail
Example	If student completes step as written, record "✓". If student omits step or performs it in error, record initials.	✓	*JH*		
1.	Gathered supplies and reviewed the new or established patient's medical history form.				
2.	Correctly prepared the patient: ❐ Greeted the patient, introduced self, escorted him or her to exam room, and verified name. ❐ Made appropriate eye contact with the patient. ❐ Established a professional and empathetic atmosphere ❐ Explained procedure to patient.				
3.	Responded to patient concerns: ❐ Showed empathy towards patient ❐ Assured the patient understands concerns by repeating them and verifying them with patient ❐ Explained procedure again to assure patient understanding ❐ Answered any questions from patient ❐ Assured patient that procedure is necessary ❐ Provided necessary follow-up contact information				
4.	Demonstrated professional behavior and exhibited appropriate conduct: ❐ Prioritized tasks; remained organized throughout task ❐ Communicated with patient appropriately and with ease throughout task ❐ Properly disposed of medical waste according to OSHA guidelines ❐ Groomed appearance and appropriate attire				

OSHA, Occupational Safety and Health Administration.

PROCEDURE 3.1 Instructing Patients How to Collect a Clean-Catch Urine Specimen

Equipment and Supplies

Sterile urine collection container, label, antiseptic towelettes

Procedure

For a Female Patient

1. Wash your hands and gather the equipment.
2. Greet and identify the patient and provide her with the clean-catch urine supplies.
3. Instruct the patient to sanitize her hands and remove her underwear.
4. Instruct the patient to spread apart her labia with one hand to expose the urinary meatus (Figure A). Tell her to keep this area spread apart with her nondominant hand during the entire cleaning procedure.
5. Instruct the patient to take one antiseptic towelette and clean one side of the urinary meatus from front to back on one side. She should clean from front to back so that microorganisms in the anal region are not spread into the urinary meatus area.
6. Instruct the patient to repeat the same procedure with another antiseptic towelette, wiping from front to back on the other side of the urinary meatus.
7. Instruct the patient to use a third antiseptic towelette to wipe from front to back directly across the urinary meatus.

8. Instruct the patient to continue to keep the labia spread apart and to void a small amount of urine into the toilet to flush away microorganisms that may be around the urinary meatus (Figure B). Tell her to be careful not to touch the inside of the sterile container at any time during the procedure.
9. Instruct the patient to collect the second part of the urine in the container (Figure C). This is the midstream flow of urine.
10. Instruct the patient to urinate the last amount of urine into the toilet. This will ensure that the first and last sections of the urine flow are not in the container, only the midstream section.
11. Instruct the patient to dry the area with a tissue and wash her hands.
12. Instruct the patient to carefully cap the specimen container and put it in a specified place if collected in the office or refrigerate it if collected at home.
13. Gloves should be worn when receiving the specimen from the patient. The sample container (not the lid) should be labeled correctly, and a requisition should be completed if required.
14. The person receiving the sample should remove the gloves and sanitize his or her hands after the urine has been placed in the testing area.
15. The procedure should be charted correctly. The charting should document that midstream clean-catch urine collection instructions were given and that the specimen was received from the patient.

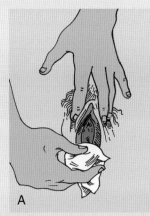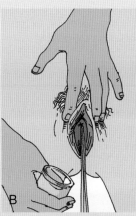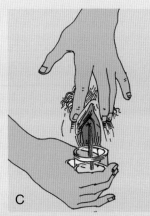

Procedure for female midstream clean-catch urine collection. **A,** Clean the labia from front to back with antiseptic. **B,** Urinate the first part into the toilet. **C,** Collect the middle of the specimen into the cup and then urinate the last part into the toilet.

For a Male Patient

1. Wash your hands and gather the equipment.
2. Greet and identify your patient and provide him with the clean-catch urine supplies.
3. Instruct the patient to sanitize his hands and remove his underwear.
4. If the patient is uncircumcised, instruct him to retract the foreskin, holding it back during the entire procedure.
5. Instruct the patient to clean the area around the penis opening (glans penis) by starting at the tip of the penis and cleaning downward (Figure D), using a separate antiseptic towelette for each side.
6. Instruct the patient to use a third antiseptic towelette to clean directly across the meatus.
7. Instruct the patient to void a small amount of the urine into the toilet to flush away microorganisms that may surround the urinary meatus (Figure E).
8. Instruct the patient to collect the second part of the urine in the container, being careful not to touch the inside of the container (Figure F).

9. Instruct the patient to void the last amount of urine into the toilet so that only the midstream section is collected.
10. Instruct the patient to dry the area with a tissue if needed.
11. Instruct the patient to carefully cap the specimen container and place it in a specified place if collected in the office or refrigerate it if collected at home.
12. Gloves should be worn when receiving the specimen from the patient. The sample container (not the lid) should be labeled correctly, and a requisition should be completed if required.
13. The person receiving the sample should remove the gloves and sanitize his or her hands after the urine has been placed in the testing area.
14. The procedure should be charted correctly. The charting should document that midstream clean-catch urine collection instructions were given and that the specimen was received from the patient.

PROCEDURE 3.1   Instructing Patients How to Collect a Clean-Catch Urine Specimen—cont'd

Procedure for male midstream clean-catch urine collection. **D,** Clean area around penis opening and across the opening. **E,** Void a small amount into the urinal or toilet. **F,** Collect the second part of urine in the container and then void the last part in the urinal. (From Stepp CA, Woods M: *Laboratory procedures for medical office personnel*, Philadelphia, 1998, Saunders.)

PROCEDURE 3.2   Instructing Patients How to Collect a 24-Hour Urine Specimen

Procedure

Sanitize your hands and assemble and label the correct specimen collection equipment. Determine that you are instructing the correct patient by having the patient state his or her name. Provide the patient with the required equipment and written instructions.

1. Wash your hands and gather the equipment.
2. Greet and identify your patient.
3. Instruct the patient to empty the bladder into the toilet after arising on the first day of the 24-hour procedure. Inform the patient not to save this specimen but to record the exact time the bladder was emptied. The purpose is to start the 24-hour period with an empty bladder and then start saving or measuring the urine formed by the kidneys after that time for 24 hours.
4. Instruct the patient that each time he or she urinates for the next 24 hours, the urine must be voided directly into the collection container, including any urine expelled during the night. It might be necessary to give female patients a large sterile container that has a wide opening in which they can void; afterward, they can pour the contents into the 24-hour jug.
5. Tell the patient to be sure to screw the lid on tightly each time and keep the container refrigerated or keep it at room temperature (preservative added) as

required for the analyte being tested. If at any time during the procedure some urine is not collected, the test must be started again. Examples include the patient forgetting to collect some urine; spilling some urine; and, if the patient is a child, wetting the bed with urine.

6. Instruct the patient that on the following morning, he or she must collect the last specimen at the same time he or she emptied the bladder on the first day. Therefore, the first morning specimen on the second day is kept, and it ends the 24-hour collection procedure.
7. Instruct the patient that on the day the procedure is completed, the container must be returned to the physician's office or to the laboratory.
8. After the patient has completed the procedure and returned the container, check the label for completeness and ask the patient whether any problems occurred during the collection procedure.
9. A requisition form must be completed and the 24-hour urine container transported to the laboratory that will perform the test.
10. Document in the patient's chart the instructions and equipment that were supplied to the patient. Also document that the specimen was sent to an outside laboratory. Include the type of specimen that was sent, the date, the time, the name of the laboratory to which it was sent, and the test that was ordered.

❖ CLIA-WAIVED TESTS

Routine Urinalysis

Urinalysis is the description and measurement of the substances found in urine. It is the most common test performed in the medical office. The specimen is easily obtained, and the testing is not difficult to perform. Urinalysis can be used for screening in a physical examination, to assist the physician in the diagnosis of pathological conditions, and to determine the effectiveness of a treatment. A routine urinalysis consists of three parts: physical analysis, chemical analysis, and microscopic analysis. Figure 3.7 is an example of a urinalysis requisition or report form containing spaces to report test results for routine, microscopic, and quantitative analyses. NOTE: The quantitative tests in the right-hand column of the requisition are not CLIA waived and are generally performed on a 24-hour collected specimen in which the total volume of the urine has been measured and recorded.

Fresh, refrigerated, or chemically preserved urine can be used when performing a routine urinalysis. Preservatives are usually used for specimens being sent to a lab a long distance away and requiring prolonged storage. Nonpreserved, fresh urine is preferred because some preservatives can interfere with the chemicals used in the testing. Urine should be tested within 2 hours of voiding, but if this is not possible, the urine should be refrigerated. Before testing, the urine must be brought to room temperature and be well mixed.

Urine that stands at room temperature for more than 2 hours may undergo the following changes:

- Bacteria will multiply, causing the urine to be cloudy. Some bacteria can break down urea to ammonia, which will change the **pH** (scale that measures acidity or alkalinity) of the urine to alkaline and can affect some chemical tests i.e., false-positive protein, false-negative result for specific gravity.
- Glucose that could be present in the urine decreases as it is metabolized by microorganisms.

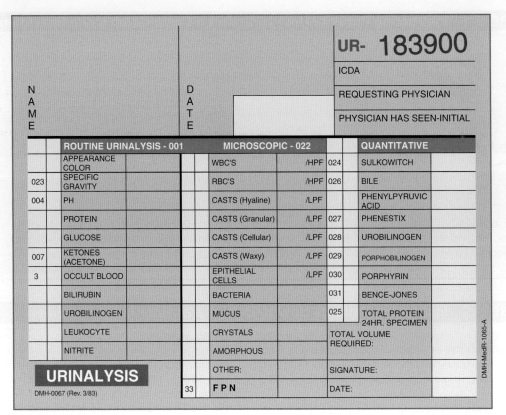

			UR- **183900**
			ICDA
N A M E	**D A T E**		REQUESTING PHYSICIAN
			PHYSICIAN HAS SEEN-INITIAL

ROUTINE URINALYSIS - 001			**MICROSCOPIC - 022**			**QUANTITATIVE**	
	APPEARANCE COLOR		WBC'S	/HPF	024	SULKOWITCH	
023	SPECIFIC GRAVITY		RBC'S	/HPF	026	BILE	
004	PH		CASTS (Hyaline)	/LPF		PHENYLPYRUVIC ACID	
	PROTEIN		CASTS (Granular)	/LPF	027	PHENESTIX	
	GLUCOSE		CASTS (Cellular)	/LPF	028	UROBILINOGEN	
007	KETONES (ACETONE)		CASTS (Waxy)	/LPF	029	PORPHOBILINOGEN	
3	OCCULT BLOOD		EPITHELIAL CELLS	/LPF	030	PORPHYRIN	
	BILIRUBIN		BACTERIA		031	BENCE-JONES	
	UROBILINOGEN		MUCUS		025	TOTAL PROTEIN 24HR. SPECIMEN	
	LEUKOCYTE		CRYSTALS			TOTAL VOLUME REQUIRED:	
	NITRITE		AMORPHOUS				
URINALYSIS			OTHER:			SIGNATURE:	
DMH-0067 (Rev. 3/83)		33	**F P N**			DATE:	

DMH-MedR-1065-A

FIG. 3.7 Urinalysis laboratory form. (From Bonewit-West K: *Clinical procedures for medical assistants,* ed 10, St. Louis, 2018, Elsevier.)

- Ketones are volatile and can evaporate yielding false-negative result.
- Cells in the urine will **lyse** (break open).
- **Casts** (elements excreted in the urine in the shape of the renal tubules and ducts) dissolve and disappear, and crystals may dissolve if the pH changes.
- **Bilirubin** (a waste product from the breakdown of hemoglobin that is metabolized by the liver), if present, will be oxidized with exposure to light.

If substances, originally present in the urine, are dissolved, eliminated, or lysed, then the microscopic testing for such analytes will result in false-negative reports.

Physical Routine Urinalysis

The physical part of a urinalysis consists of observing the color, odor, and appearance (transparency) of a urine specimen. To determine the color and appearance, the urine must be viewed through a clear container. NOTE: In the past, the urine would also be tested for pH and specific gravity during the physical analysis. These two tests are now included in the chemical analysis of urine because they are measured using the same test strips as the chemical analytes.

Color. The color of normal urine (Figure 3.8) is typically described as *straw colored (light yellow),* to *yellow,* to *amber (dark yellow).* Varying amounts of a normal pigment called *urochrome* give the urine its characteristic shades of yellow. Whereas concentrated urine with less water and more substances is dark yellow to amber, more diluted urine is a lighter yellow or straw color. The first morning specimen is most

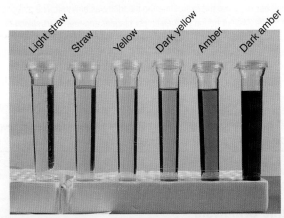

FIG. 3.8 Normal colors of urine with their various descriptions. (From Bonewit-West K: *Clinical procedures for medical assistants,* ed 10, St. Louis, 2018, Elsevier.)

concentrated (dark yellow); the urine becomes more dilute (lighter in color) as the day progresses and more fluid is consumed.

Sometimes additional substances may cause a change in the color of urine, but this is not necessarily associated with disease. Such color changes may be caused by food dyes, some medications, and vitamins.

The colors in the following list, however, may be indications of a pathologic condition. The following are abnormal urine colors and their possible causes:

- Yellow-brown—caused by bilirubin resulting from excessive RBC destruction or bile duct obstruction

- Orange-yellow—caused by bilirubin or urobilinogen resulting from a reduction in the functioning of liver cells or excessive RBC destruction, medications such as rifampin, Pyridium, Azulfidine; and dehydration
- Reddish-orange—medications such as rifampin or Pyridium
- Green—caused by biliverdin resulting from the oxidation of bilirubin; UTI caused by *Pseudomonas* bacteria; medications such as amitriptyline, Indocin, or Diprivan; and food dyes
- Red or pink—beets, blackberries, rhubarb ingestion; medications such as rifampin or Pyridium; laxatives containing senna; hematuria caused by UTI, kidney stone, or tumors or in long distance runners
- Dark red—caused by erythrocytes (RBCs) resulting from the bleeding of urinary structures, the occurrence of the menstrual cycle, or the presence of hemoglobin from the breakdown of erythrocytes
- Red-brown—caused by erythrocytes and hemoglobin or myoglobin (from skeletal or cardiac muscle breakdown)
- Clear red—caused by hemoglobin and porphyrin products
- Cloudy red—caused by intact erythrocytes
- Black on standing—alkaptonuria due to excretion of homogentisic acid

Odor. A fresh urine specimen has a slight aroma. Odor is not normally recorded in a urinalysis, but some characteristic odors may indicate certain conditions.

- An *ammonia odor* may indicate bacteria in the urine. Also, if urine is left standing, urea converts to ammonia.
- A *sweet* or *fruity odor* may be an indication of the presence of ketones. Ketones are an intermediate product of fat metabolism found in patients with uncontrolled diabetes and patients consuming low-carbohydrate diets.
- A *foul odor* is characteristic of a UTI. The longer the urine stands, the worse the odor becomes. The decomposition of leukocytes (white blood cells) causes the foul odor.
- A *musty* or *mousy odor* can be caused by certain foods, such as asparagus, or by an inherited metabolic condition, phenylketonuria (PKU), that occurs in newborns.

Appearance. The appearance part of a physical urinalysis evaluates the transparency of the urine. This can be performed accurately only if the urine is in a clear container; it is usually done at the same time the color is evaluated. The urine should be well mixed before assessment of transparency. The terms used to describe the appearance of urine are *clear, hazy (slightly cloudy), cloudy,* and *turbid (very cloudy)* (Figure 3.9).

Some of the substances that may cause a freshly voided urine specimen to appear cloudy are bacteria, yeast, blood cells, casts, mucous threads, and sperm. These substances could be clinically important and are evaluated further in the chemical and microscopic parts of the urinalysis. Urine that is clear when voided may become cloudy as it is allowed to stand. Dissolved substances crystallize as urine cools, causing the cloudy appearance.

Chemical Urinalysis

The second part of a urinalysis is the chemical testing, which helps diagnose pathologic conditions. A reagent strip is a thin plastic strip containing pads impregnated with chemical reagents that test for specific substances. When each reagent

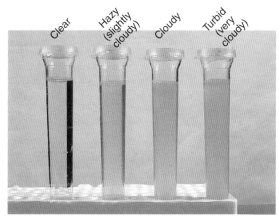

FIG. 3.9 Appearance of urine showing clear to turbid (very cloudy) characteristics. (From Bonewit-West K: *Clinical procedures for medical assistants,* ed 10, St. Louis, 2018, Elsevier.)

pad reacts with its specific analyte, a color change occurs. The greater the amount of a particular analyte that is present in urine, the darker the color will be on the reagent pad. This is referred to as *semiquantitative testing.* Whereas a *qualitative* test indicates whether a particular analyte is present, *semiquantitative* testing determines the approximate quantity of an analyte. *Quantitative* testing measures the exact amount of a substance and usually requires more complex equipment and procedures that are not usually available in a physician's office. Reagent strips provide both qualitative and semiquantitative measurements, with results recorded in ranges such as trace, 1+, 2+, and 3+; small, moderate, and large; and negative and positive.

Reagent strips are also time dependent, which means that each test on a strip must be read at a specific time. The tests on the strips are referred to as *screening tests.* If a result is abnormal, then additional testing may be performed to confirm the presence of the abnormal analyte. Some of these confirmatory tests will be reviewed when individual analytes are discussed.

Urinalysis chemistry strips (Figure 3.10A-B) have multiple reagent pads on each strip. The most commonly used testing strip consists of reagent pads for specific gravity, pH, glucose, ketones, bilirubin, urobilinogen, blood, protein, nitrite, and leukocytes. Some physician offices may use a test strip with fewer test pads more appropriate for their medical practice. For example, an obstetrician may use a two-pad test strip to monitor pregnant patients for only glucose and protein levels.

The color comparisons provided by the manufacturer may indicate more than one set of units for reporting positive results for specific analytes. The physician will indicate to the medical assistant which set of reporting units is to be used. For example, positive glucose results could be reported as *0.25% to 2% or more* or as *100 to 2000 mg/dL or more.*

Chemical urinalysis—quality assurance. The following guidelines help ensure high-quality results when performing urinalysis testing with a reagent strip:

- The reagent strip bottle must be kept tightly closed when not in use because moisture from air, light, and aerosols can affect the accuracy of the testing.

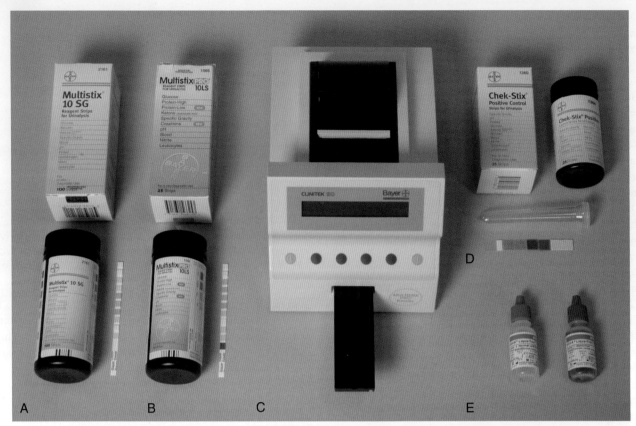

FIG. 3.10 Urinalysis chemistry supplies. *(A)* Multistix 10 SG urinalysis chemistry reagent strips; *(B)* Multistix Pro10LS urinalysis chemistry reagent strips that also test for microalbumin; *(C)* Clinitek instrument; *(D)* Chex-Stix positive control strips; *(E)* KOVA normal and abnormal controls.

- The pads on the strip should not be touched or placed on any surface.
- Keep the strips in a cool, dry place but do not refrigerate them.
- Do not use an expired bottle (the expiration date is displayed on the bottle).
- Any bottle that has been open longer than 2 months should not be used. Repeated exposure to air can change the accuracy of the strips. Be sure to note the written date on the label indicating when the bottle was opened.
- Do not combine strips from different bottles.
- Follow all directions from the manufacturer.
- Mix the urine specimen well and bring it to room temperature before testing.
- Make sure that all pads are covered with the specimen.
- Do not leave the strip in the urine too long because this can cause the chemical in the pads to leach (wash out) into the urine.
- When taking the strip out of the urine, remove excess urine by pulling the back side of the strip against the edge of the container and then briefly blot the edge of the strip against absorbent paper.
- Hold the strip horizontally to keep the colors on one pad from running into another while you are comparing the colors to the reference testing chart. Do not touch the bottle

with the strip while comparing (see Procedure 3.3). NOTE: There are plastic charts available from the manufacturer that can be cleaned and disinfected should they become contaminated.
- Record observed results for each analyte on the lab log and requisition/report.

Reagent strip quality control. To ensure the accuracy of results, quality control procedures must be followed when performing chemical tests on urine. Quality control determines whether the reagent strips are working properly and whether the test is being correctly performed and accurately interpreted.

Several reagent control methods can be used (Figure 3.10D-E). One method is to use a control strip containing synthetic ingredients *(D)*. The strip is placed in water to dissolve the ingredients, and this solution is then tested as a urine specimen. Another method is to use a dehydrated urine control, which can be purchased from the manufacturer in normal and abnormal levels *(E)*. The controls are rehydrated according to the manufacturer's directions, and then a chemical examination is performed in the same way a patient's urine sample would be examined.

With any quality control method, the results obtained must be compared with the manufacturer's ranges that accompany the controls, and the results must be logged in quality control record books. If the results do not fall within the quality control ranges, then appropriate steps must be taken to determine the cause. No patient testing should be performed until the quality control results fall within the acceptable ranges.

Proficiency checklists (also referred to as *procedure sheets*) for any new laboratory test must be documented for each person performing the test. In this case, each person would run the test using the urinalysis controls, write the results on the laboratory log, and then check to see if the results fall within the manufacturer's control range before testing patients. The procedure sheets for urinalysis along with the log sheets for both control results, and patient results are available in the workbook and the website.

Automated clinitek method. Urine analyzers are available that automatically read the chemistry strips (Figure 3.11). The Clinitek analyzer, for example, runs the chemical analysis according to the principle of reflectance photometry. A microprocessor in the machine controls the movement of the strip into the reflectometer, where a light of specific wavelengths is beamed onto the strip. The light that is reflected is measured, converted into a digital reading, and printed.

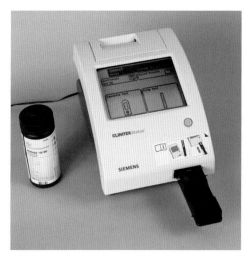

FIG. 3.11 Clinitek urine analyzer with tray for measuring reagent strips. (Photo by Zack Bent.)

In the automated method, the timing and color interpretation are consistent and do not vary among individual readers as the visual interpretation of color does. A disadvantage of this method is that if the urine contains a large amount of pigment, the machine cannot recognize this and will give false results based on the pigment rather than the presence of analytes.

Urine Test Strips

The routine tests included in a chemical examination of urine are specific gravity, pH, glucose, ketones, bilirubin, urobilinogen, blood, protein, nitrites, and leukocytes. These tests can provide the physician with information about the status of the patient's acid–base balance, carbohydrate metabolism, liver and kidney functions, and possible UTIs.

Specific gravity. To measure the specific gravity of urine, the weight of the urine is compared with the weight of an equal volume of water, which has a standardized specific gravity of 1.000. Specific gravity measures the amount of particles that are dissolved in the urine, which indicates the ability of the kidneys to concentrate the urine.

Pathologic conditions that *increase* urine concentration and raise specific gravity include adrenal insufficiency, congestive heart failure, hepatic disease, and glycosuria (glucose in the urine) seen both in diabetes mellitus and in dehydration caused by fever, vomiting, and diarrhea.

Pathologic conditions that *decrease* urine concentration include chronic renal insufficiency, diabetes insipidus, and malignant hypertension.

The normal range for urine specific gravity is 1.003 to 1.030, but the range is usually between 1.010 and 1.025. The first morning urine is more concentrated and therefore has a higher specific gravity. Urine becomes more dilute as fluids are consumed throughout the day, so subsequent urine samples have a lower specific gravity.

pH. The pH of a substance measures its level of acidity or alkalinity (Figure 3.12). A pH of 7 is neutral, 0 to 6 is acidic, and 8 to 14 is alkaline. The lungs and kidneys are responsible for maintaining the body's acid–alkaline balance in the blood. The blood pH

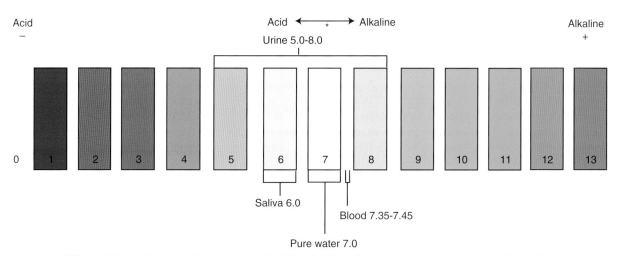

FIG. 3.12 The pH scale. (From Stepp CA, Woods M: *Laboratory procedures for medical office personnel,* Philadelphia, 1998, Saunders.)

must be in a range of 7.35 to 7.45. If the blood pH is less than 7.35, acidosis occurs, and if the pH is greater than 7.45, alkalosis occurs. Both acidosis and alkalosis in the blood are critical conditions.

Normal urine pH has a variable range of 5.0 to 8.0. The average is 6.0, slightly acidic. The pH of urine is determined by measuring the amount of hydrogen ions present. The pH should be measured by testing a freshly voided specimen because urea is converted to ammonia by bacteria in urine that has been standing at room temperature. This conversion causes the urine to become alkaline. Freshly voided urine that is alkaline, however, may for example, indicate a bacterial UTI.

Glucose. Glucose is not normally found in urine. In the glomerulus of the nephron, glucose is filtered into a glomerular filtrate, and in the renal tubules, this substance is reabsorbed into the blood. However, if a large amount of glucose is present in the blood, glucose in the tubules cannot be reabsorbed because the renal threshold level has been reached. For glucose, the renal threshold level is between 160 and 180 mg/dL.

Glucose is the only sugar that is routinely tested for in urine and when present, is referred to as glycosuria or glucosuria. The reagent strip method of testing is an enzymatic reaction using the enzyme glucose oxidase that is specific for glucose. The presence of glucose in the urine may indicate diabetes mellitus, but it may also occur after vigorous exercise or during acute emotional stress. False-positive results can also be obtained in the presence of large quantities of aspirin, ascorbic acid (vitamin C), and any medication containing levodopa.

Other sugars that can be found in urine are lactose, fructose, galactose, and pentose. The presence of these substances may be tested by using the Clinitest (Bayer Corp.) procedure that identifies the presence of reducing substances (substances that easily lose electrons). Children younger than 2 years of age are tested for reducing substances (i.e., other sugars) to screen for inborn errors of metabolism such as galactosemia. However, this practice is less useful today than in the past because most states have mandatory testing for galactosemia for all newborns, which is part of the Newborn Screening Panel. If the galactose test result is positive, it is confirmed by genetic testing.

Galactosemia is a rare metabolic condition in which the body is not able to convert galactose to glucose, resulting in the excretion of galactose in the urine. In infants, this condition results in the failure to thrive because of anorexia, vomiting, and diarrhea. In addition, enlargement of the liver and spleen; cirrhosis; cataracts; mental retardation; and, in extreme cases, permanent brain damage or even death can occur. A positive Clinitest result and a negative glucose strip test result in a pediatric urine analysis could indicate galactose in the urine.

Lactose may be found in the urine of pregnant women, and in rare instances, fructose and pentose can be found in urine because of high consumption of honey or fruit (Procedure 3.5).

Ketones. Ketones are products of fat metabolism that are then oxidized by the muscles. The body normally uses carbohydrates for energy, but if the body is deficient in carbohydrates, it metabolizes fats. Excessive fat metabolism can lead to the production of large amounts of ketones that the muscles cannot oxidize. The excess ketones accumulate in tissues and blood and subsequently in the urine, a condition called ketonuria.

Ketones and glucose in the urine may be associated with uncontrolled diabetes mellitus. The glucose levels in the blood and urine of a person with diabetes are high because insulin is either absent or not working correctly and the glucose cannot be metabolized for energy. Fats are then metabolized for energy, and ketone blood levels increase, causing ketones to spill over into urine. In addition, ketones are acid compounds; therefore, ketonuria is correlated with a low pH (acid) urine. If glucose, ketones, and acidity are all present in the urine, this may indicate a condition known as *ketoacidosis,* which may lead to diabetic coma.

Other conditions that may lead to ketonuria are fevers, starvation, anorexia, prolonged vomiting, and diets high in fat and low in carbohydrates. NOTE: These conditions generally do not have glucose present.

Ketones evaporate at room temperature; therefore, the urine specimen must be tested immediately or capped tightly and refrigerated. If the reagent strip is positive for ketones, the confirmatory test Acetest (Bayer Corp.) can be performed to confirm the presence of ketones.

NOTE: Because of the increased sensitivity and specificity of automated semiquantitative analyzers, there no longer exists a rationale to continue the use of confirmatory testing for ketones (Acetest) and bilirubin (Ictotest, discussed later).

Bilirubin. The life span of an RBC is 120 days, after which the red cell lyses and releases hemoglobin. Heme, a product of hemoglobin decomposition, subsequently breaks down to form bilirubin. Bilirubin is an intensely yellow (yellow-orange) pigmented substance that is not soluble in water and must attach to a protein, usually albumin, to be transported through blood. Attached to protein, bilirubin does not pass through the glomerulus because of its large size. Instead, it enters the liver. In the liver, it becomes water soluble (conjugated to glucuronic acid), enters the gallbladder, and is excreted into bile in the gallbladder and eventually into the small intestine, where it becomes a substance called *urobilinogen.* (See Figure 5.6 for a graphic representation of this process.)

Bilirubin is normally not found in urine. Bilirubin levels are elevated if conditions such as hepatitis, excessive hemolysis (red cells breaking open and releasing hemoglobin), liver damage, and obstruction of the bile duct are present. The yellow-orange color is called *jaundice* when it is found in the skin, mucous membranes, sclera of the eye, plasma, and urine. The color of urine containing bilirubin can be yellow-orange to yellow-brown. A yellow foam forms when it is shaken. If the reagent strip is positive for bilirubin, an Ictotest (Bayer Corp.) can be performed to confirm the presence of bilirubin. As noted in the discussion of ketones, the use of Ictotest is no longer recommended.

Urobilinogen. Urobilinogen results from the breakdown of bilirubin in the colon by bacteria. The circulatory system reabsorbs approximately half of the urobilinogen that forms in the intestines, and the remaining half then travels to the liver, where it is sent to the intestines and excreted in the feces. It either remains in this form or is further oxidized to urobilin by intestinal flora. Feces derive their color from bile, stercobilin, and urobilin. Small amounts of urobilinogen may be present in the urine (1%), but most is excreted in the feces.

Urine urobilinogen levels may be increased in conditions such as excessive hemolysis of RBCs, cirrhosis, infectious mononucleosis, and congestive heart failure.

Blood. Three types of blood components give a positive reagent strip reaction for blood: intact RBCs (nonhemolyzed), hemoglobin (from lysed RBCs), and myoglobin. The presence of intact RBCs in urine is called hematuria and usually occurs in UTIs associated with bleeding, such as cystitis and urethritis. Kidney stones, tumors, and lesions may also cause bleeding.

If a female patient is having a menstrual period, a clean-catch, midstream urine specimen is recommended, and her menstrual status should be noted on the requisition. In general, if small amounts of blood and protein are detected on the urine dipstick, it may be necessary to repeat the urinalysis in 1 or more weeks, after the menstrual cycle is complete, to rule out possible infection.

Hemoglobin in the urine, *hemoglobinuria,* is caused by blood transfusion reactions, malaria, drug reactions, snakebites, and severe burns. Because it is the result of hemolyzed RBCs that are no longer visible, it is referred to as "occult (hidden) blood." Myoglobin, an oxygen-storing pigment of muscle tissue, can be found in urine after massive muscle injury, physical trauma, or electrical injury.

Protein. Protein molecules are normally too large to pass through the glomerulus. One of the first signs of renal disease is proteinuria, the presence of large amounts of protein in the urine. Sometimes protein is temporarily found in the urine and may not be pathogenic—for example, during fever, exposure to heat or cold, excessive exercise, and emotional stress. However, large amounts of protein repeatedly excreted in the urine over a period of time indicate renal disease. In pathologic conditions, albumin is the protein found in urine. Other types of protein that can be found in urine are listed in Table 3.2. Proteinuria may occur because of damage to the glomerulus or an imperfection in the reabsorption ability of the renal tubules.

In addition, pregnant women are routinely checked for protein in the urine because it may be a sign of preeclampsia.

Correlating protein level with specific gravity is important because urine with a low specific gravity (very dilute) showing a trace or small amount of protein may be a significant abnormal result.

A microalbumin test can detect very small amounts of albumin excreted in urine. Normal excretion of protein in a 24-hour urine is less than 30 mg/day. Microalbuminuria is excretion of 30 to 300 mg of protein a day. The microalbumin test can be used to detect early signs of kidney damage in patients who are at risk of developing kidney disease (i.e., type 1 diabetes, type 2 diabetes, high blood pressure). Annual screening for microalbuminuria helps identify patients with nephropathy at an early stage. Frequency of testing for microalbumin depends on the patient's health conditions and signs of kidney damage. Because urine concentration is so variable, it is recommended that the urine be standardized by performing a ratio of microalbumin to the creatinine concentration, which is excreted at a constant rate. Less than 3.4 mg/mmol (millimole) is considered negative, and levels between 3.4 and 33.9 mg/mmol indicate microalbuminuria. Bayer Corp. has developed microalbumin/creatinine ratio test strips that can be visually read or measured on the Clinitek instrument. The Multistix Pro10LS is a urinalysis strip that measures a protein/creatinine ratio (see Figure 3.10B).

Microalbumin screening is critical for the following conditions:
- Diabetes mellitus
- Hypertension
- Heart attack
- Stroke
- Pregnancy

Bence Jones protein is another protein found in the urine of patients with multiple myeloma, a malignant cancer of the bone marrow. Bence Jones protein precipitates out at temperatures between 45° and 55°C and then redissolves when boiled.

Nitrites. Some urinary tract bacteria can convert nitrate, which is found normally in the urine, to nitrite. The first morning specimen is recommended for this test because the urine must stay in the bladder for at least 4 to 6 hours to allow any bacteria that may be present sufficient time to convert nitrates to nitrites. Urine should not be left standing because bacterial contamination may convert nitrate to nitrite and give a false-positive reaction. A negative nitrite test does not necessarily mean that no bacterial infection is present. Some bacteria cannot convert nitrates to nitrites, or possibly the urine did not stay in the bladder for 4 to 6 hours. A positive nitrite test result is correlated with a positive leukocyte test and then confirmed with a bacterial culture to determine the quantity and identification of the organisms. The most common organism that causes UTIs, *Escherichia coli,* does convert nitrates to nitrites.

Leukocytes. Another test on the reagent strip determines the presence of leukocytes, or white blood cells (WBCs). The strip tests for esterase, which is produced by lysed granulocytic WBCs (cells broken open). The presence of WBCs usually indicates a UTI and should be correlated with a nitrite test.

Microscopic Urinalysis

The microscopic examination of urine consists of examining, counting, and categorizing the solid material seen under the microscope. A standardized method called the *KOVA System* is

TABLE 3.2	**Proteins Found in Urine**
Protein	**Associated Causes or Conditions**
Albumin	Strenuous physical exercise
	Emotional stress
	Pregnancy-preeclampsia
	Infection
	Glomerulonephritis
	Neonates (first week)
Globulins	Glomerulonephritis
	Renal tubular dysfunction
Hemoglobin	Hematuria
	Hemoglobinuria
Fibrinogen	Severe renal disease
Nucleoprotein	White blood cells in urine
	Epithelial cells in urine
Bence Jones	Multiple myeloma
	Leukemia

Patient:					Date/Time Spec. Collected:									
Doctor:			DOB:		Date/Time Spec. Completed:									
		TEST	**REFERENCE**	**RESULT**	**TEST**	**REFERENCE**	**RESULT**		**TEST**	**REFERENCE**	**RESULT**	**TEST**	**REFERENCE**	**RESULT**
☐	VOID	Color	Yellow		Blood	Neg			WBC	0-5 HPF		Bact.	0-5	
☐	CC	Char.	Clear		pH	5.0-8.0			RBC	0-3 HPF		Mucus	0	
☐	CATH	Glucose	Neg		Protein	Neg	MICRO		Epith.	D		Casts	0	
☐	TURBID	Bilirubin	Neg		Urobili	0.2-1.0 EU			Cryst.	0-3 HPF				
☐	HAZY	Ketone	Neg		Nitrite	Neg	OTHER:							
☐	CLEAR	Sp. Gr	1,000-1,030		Leuk	Neg								

FIG. 3.13 Example of a urinalysis form to be completed and inserted into the patient record. NOTE: The physician or laboratory technician will fill out the microscopic results on the right side of the report form.

used to prepare the microscopic slide. It consists of centrifuging a standard amount of urine for a specific time with a specific centrifugal force. After centrifugation the urine separates into sediment, the material at the bottom of the centrifuged tube of urine, and supernatant, the liquid portion of urine on top of the spun sediment. The supernatant is poured off, and the sediment is stained and poured onto a slide or transferred into a KOVA slide chamber. The slide is then placed under the microscope and focused in preparation for the analysis by the physician or trained professional (see Procedure 3.6 at the end of this section).

Becoming proficient at urinalysis physical and chemical testing and preparing a urine for microscopic testing. Now that you have learned how to describe the physical characteristics of urine and how to measure the specific gravity, pH, and various urine analytes, you are ready to perform a urinalysis and record your results on a form such as that shown in Figure 3.13.

NOTE: You may also prepare the urine for a microscopic evaluation by the physician or medical laboratory technician who will complete the microscopic results on the right side of the report form. (See Procedure 3.6.) The proficiency check-off sheets, report forms, and logs are all located in your workbook.

The following are additional ways to increase your knowledge:
1. Answer the questions at the end of this chapter and in Chapter 3 in the workbook.
2. View the online anatomy animations and the procedural video on Urinalysis on Evolve to see demonstrations of the skills.
3. Perform the online lesson entitled "How to Obtain a Urine Specimen: Performing a Urinalysis" to prepare for your lab.
4. Study Procedure 3.3: Manual Chemical Reagent Strip Procedure in the text and workbook before your laboratory class.
5. Study Procedure 3.4: Clinitek Analyzer Method for Chemical Reagent Strip and Procedure 3.5: Clinitest Procedure for Reducing Substances Such as Sugars in the Urine before class.
6. Study Procedure 3.6: Procedure for the Preparation and the Microscopic Examination of Urine then prepare a slide for urine microscopic examination

PROCEDURE 3.3 Manual Chemical Reagent Strip Procedure

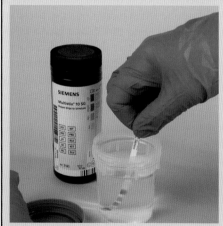 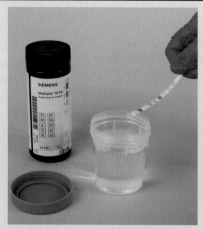 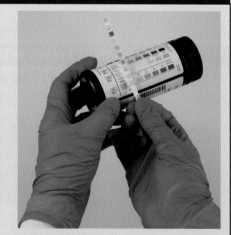

A, Urinalysis chemistry procedure. Dip the reagent strip in the urine, making sure all the reagent pads are wet.

B, Slide the back of the reagent strip on the urine cup as it is removed to eliminate excess fluid and then blot the edge of the strip against absorbent paper.

C, Compare each color pad on the strip to the reference chart starting with the first pad (glucose) and its corresponding row on the bottom of the chart.

PROCEDURE 3.3   Manual Chemical Reagent Strip Procedure—cont'd

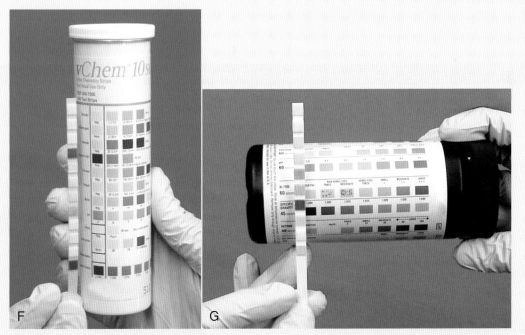

D-E, The two color charts provided to show the variation in reporting parameters that exist among manufacturers. The Iris vChem 10sg strip and its corresponding color chart (D) and the Siemens/Bayer Multistix 10 SG Reagent strip and its color chart (E). (D, Courtesy of Beckman Coulter. All rights reserved. E, © Siemens Healthineers 2018. Used with permission.)

F-G, Proper orientation of the reagent strip to the color chart is critical when reading results. These figures illustrate the differences involved in properly orienting reagent strips to the manufacturer's color chart. The Iris vChem 10sg method (F) and the Bayer (or Siemens) Multistix 10 SG method (G). (From Brunzel NA: *Fundamentals of urine and body fluid analysis*, ed 4, St. Louis, 2018, Elsevier.)

Continued

PROCEDURE 3.3 Manual Chemical Reagent Strip Procedure—cont'd

Purpose

Testing for chemical substances in a urine specimen

Equipment and Supplies

Gloves, reagent strips, timing device, reference chart, patient's requisition

Procedure

1. Sanitize and glove your hands and assemble the equipment. Check the expiration date and the date the reagent bottle was first opened located on the reagent strip bottle. Do not use them if expired.
2. Have the patient produce freshly voided urine in the appropriate container. The sample must come to room temperature, if necessary. Be sure to mix the urine sample before testing. (NOTE: Urine is usually poured into a conical tube to make it easier to determine the color and appearance. This type of tube is used for centrifugation in the microscopic part of the urinalysis, and it also keeps the original container sterile if a urine culture is necessary.)
3. NOTE: Perform quality control testing using manufacturer's controls *before* testing patients. Record and compare the control results to ensure accuracy by checking the results against the manufacturer's control values.
4. After you remove the strip from the bottle, close it immediately. Do not touch the pads.
5. Make sure the pads are completely covered with urine but do not immerse the strip for more than a few seconds (Figure A).
6. Pull the nonpad side of the strip along the edge of the container (Figure B) and then briefly blot the edge of the strip against absorbent paper.
7. Hold the strip parallel to the color chart (in a horizontal position) so that the reagents in the pads do not interact (Figure C). To keep from contaminating the chart, do not place the strip on it.

8. The reagents in the pads are time dependent, so read each test on the strip at its particular time and compare it with the reference chart (Figure D-G). Start with the pad that corresponds with the bottom row of the color chart. The 10 tests on Multistix 10 SG reagent strips and their reading times are as follows:
   - Glucose: 30 seconds
   - Bilirubin: 30 seconds
   - Ketones: 40 seconds
   - Specific gravity: 45 seconds
   - Blood: 60 seconds
   - pH: 60 seconds
   - Protein: 60 seconds
   - Urobilinogen: 60 seconds
   - Nitrite: 60 seconds
   - Leukocytes: 2 minutes
9. After you have read all the pads, discard the strip in a biohazard bag.
10. Remove the gloves and sanitize your hands.
11. Document the procedure, indicating the results, the brand name of the test strip used, the date, the time, and the name of the person testing in the patient's chart (or record results on the preprinted patient's requisition or report).
12. Pour the remaining urine down the sink and place the container in the biohazard waste container. Be sure to have a stream of water started before pouring the urine down the sink to keep from splattering the sample. NOTE: If the results of a urine test are abnormal, do not discard the specimen until the physician approves because he or she may want to order additional tests on the specimen.

PROCEDURE 3.4 Clinitek Analyzer Method for Chemical Reagent Strip

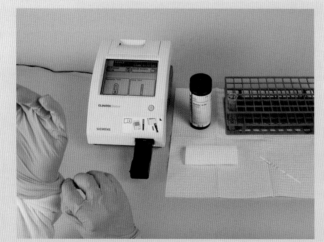

A, Prepare the following: gloves, Clinitek analyzer, absorbent paper, Multistix 10 SG reagent strips or Multistix Pro10LS strips, patient's urine, and control specimen.

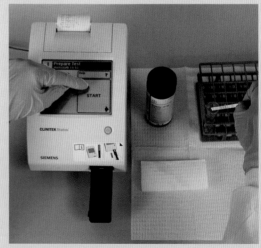

B, Follow the prompts on the instrument monitor or the manufacturer's flow sheet. IMPORTANT NOTE: Before pressing the "start" command, have your test strip ready to dip into the urine.

PROCEDURE 3.4 Clinitek Analyzer Method for Chemical Reagent Strip—cont'd

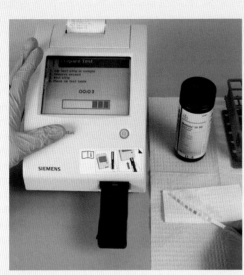

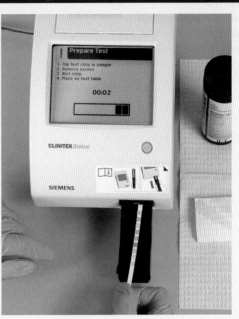

C, Immediately after pressing "start," you have 8 seconds to dip the strip in the urine, remove excess urine from the back of the strip, turn the strip sideways, and blot on the paper.

D, Place the strip in the proper position on the tray (within the 8 seconds). NOTE: This strip still needs to be straightened.

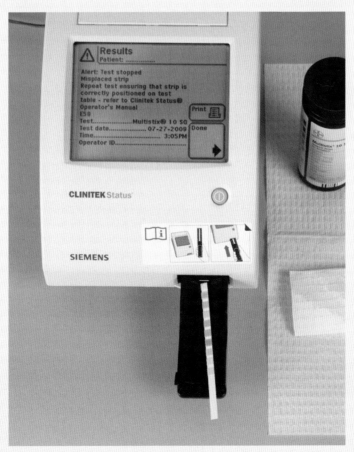

E, If the reagent strip was placed incorrectly, an error message will appear, and the tray will push the sample out. You will need to start the test again with a new strip.

Continued

PROCEDURE 3.4   Clinitek Analyzer Method for Chemical Reagent Strip—cont'd

Equipment and Supplies

Gloves, Multistix 10 SG reagent strips or Multistix Pro10LS strips, absorbent paper, Clinitek analyzer (Figure A)

Procedure

1. Assemble the equipment. Sanitize and glove your hands. Check the expiration date on the reagent strip bottle. Do not use if expired.
2. Be sure to mix the room temperature urine sample and pour it into a conical tube before testing.
3. NOTE: Perform quality control using a manufacturer's liquid control. Record the results and check for accuracy.
4. After you remove the strip from the bottle, close it immediately. Do not touch the reagent pads.
5. Follow the instructions on the instrument monitor or the manufacturer's flow sheet.
   - Enter technician identification.
   - Enter patient information.
   - Before pressing the "start" command, have your test strip ready to dip into the urine (Figure B).
6. After pressing start, you will have 8 seconds to do the following:
   - Dip the strip into the urine, making sure all the pads are completely covered with urine, but do not immerse the strip for more than a few seconds.
   - Remove excess urine from the strip by pulling the nonpad side of the strip along the edge of the container.
   - Blot the edge of the strip against absorbent paper briefly (Figure C).
   - Place the strip in the Clinitek tray, making sure it is placed correctly (Figure D).
7. When the instrument completes its 8-second countdown, it will pull the specimen into the analyzer. NOTE: If the reagent strip was placed incorrectly, an error message will appear, and the tray will push the sample out (Figure E). The reagent strip must be discarded, the instrument will need to be reset, and a new reagent strip must be used to run the test again.
8. While the instrument is measuring each of the timed reagent pads, you will be prompted to record the color and transparency of the urine specimen.
9. When the test is complete, the analyzer will eject the sample tray and print the date, the time, the patient's name, the name of the person performing the test, the results of the 10 tests, and the color and transparency of the specimen.
10. Discard the strip in the appropriate biohazard waste container. Gently wipe off the tray with gauze or paper towel. Pour the remaining urine down the sink, if no additional tests will be ordered, and place the container in the biohazard waste container. Be sure to have a stream of water started before pouring the urine down the sink to keep from splattering the sample.

PROCEDURE 3.5   Clinitest Procedure for Reducing Substances Such as Sugars in the Urine

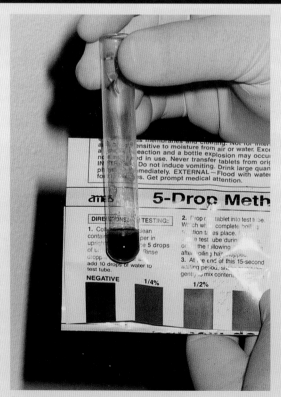

A, Comparison chart for measuring the color results of the Clinitest sugar test. The specimen result is blue, which would be negative for sugar. (From Proctor D, Adams A: *Kinn's the medical assistant: an applied learning approach,* ed 12, St. Louis, 2014, Saunders.)

Equipment and Supplies

Bottle of Clinitest tablets, Clinitest glass tube, tube of water with pipette, urine sample with pipette, Clinitest reference chart

Procedure

1. Gather equipment, sanitize your hands, and put on gloves.
2. Add 5 drops of urine to 10 drops of water in a Clinitest tube.
3. Place the tube in a rack. Put a Clinitest tablet into the lid of the bottle so that you do not touch it; the tablet could become caustic if it becomes moist. Tap the tablet into the tube.
4. The boiling reaction that occurs is very hot. Observe it for any color change. Observe for the "pass-through effect" that results with color changes occurring during the reaction to bright orange and then back to dark blue, appearing negative when the reaction is completed and results are determined. It is critical to watch for this phenomenon to prevent reporting a false-negative result. The pass-through effect occurs as a result of very high concentrations of reducing substances in the urine. If this does occur, results should be recorded as greater than 2% if using the 5-drop method or as greater than 5% if using the 2-drop method. The final color of either method should not be compared with the color chart when the pass-through effect takes place.
5. Mix the tube 15 seconds after the boiling has stopped to blend the contents.
6. Compare the color of the reaction with the Clinitest chart (Figure A) for the 5-drop method and record the results. If the rapid pass-through effect has occurred and you briefly see an orange color, the test must be reported as positive. Refer to step 4.
7. Discard the equipment in the appropriate biohazard waste container. The remaining urine should be rinsed down the sink, and the container should be placed in a biohazard waste container. Be sure to have a stream of water started before pouring the urine down the sink to keep from splattering the sample.
8. Disinfect the work area.
9. Remove gloves and sanitize your hands.
10. Correctly document the results in the patient's chart.

PROCEDURE 3.6 **Procedure for the Preparation and the Microscopic Examination of Urine**

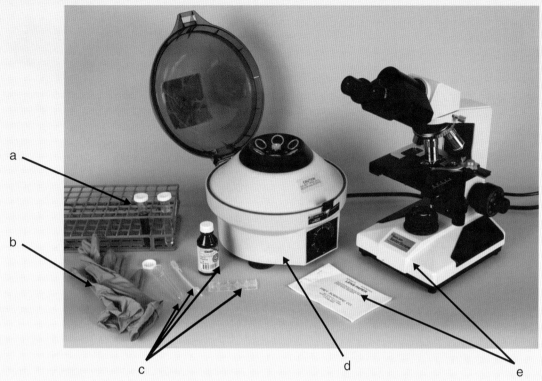

A, *(a)* Specimen (freshly voided urine) in tube holder, *(b)* gloves, *(c)* KOVA system (cap and tube, pipette, stain, slide), *(d)* centrifuge, *(e)* microscope and lens paper.

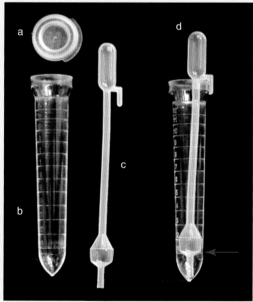

B, The KOVA System consists of a KOVA cap *(a)*, a KOVA tube *(b)*, and a KOVA Petter *(c)*. The clear plastic centrifuge tube is filled to the appropriate graduation mark with well-mixed urine and is capped. After centrifugation, the specially designed KOVA Petter is gently slid into the tube, and the end is firmly seated into the base *(d)*. The bulblike end fits snuggly, such that all but 1 mL of urine can be easily decanted *(red arrow)*. The retained supernatant urine is used to resuspend the sediment for the microscopic examination. (From Brunzel NA: *Fundamentals of urine & body fluid analysis,* ed 4, St. Louis, 2018, Elsevier.)

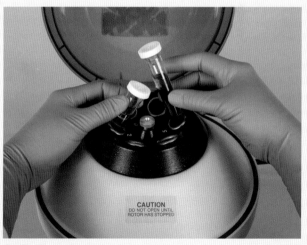

C, Place a centrifuge tube with urine and a centrifuge tube with the same amount of water or urine directly opposite each other to balance the centrifuge. Spin for 5 minutes at 1500 rpm.

Continued

PROCEDURE 3.6   Procedure for the Preparation and the Microscopic Examination of Urine—cont'd

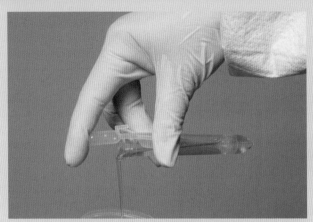

D, After centrifuging, place the pipette in the spun specimen to hold back the sediment and pour off the supernatant.

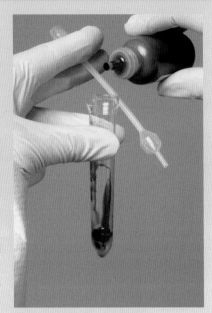

E, Add stain to the sediment and mix well.

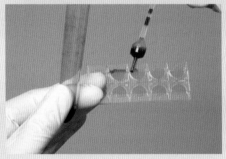

F, Fill the slide wells with the well-mixed stained sediment.

Equipment and Supplies
Specimen (freshly voided urine), KOVA system (cap, pipette, slide, stain), test tube holder, centrifuge, microscope (Figure A)

Preanalytical: Microscopic Setup
1. Sanitize your hands and collect the equipment.
2. Put on gloves and mix the urine. Allow it to come to room temperature if needed.
3. Pour the well-mixed urine specimen to the 12-mL mark in a urine centrifuge tube and cap it.
4. Centrifuge the tube for 5 minutes at 1500 rpm, which will cause the solid particles in the urine to settle to the bottom of the tube (Figure B).
5. After centrifugation is completed, carefully remove the spun tube from the centrifuge so that the sediment is not disturbed.
6. After removing the cap, place the KOVA pipette into the bottom of the tube. Seat the tube firmly, hooking the clip on top of the pipette over the outside of the tube.
7. Pour off (decant) the supernatant by inverting the tube (Figure C). With the KOVA pipette method, approximately 1 mL of sediment will remain in the tube.
8. Remove the pipette from the tube and add 1 drop of stain so that the structures may be seen more easily (Figure D). Reinsert the pipette into the tube and mix the urine sediment and stain by gently squeezing on the pipette bulb.
9. Transfer 1 drop of the stained sediment mixture to the KOVA slide by placing the tip of the pipette onto the open area of one of the sections and

squeezing the bulb until the well is filled (Figure E). Do not overfill or underfill the well. Return the pipette to the urine tube after the well is filled. To allow the sediment to settle, let the filled well sit for 1 minute before performing the microscopic examination. NOTE: An alternative method is to place a drop of mixed sediment onto a glass slide and place a glass coverslip over the drop of urine.
10. Place the filled well (or slide) on the mechanical stage of the microscope and focus on low power with the coarse adjustment. With the fine adjustment knob, bring the specimen into sharp focus. Adjust the light source as needed for low power.

Analytical Interpretation of the Sediment on the Slide (Performed by a Physician or Laboratory Technician)
1. Scan the specimen under low power for casts, particularly at the edge of the slide.
2. Change the objective to high power by rotating the nosepiece and clicking it into place. Bring the specimen into sharp view by focusing with the fine adjustment. The coarse adjustment should not be used for focusing the high power objective because the objective could strike the slide. The intensity of the light source will need to be adjusted for the high power objective.
3. Use high power to examine the specimen, viewing 10 to 15 fields. Casts are counted on low power but identified on high power. All other substances seen should be counted and identified on high power.
4. Record the results for each field.

Postanalytical: Cleanup and Recording of Results
5. The medical assistant may be asked to turn off the microscope and discard the plastic KOVA slide, pipette, and capped centrifuge tube in the biohazard waste container. Rinse the remaining urine down the sink and place the container in a biohazard waste container.
6. Remove the gloves and discard them in a biohazard waste container. Sanitize your hands.
7. Record the physician's calculated results of each finding on the patient's requisition form and chart.

❖ADVANCED CONCEPTS

Medical assistants prepare the urine microscopic slide, and either medical technologists or physicians interpret the results. The medical assistant should be familiar with the terminology of the microscopic findings and the basic shapes of the elements found in the urinary sediment in order to understand the complete urinalysis report. The sediment is examined under the microscope for the presence of cells, casts, crystals, and other substances. First, the presence of casts is viewed using the low power objective of the microscope; then all other substances are observed on high power. NOTE: See the "urinalysis videos" online showing actual microscopic views of cells; casts; and some of the crystals, parasites, and fungi. Compare the videos with the Microscopic Urinalysis Atlas below (Figure 3.14).

Microscopic Elements in Urine and Their Significance
Cells (See First Row of the Atlas—Figure 3.14)
The following cells may be found and reported during a microscopic examination.

Red blood cells. Hematuria is the abnormal presence of RBCs in the urine (#1 in the Microscopic Urinalysis Atlas; see Figure 3.14). RBCs are round, biconcave, nonnucleated, colorless

MICROSCOPIC URINALYSIS ATLAS

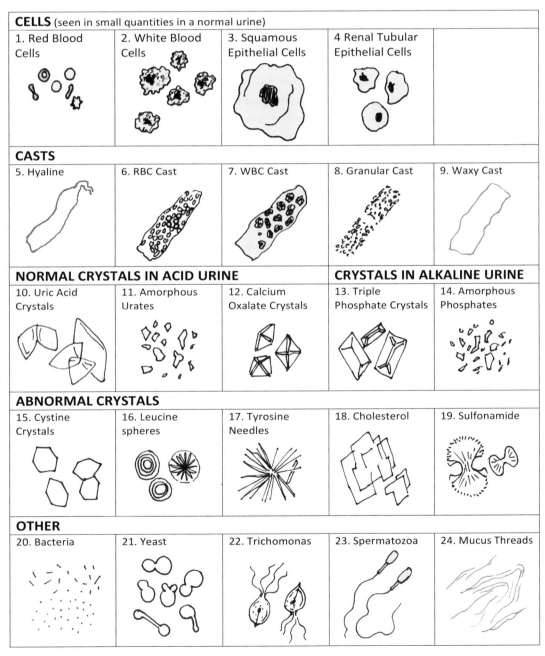

FIG. 3.14 The microscopic elements in urine and their significance. (Courtesy of Gala Bent.)

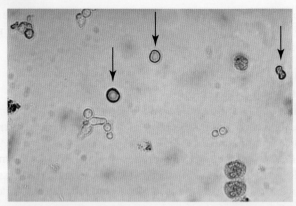

FIG. 3.15 Three red blood cells: Two viewed from above appear as biconcave disks, and one viewed from the side appears hourglass-shaped *(arrows)*. Also present are budding yeast and several white blood cells. (From Brunzel NA: *Fundamentals of urine & body fluid analysis,* ed 4, St. Louis, 2018, Elsevier.)

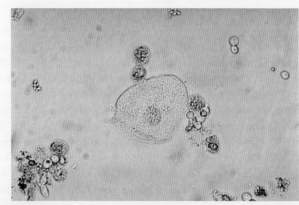

FIG. 3.16 Several white blood cells with characteristic cytoplasmic granules and lobed nuclei surrounding a squamous epithelial cell. Budding yeast cells are also present. (From Brunzel NA: *Fundamentals of urine & body fluid analysis,* ed 4, St. Louis, 2018, Elsevier.)

disks. They are highly refractile in unstained urine and can be difficult to differentiate from other structures, such as yeasts and oil droplets. Yeast usually shows budding, but RBCs do not (Figure 3.15). RBCs shrink in concentrated urine and are referred to as *crenated.* RBCs will swell and hemolyze in diluted urine. If the RBCs have been hemolyzed (broken open), they will not be seen on the microscopic examination, but the hemoglobin will be detected on the blood pad of the chemical strip test. A few RBCs, 1 to 2 per high power field (hpf), can be normal. Bleeding, damage to the glomerulus (e.g., inflammation of the glomerulus, or glomerulonephritis), and vascular injury are associated with the presence of RBCs in the urine. See microscopic Figure 3.15.

White blood cells. The condition pyuria, or WBCs in the urine, usually indicates the presence of an infection in the genitourinary system (#2 in the Microscopic Urinalysis Atlas; see Figure 3.14). WBCs are larger than RBCs, approximately 12 micrometers in diameter. The most common WBC found in the urine is the neutrophil, which possesses a multilobed nucleus and granules. A urine microscopic examination normally contains 0 to 5 WBCs/hpf. Pyuria can be temporary or caused by fevers or strenuous exercise, but the presence of WBCs can be a factor in pyelonephritis, cystitis, prostatitis, and urethritis.

Epithelial cells. Another type of cell that can be found in the urine is the epithelial cell. Several types exist.

Squamous epithelial cells (see #3 in the Microscopic Urinalysis Atlas; see Figure 3.14) are the most frequently seen and least significant of the epithelial cells found in urine. They are derived from the lining of the vagina and the lower portion of the male and female urethras. These cells are large and have abundant, irregular cytoplasm with a central nucleus the size of an RBC. See microscopic Figure 3.16.

Transitional or *caudate epithelial cells* come from the lining of the renal pelvis, bladder, and upper urethra. They are spherical, polyhedral, or caudate (having a tail), with a central nucleus, and are smaller than squamous epithelial cells. They can be found in pairs and small clumps after catheterizations. The presence of large numbers of transitional epithelial cells may indicate a pathologic condition.

Renal tubular epithelial cells (RTEs) (#4 in the Microscopic Urinalysis Atlas; see Figure 3.14) are the most significant of the epithelial cells. The presence of increased amounts (>2/hpf) indicates tubular necrosis. The size and shape of these cells vary depending on their origin. These cells are round to oval, sometimes rectangular to columnar, and slightly larger than WBCs, and they can be distinguished from leukocytes by the presence of a single round, eccentric nucleus. Renal tubule cells are present in microscopic urine in conditions such as pyelonephritis, toxic reaction, viral infections, allograft rejection, and secondary effects attributable to glomerulonephritis.

Casts (See Second Row of the Atlas—Figure 3.14)

Casts are formed primarily within the lumen of the distal convoluted tubules and the collecting ducts. They provide a microscopic view of conditions within the nephron. Their shapes usually contain parallel sides and rounded ends. The main component of a cast is a gel-like protein. Four factors can lead to cast formation: decreased urine flow, increased acidity (low pH), increased concentration (high specific gravity), and increased plasma protein. When these factors are present, a cast is formed in the following manner:

1. Protein aggregates into individual protein fibrils that attach to renal tubule cells.
2. The protein fibrils interweave, forming a loose fibril network that becomes a solid structure.
3. Urinary components, such as RBCs or epithelial cells, may attach to the solid structure.
4. The protein fibril structure detaches from the epithelial cells lining the renal tubules and is excreted as a cast.

Casts are observed and counted on low power, but they are identified on high power. They tend to migrate to the edges of the slide, so this area must be examined. Fresh urine should be examined because casts dissolve in alkaline urine that has been standing.

Hyaline casts. The hyaline cast (#5 in the Microscopic Urinalysis Atlas; see Figure 3.14) is the most frequently seen cast. It consists almost entirely of protein and appears colorless in unstained urine. Because the hyaline cast has a refractive index very similar to that of urine, it must be examined with the light subdued. This cast can normally be found in the urine (0–2/hpf). Conditions such as strenuous exercise, dehydration, heat exposure, and emotional stress can cause hyaline casts to be present in the urine. See microscopic Figure 3.17. These casts can also be found in pathologic conditions such as acute glomerulonephritis, pyelonephritis, chronic renal disease, and congestive heart failure.

Red blood cell casts. An RBC cast (#6 in the Microscopic Urinalysis Atlas; see Figure 3.14) contains RBCs, is refractile, and is yellow-orange to orange-red in color. RBC casts are primarily associated with glomerulonephritis. As they age, the RBCs lyse. and the cast becomes a hemoglobin cast. A hemoglobin cast has the same color as an RBC cast but without visible intact cells.

White blood cell casts. White blood cell casts (#7 in the Microscopic Urinalysis Atlas; see Figure 3.14) most frequently contain neutrophils, one type of WBC, that are refractile because of the presence of granules and multilobed nuclei. They indicate infection or inflammation within the nephron, mostly seen in pyelonephritis.

Renal epithelial cell casts. Renal epithelial cell casts contain renal tubule epithelial cells and can be very difficult to differentiate from WBC casts. They are found in conditions such as heavy metal and chemical- or drug-induced toxicity, viral infection, and allograft rejection.

Granular casts. Granular casts (#8 in the Microscopic Urinalysis Atlas; see Figure 3.14) contain granules throughout the matrix. They can appear as coarse or finely granular, but distinguishing between the two is not necessary. When urinary flow diminishes, a granular cast may form as a result of the disintegration of cellular casts and tubule cells or protein aggregates filtered by the glomerulus. Granular casts result from stress and strenuous exercise but can also be found in conditions such as nephrotic syndrome, orthostatic proteinuria, and congestive heart failure.

Waxy casts. Waxy casts (#9 in the Microscopic Urinalysis Atlas; see Figure 3.14) are very refractile and are homogeneously smooth, with ends that are blunt and cracked. These casts appear dark pink, if stained, and represent extreme urine stasis (stoppage of urine), signifying chronic renal failure.

Crystals (See Third and Fourth Rows of the Atlas)

Crystals are formed by the precipitation of urine salts when changes in pH, temperature (crystals form readily at low temperatures), or concentration occur. The most important aid in the identification of urine crystals is based on the urine pH. Although most crystals are normal when found in acidic and alkaline urine, the few abnormal crystals cited next may represent disorders such as liver disease, inborn errors of metabolism, or renal damage caused by the crystallization of iatrogenic compounds (caused by treatment or diagnostic procedures) and must be detected and reported. Crystals are counted and identified under high power and reported as few, moderate, and many.

Crystals in acidic urine. The most common crystals normally seen in acid urine are uric acid crystals, amorphous urates, acid urates, and calcium oxalate.

Uric acid crystals (#10 in the Microscopic Urinalysis Atlas; see Figure 3.14) are typically four-sided and flat yellow to reddish brown. They can be seen in a variety of shapes, such as rhombic, wedge, and rosette. Although these crystals are usually normal, they can be seen in patients with leukemia who are receiving chemotherapy and sometimes in patients with gout. See microscopic Figure 3.18.

Amorphous urates (#11 in the Microscopic Urinalysis Atlas; see Figure 3.14) are yellow-brown granules often found in clumps that give the urine a macroscopic (i.e., sufficiently large to see with the eyes) pink "brick dust" color. See microscopic Figure 3.19.

Acid urates are found in urine at pH levels below 7 and are frequently seen in urine that has been refrigerated.

Calcium oxalates (#12 in the Microscopic Urinalysis Atlas; see Figure 3.14) are frequently found in acid urine but can also be found in neutral and rarely in alkaline urine. They are commonly seen as colorless octahedron crystals that resemble envelopes (they have the appearance of an × on

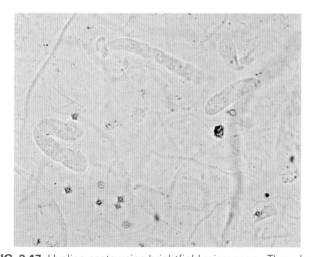

FIG. 3.17 Hyaline casts using brightfield microscopy. Three hyaline casts and mucus threads are present. Red blood cell under hyaline cast at the upper right; four calcium oxylate crystals under cast on the left. (From Brunzel NA: *Fundamentals of urine & body fluid analysis,* ed 4, St. Louis, 2018, Elsevier.)

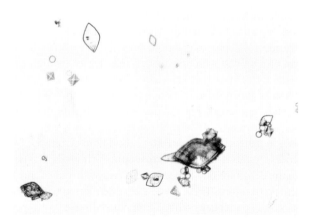

FIG. 3.18 Uric acid crystals (diamond shaped) and a few calcium oxalate crystals. Note the darker coloration as the crystals layer and thicken. (From Brunzel NA: *Fundamentals of urine & body fluid analysis,* ed 4, St. Louis, 2018, Elsevier.)

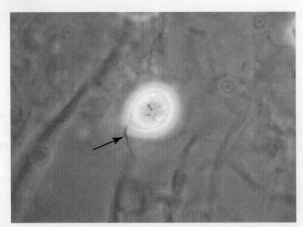

FIG. 3.19 A trichomonad in urine sediment. Because of their rapid flitting motion, only one of the flagella is visible in this view *(arrow)*. Mucus, white blood cells, and other trichomonads are present but are not in focus at this focal plane. (From Brunzel NA: *Fundamentals of urine & body fluid analysis,* ed 4, St. Louis, 2018, Elsevier.)

them). The presence of calcium oxalate crystals in fresh urine may indicate the formation of renal calculi (kidney stones). They are also associated with foods high in oxalic acid, such as tomatoes and asparagus, and ascorbic acid (oxalic acid is an end product of ascorbic acid).

Crystals in alkaline urine. The majority of normal crystals seen in alkaline urine are phosphates and include triple phosphate, and amorphous phosphate.

Triple phosphate crystals (#13 in the Microscopic Urinalysis Atlas; see Figure 3.14) resemble coffin lids and have no clinical significance. They are found in very alkaline urine that contains urea-splitting bacteria.

Amorphous phosphate crystals (#14 in the Microscopic Urinalysis Atlas; see Figure 3.14) are found in urine with a pH greater than 7. They are yellow-brown granules with no distinctive shape. These crystals, which form when urine cools to room temperature, have a macroscopic appearance of white turbidity.

Abnormal crystals in acidic urine. Most abnormal crystals are found in acid urine and only rarely in neutral urine.

Cystine crystals (#15 in the Microscopic Urinalysis Atlas; see Figure 3.14) appear as colorless, refractile, hexagonal plates and can be confused with uric acid crystals. Differentiation can be made by the fact that uric acid crystals are very birefringent under a polarized microscope. However, only thick cystine crystals have polarizing abilities. Positive identification can be made with a cyanide-nitroprusside test. These crystals may be seen in patients with a hereditary condition, cystinuria.

Leucine crystals (#16 in Microscopic Urinalysis Atlas; see Figure 3.14) are oily-appearing spheres with radial and concentric striations. These crystals are often found with tyrosine crystals in patients who have severe liver disease.

Tyrosine crystals (#17 in the Microscopic Urinalysis Atlas; see Figure 3.14) resemble fine needles in sheaves or rosettes and are found in conjunction with leucine. They may occur in patients with inherited disorders of amino acid metabolism.

Bilirubin crystals are seen in hepatic disorders and appear as clumped needles or granules with the characteristic yellow color of bilirubin. They should not be reported in the absence of bilirubin.

Cholesterol crystals (acid pH) are rarely seen because lipids do not usually crystallize, but they can be found in urine that has been refrigerated. They appear as rectangular plates with a notch in one or more corners (#18 in the Microscopic Urinalysis Atlas; see Figure 3.14). Along with fatty casts and oval fat bodies (discussed later in this chapter), cholesterol crystals are characteristic of disorders such as nephrotic syndrome.

Sulfonamide (#19 in the Microscopic Urinalysis Atlas; see Figure 3.14) and *ampicillin crystals* are formed after inadequate hydration in patients being treated with these antibiotics.

Other Substances (See Fifth Row of the Atlas)

Bacteria. Because bacteria (#20 in the Microscopic Urinalysis Atlas; see Figure 3.14) are normally not found in the urine, the presence of bacteria could indicate either contamination of the specimen or the presence of a UTI. WBCs present with bacteria could signify a UTI. Because contaminant bacteria reproduce rapidly if the urine is kept at room temperature for a prolonged period, testing and microscopic examination should be performed on fresh urine. Bacteria are very tiny and must be viewed with high power. They appear as either rod shaped (bacilli) or round (cocci) and are reported as few, moderate, or many, or as 1+, 2+, 3+, or 4+.

Yeast. Yeasts (#21 in the Microscopic Urinalysis Atlas; see Figure 3.14) are small, oval organisms that may bud. Differentiating them from RBCs is sometimes difficult, but the budding characteristic is helpful. *Candida albicans* is a yeast that may be found in the urine of women who have a vaginal infection (candidiasis), in patients with diabetes mellitus, and in immunocompromised patients. Yeasts are reported in the same way as bacteria.

Parasites. *Trichomonas vaginalis* (#22 in the Microscopic Urinalysis Atlas; see Figure 3.14) is the most frequently seen parasite in urine specimens. It is a pear-shaped flagellate with an undulating membrane and a characteristic rapid darting movement that helps identify it in a wet preparation. See figure 3.19. *T. vaginalis* is a sexually transmitted parasite that causes vaginal inflammation in women and infection of the urethra and prostate in men. It is reported as rare, few, moderate, or many per high power field.

Sperm. Spermatozoa, or sperm (#23 in the Microscopic Urinalysis Atlas; see Figure 3.14), can be found in both male and female urine after sexual intercourse. They have oval, slightly tapered heads and long, flagella-like tails. Spermatozoa are reported as 1+, 2+, 3+, or 4+.

Mucus. Mucus (#24 in the Microscopic Urinalysis Atlas; see Figure 3.14) is a protein whose major constituent is Tamm-Horsfall protein. It is produced by the glands and epithelial cells of the lower genitourinary tract and renal tubular epithelial cells. Microscopically, mucus appears as threadlike structures. To see mucus, the microscope light must be subdued. The presence of mucus in the urine has no clinical significance.

Artifacts. Artifacts that may be found in the urine may include fecal contamination, starch granules from gloves, air bubbles, pollen grains, hair, and clothing and diaper fibers.

REVIEW QUESTIONS*

1. A patient's urine specimen is orange-yellow (or greenish). Which of the following substances would be found in the urine?
   a. Glucose
   b. Ketones
   c. Bilirubin
   d. Nitrate

2. Which substance would be found in normal urine that gives the urine its yellow color?
   a. Hemoglobin
   b. Urochrome
   c. Porphyrin
   d. Myoglobin

3. Which four conditions are conducive to cast formation?
   a. High pH (alkaline), increased plasma proteins, increased rate of urine flow, and low specific gravity
   b. Low pH, increased plasma proteins, decreased rate of urine flow, and low specific gravity
   c. Low pH, decreased plasma proteins, decreased rate of urine flow, and high specific gravity
   d. Low pH (acidic), increased plasma proteins, decreased rate of urine flow, and high specific gravity

4. In a 24-hour urine specimen collection method, which of the following is correct?
   a. All the urine for a 24-hour period is collected, including the first morning sample of the first day.
   b. When the patient is collecting a urine sample, the first third should go into the toilet.
   c. The first specimen of a 24-hour urine is collected.
   d. The last specimen of a 24-hour urine is collected.

5. Which of the following values would represent a dilute specific gravity?
   a. 1.015
   b. 1.005
   c. 1.020
   d. 1.025

6. The correct flow of urine is
   a. glomerulus, glomerular capsule, renal tubules, urinary bladder, renal pelvis, ureter, urethra, and urinary meatus.
   b. glomerulus, glomerular capsule, renal pelvis, renal tubules, ureter, urinary bladder, urethra, and urinary meatus.
   c. glomerulus, glomerular capsule, renal tubules, renal pelvis, urinary bladder, ureter, urethra, and urinary meatus.
   d. glomerulus, glomerular capsule, renal tubules, renal pelvis, ureter, urinary bladder, urethra, and urinary meatus.

7. Which of the following substances is observed and counted on low power?
   a. Crystals
   b. Casts
   c. Yeasts
   d. Bacteria

8. Which casts are occasionally found in healthy people?
   a. Renal epithelial casts
   b. White blood cell casts
   c. Hyaline casts
   d. Waxy casts

9. Triple phosphate crystals resemble
   a. envelopes.
   b. dumbbells.
   c. rosettes.
   d. coffin lids.

10. Which is the most common parasite found in the urine?
    a. *Candida albicans*
    b. *Trichomonas vaginalis*
    c. *Enterobius vermicularis*
    d. *Escherichia coli*

Educating a female patient in the correct midstream clean-catch method of collection includes some of the steps below. Write "C" if the step is correct and "I" if the step is incorrect. If the step is incorrect, explain why.

11. The patient should wash her hands.
12. The patient should spread the labia and hold them apart during the procedure with her nondominant hand.
13. The patient should clean one side with a towelette, wiping from back to front.
14. The patient should repeat step 3 (step 13 above) on the other side with the same towelette.
15. The patient should urinate the first third of the urine into the toilet, catch the second third in the sterile cup, and urinate the last third in the toilet.
16. The medical assistant should disinfect the outside of the container.

*Answers to these Review Questions are located in the Appendix on p. 278.

WEBSITES

National Kidney Foundation:
www.kidney.org/
National Institute of Diabetes & Digestive & Kidney Diseases (NIDDK):
www.niddk.nih.gov

National Kidney Disease Kidney Education Program (NIH):
www.nkdep.nih.gov/index.htm
"Bladder Diseases" from Medline Plus (NIH and the U.S. National Library of Medicine):
www.nlm.nih.gov/medlineplus/bladderdiseases.html

4 CHAPTER

Blood Collection

OBJECTIVES

After completing this chapter, you should be able to do the following:

1. Define and match key terms and abbreviations in this chapter.

Fundamental Concepts: Theory, Safety, and Patient Preparation

2. Identify the cardiovascular anatomic structures and state their functions and relationships to blood collection.
3. Discuss the Needle Stick Safety and Prevention Act and list the ways an employer complies with the Act.
4. Perform the appropriate steps for patient preparation, emphasizing the importance of correctly identifying the patient.

Blood Collection Procedures: Capillary Puncture and Venipuncture

5. Do the following regarding capillary puncture procedures:
   - Perform the proper procedure for capillary puncture according to the stated task, conditions, and standards listed in the Learning Outcome Procedure Sheets in the student workbook, demonstrating an understanding of site selection, equipment, and complications of this procedure.
   - Perform or describe a simulated heel stick and neonatal blood screening collection onto a card according to the stated task, conditions, and standards listed in the Learning Outcome Evaluation in the student workbook.
   - Relate the most current Occupational Safety and Health Administration (OSHA) safety guidelines for capillary puncture methods and maintain a safe work environment by following the most current guidelines for disposing used equipment and cleaning and disinfecting the work area.

6. Perform the following regarding venipuncture procedures:
   - Evaluate a patient's venipuncture site availability and determine the correct venipuncture method that should be performed.
   - Describe the vacuum tube, syringe, and butterfly venipuncture equipment and explain the order of draw for multiple-tube orders.
   - Perform a Vacutainer venipuncture, syringe venipuncture, and butterfly venipuncture according to the stated task, conditions, and standards listed in the Learning Outcome Evaluation in the student workbook.
   - Relate the most current OSHA safety guidelines for the various venipuncture methods and maintain a safe work environment by following the most current guidelines for disposing used equipment and cleaning and disinfecting the work area.

Advanced Concepts: Specimen and Patient Care

7. Describe or perform the proper way to process blood specimens, including how to centrifuge a serum specimen and a plasma specimen in a serum separator tube and a plasma separator tube. Also, determine specimen acceptability.
8. Identify patient issues and complications that may occur during phlebotomy procedures and discuss and demonstrate the appropriate steps to take when they occur; also discuss the importance of risk management as it pertains to blood collection procedures.
9. Demonstrate the following (affective) behaviors:
   - Explain to a patient the rationale for performance of a procedure.
   - Show awareness of a patient's concerns related to the procedure being performed.
   - Incorporate critical thinking skills when performing venipuncture and capillary puncture.

KEY TERMS

antecubital space: depression area in front of the elbow

anticoagulant: a natural or synthesized chemical that prevents blood from clotting

arteries: blood vessels with a pulse that carry blood away from the heart

blood culture: a test to detect bacteria or organisms growing in the blood

buffy coat: narrow middle layer of white blood cells and platelets in a centrifuged whole blood specimen

capillaries: network of microscopic blood vessels connecting arterioles and venules that contain a mixture of arterial and venous blood

capillary action: process by which blood flows freely into a capillary tube in microcollection procedures

capillary puncture: skin puncture or "stick" (typically finger-sticks on adults and heel sticks on infants)

cyanotic: a condition in which the skin and mucous membranes are blue; caused by an oxygen deficiency

edema: abnormal collection of fluid in interstitial spaces that causes swelling

EDTA (ethylenediaminetetraacetic acid): a synthesized anticoagulant that also preserves the blood cells

evacuated tube: tube with air removed to produce a vacuum (e.g., Vacutainer tube used in collecting blood)

hematoma: tumor or swelling of blood in the tissues (resulting in bruising during blood collection procedures)

hemoconcentration: condition in which the blood concentration of large molecules such as proteins, cells, and coagulation factors increases due to decreased plasma volume

hemolysis: the breaking open or rupture of red blood cells and the release of hemoglobin

heparin: a natural anticoagulant that prevents the blood from clotting

humors: fluid or semifluid substances found in the body

interstitial fluid: all the fluid except blood that is found in the space between tissues; also referred to as tissue fluid

lancets: capillary puncture devices

lumen: inner tubular space of a needle, vessel, or tube

mastectomy: removal of the breast

microcollection: collecting a small amount of blood by capillary puncture of the finger or heel

neonate: a newborn child

osteomyelitis: inflammation of the bone; caused by bacterial infection

palpating: gently touching and pressing on an area to feel texture, size, consistency, and direction

petechiae: tiny purple or red skin spots caused by small amounts of blood under the skin; found in patients with coagulation problems; the condition can lead to excessive bleeding during phlebotomy procedures

phlebotomy: blood collection; derived from the Greek words *phlebo,* meaning vein, and *tomy,* meaning to cut

plasma: liquid part of whole blood

serum: liquid part obtained when blood is clotted; lacks the clotting factors

stat: needed immediately

syncope: fainting

tourniquet: a band placed above the venipuncture site to make the vein more prominent

veins: blood vessels with valves that carry blood toward the heart

ABBREVIATIONS

CLSI: Clinical Laboratory Standards Institute
PKU: phenylketonuria (an inherited metabolic disorder)

PST: plasma separator tube
SST: serum separator tube

❖ FUNDAMENTAL CONCEPTS: THEORY, SAFETY, AND PATIENT PREPARATION

One of the skills that medical assistants perform routinely is blood collection, or phlebotomy. The word *phlebotomy* means cutting into a vein, and *phlebotomist* is the term for the professional who performs phlebotomy. The history of blood collection dates to before the fifth century BC. At that time, all medical treatment was based on four body humors (fluid or semifluid substances found in the body): blood, phlegm, yellow bile, and black bile. Techniques such as purging, starving, vomiting, and bloodletting were used. By the Middle Ages, barbers, along with surgeons, practiced the art of bloodletting. The red stripe on the barber's pole represented blood, the white stripe represented the tourniquet, and the pole symbolized the stick squeezed by the patient to dilate the vein. Bloodletting flourished into the 18th and early 19th centuries. In 1799, George Washington died after 9 pints of blood were taken in a 24.hour period in an attempt to cure his throat infection.

Today phlebotomy is primarily performed by trained professionals. Before studying the procedures involved with blood collection, the function and structures of blood vessels must be understood.

Function and Structures of Blood Vessels

Blood vessels are part of the cardiovascular system. They make up a *closed-circuit system* (Figure 4.1) in which blood is pumped from the heart to the blood vessels and then returns to the heart. In general, all blood vessels except capillaries have three layers (Figure 4.2). These layers surround the area through which the blood flows and are called the *outer (tunica adventitia), middle (tunica media),* and *inner layers (tunica intima).*

Types of Blood Vessels

Blood vessels are classified as arteries, arterioles, capillaries, venules, and veins. Arteries have all three layers, and their function is to carry blood away from the heart. Each artery has a thick middle muscle layer that allows the vessel to expand and contract as blood pressure rises and falls. Arteries have a pulse and are located deeper than veins. They branch into arterioles, which are smaller blood vessels. Arterioles also have three layers, but the layers are thinner than those found in arteries. Arterioles then branch into capillaries. Capillaries are microscopic blood vessels composed of one layer of simple squamous epithelial cells. Substances are exchanged between blood and the surrounding tissue in the capillaries. Capillary blood is a mixture of arterial and venous blood. Capillaries join venules, which are composed of three thin layers, and the venules unite to form veins. Veins carry blood toward the heart and contain valves that prevent backflow of blood. Veins have three layers but thinner walls and less muscle than arteries.

A difference in the feel of veins and arteries can be detected when palpating (gently touching and pressing on an area to feel texture, size, consistency, direction, and movement). Arteries

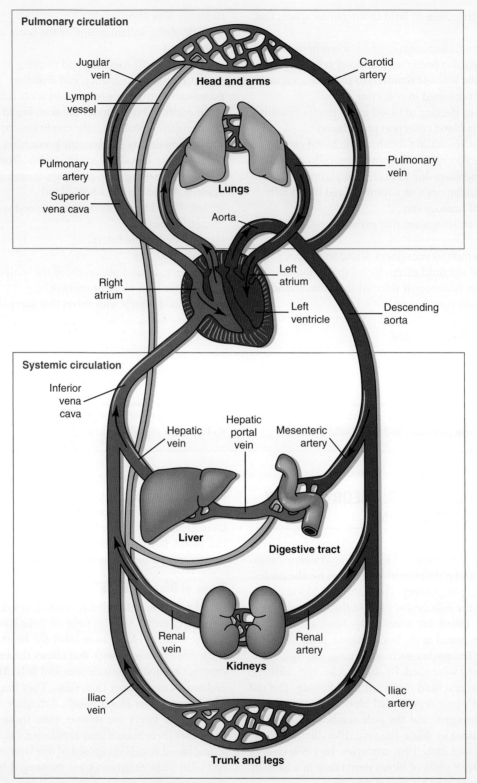

FIG. 4.1 Closed circuit system. Blood flows to the right atrium and then to the right ventricle, pulmonary artery, lungs, and pulmonary veins; then it flows to the left atrium, left ventricle, aorta, arteries, arterioles, capillaries, venules, veins, superior vena cava and inferior vena cava; and then back into the right side of the heart to repeat the sequence. (From Warekois R, Robinson R: *Phlebotomy: worktext and procedures manual,* ed 3, St. Louis, 2012, Saunders.)

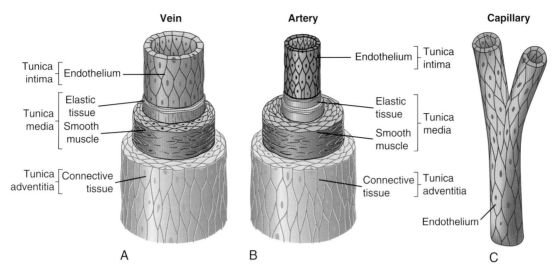

FIG. 4.2 Layers of the vein (**A**), artery (**B**), and capillary (**C**). (From Warekois R, Robinson R: *Phlebotomy: worktext and procedures manual,* ed 3, St. Louis, 2012, Saunders.)

have palpable pulses that when counted for 1 minute provide the patient's pulse rate (which is the patient's heart rate in beats per minute). Veins feel spongy and do not have a pulse. Veins are the vessels most often used in blood collection because they are closer to the surface than arteries and are safer and easier to access.

Most blood tests are performed on venous or capillary blood. The differences in the blood composition of these vessels should be understood.

Comparison of Blood Analytes in Capillary and Venous Blood

The composition of capillary blood is different from that of venous blood. Some of the differences are listed in Table 4.1. Capillary blood has higher amounts of hemoglobin and glucose than venous blood, but venous blood has higher amounts of potassium, calcium, and total protein.

Because capillary and venous blood specimens may yield different test results, performance of a capillary technique must always be reported. In addition, if an analyte from Table 4.1 needs to be retested, the same blood collection technique must be used (e.g., venipuncture versus capillary). This is especially significant when comparing glucose concentration results during a glucose tolerance test, which requires the completion of multiple glucose tests during a 2- to 3-hour time frame.

TABLE 4.1 Comparison of Capillary and Venous Blood Analyte Values

Capillary Blood Results	Venous Blood Results
Hemoglobin: higher	Potassium: higher
Glucose: higher	Total protein: higher
	Calcium: higher

Most Commonly Used Veins

The veins most commonly used when performing venipuncture are found in the antecubital space of the arm, the area in front of the elbow (Figure 4.3). There are three veins to locate. They are the median cubital vein, the cephalic vein, and the basilic vein. The median cubital is large and is the most commonly used vein. It is located in the middle of the antecubital space and is well anchored above the lower arm muscle. The second vein of choice is the cephalic vein, on the thumb side of the arm. This vein is not well anchored and may move, but in an obese person, it may be the only vein that can be found. (NOTE: When locating the cephalic vein, it helps to turn the lower arm so that the thumb of the hand is turned up, causing the cephalic vein to be on the upper surface of the arm, rather than on the lateral side.) The basilic vein is the least well anchored and is the last choice of the three. It is located on the little-finger side near the brachial artery. Its position increases the risk of puncturing the artery if the needle is inserted too deeply.

Federal Law Concerning Safety Equipment

According to the Centers for Disease Control and Prevention, health care workers receive approximately 600,000 percutaneous injuries annually from contaminated sharps. Because of concern over this issue and the development of technologies for protection, the Needlestick Safety and Prevention Act was passed by Congress, which directed the Occupational Safety and Health Administration (OSHA) to revise the Bloodborne Pathogens Standard to require employers to identify and use safer medical devices. Federal Bill HR 5178 was signed by President Bill Clinton on November 6, 2000, with an April 18, 2001, compliance date. An employer is in compliance with this law by performing the following actions:

- Creating and updating a bloodborne pathogen exposure control plan
- Evaluating and implementing safer medical devices for eliminating or minimizing occupational exposures

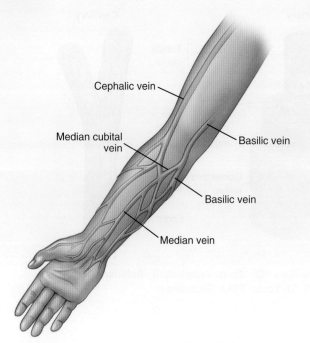

FIG. 4.3 The veins of the forearm. (From Hunt SA: *Saunders medical assisting,* St. Louis, 2002, Saunders.)

- Including health care workers who are using the devices in the evaluation and selection process
- Consistently monitoring the effectiveness of devices
- Maintaining a detailed sharps injury log, which gives a description of each exposure incident

Various current safety devices are discussed with each blood collection procedure described in this chapter.

Procedure Preparation

All blood-collecting procedures have the same preparation steps in common. These steps include having a properly completed requisition form, correctly identifying the patient, and appropriately positioning the patient. Understanding the role these steps play in the overall procedure is important.

Proper Completion of Requisitions

Requisitions are generated by a physician's order. They can be either handwritten or computer generated. The following information must be verified and included on a requisition or electronic record before obtaining the blood specimen:

- Patient's name
- Patient's identification number
- Patient's date of birth
- Name of the test ordered
- Name of the physician ordering test
- Date and time of collection
- Timing of the test (e.g., routine, stat, timed test)
- Other information, such as whether the patient is in a fasting state
- Insurance or billing information (e.g., if it is being sent to a laboratory for testing)

The requisition or electronic record must be entirely completed because it is used to correctly identify the patient and to determine how and when the specimen sample is to be collected.

Proper Identification of the Patient

The patient should always be greeted in a professional manner, and the medical assistant should introduce himself or herself to the patient. A brief explanation of the procedure being performed should be given. If the patient has any questions concerning the tests that have been ordered, the medical assistant should tactfully direct the patient to the physician.

One of the most critical steps in any phlebotomy procedure is to identify the patient correctly. The most serious laboratory error is the misidentification of a patient. To avoid this error, a three-way identification system should be used. This system consists of matching the patient's name and date of birth with the information on the test requisition, plus one more type of identification, such as a driver's license, address or zip code, phone number, or a chart number (outpatient) or hospital identification number on the patient's wrist (inpatient). When determining the patient's name, do not ask, "Are you Mrs. Smith?" Often patients may not hear the question, or they may be taking medication and mistakenly answer yes to the wrong name. It is better to ask, "Will you please spell your last name for me?"

For some tests, the patient needs to be fasting. The proper way to determine this is to ask if the patient has had anything to eat or drink for 12 to 14 hours before the phlebotomy procedure. Do not ask patients if they have fasted. Some patients do not understand this concept and may answer yes even if they have had coffee, chewed gum, or done other things that could affect the testing. If the patient is not in a fasting state, it is important to note on the requisition and the patient's chart the time and the type of food constituting the patient's last intake. Also, the physician or lab should be consulted to determine if the test will need to be rescheduled for a time when the patient is in the proper fasting state needed for the ordered test.

A patient has the right to refuse a blood collection procedure, in which case the physician should be notified.

Proper Patient Positioning

The patient must be properly positioned for a phlebotomy procedure. A semi-reclining position on an examination table is preferred. However, having the patient sit in an elevated chair with an armrest (Figure 4.4) is also appropriate. This elevated phlebotomy chair can help protect the patient from falling if he or she faints, and it allows the vessels in the arm to expand to their maximum volume when the arm is extended downward. This position is also the best way to collect multiple tubes that need to be filled from the bottom up. Never have the patient sit on a stool or stand up when drawing blood because the patient could be injured if fainting occurs.

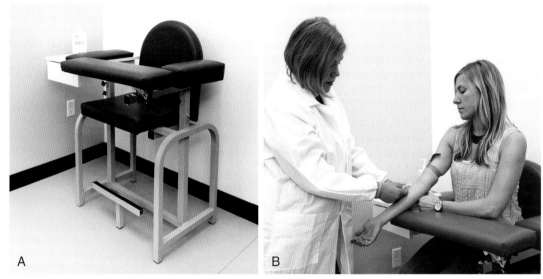

FIG. 4.4 A, Elevated phlebotomy chair allows phlebotomist to ergonomically stand upright. B, Patient extending arm downward allows the tubes to fill from the bottom up. (Photos by Zack Bent.)

BLOOD COLLECTION PROCEDURES: CAPILLARY PUNCTURE AND VENIPUNCTURE

Capillary Puncture

Although venipuncture is usually the most common blood collection method used, the capillary puncture is becoming very common in point-of-care testing (POCT) procedures. The physician typically determines if this method should be used based on the test ordered on the requisition.

Capillary puncture, also called *skin puncture* or "stick," is a method of collecting blood by puncturing the skin through the epidermis into the dermal layer. The composition of blood analytes from a skin puncture is not the same as that of venous blood. Because capillaries are the bridge between arteries and veins, a skin puncture draws blood from arterioles, venules, and capillaries as well as interstitial fluid (all the fluid except blood found in the space between tissues, also called *tissue fluid*). Blood from skin punctures is also more like arterial blood than venous blood because arteries exert more pressure into the capillaries than the veins. Because of these differences in composition (venous blood compared with capillary blood), the requisition must state that a capillary puncture procedure was performed.

The capillary puncture method is the method of choice in the following situations:
- When only a small amount of blood is needed as in point-of-care, CLIA-waived testing
- When the patient has burns, skin irritation, or small or fragile veins on the arms
- With cancer, geriatric patients, or obese patients, whose blood may be difficult to draw
- With children because the risk of venipuncture removing excessive amounts of blood may cause anemia
- When minimal blood volume reduction is critical for neonate (a newborn child) safety (e.g., a 10-mL sample

of blood is 5% to 10% of the total blood volume in a neonate's body)

The capillary puncture method should *not* be used in the following circumstances:
- If the test requires a large amount of blood, as in a sedimentation rate, coagulation test, or a blood culture (a test to detect bacteria or organisms growing in the blood)
- If the patient has poor peripheral circulation in the hands and feet
- If interstitial fluid from edema (swelling) could dilute the test, causing inaccurate results

Equipment Used in Capillary Puncture

Capillary puncture devices. Many types of capillary puncture devices, lancets, are available. The safest and most current are *retractable nonreusable lancets* (Figure 4.5) that are made with locks that prevent reuse. These retractable devices are color coded by their manufacturers according to the depth of

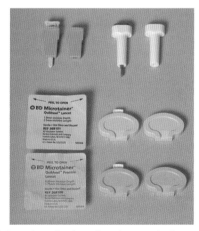

FIG. 4.5 Adult and pediatric safety lancets before and after use.

the puncture. Punctures performed on neonates and infants are implemented with the lancet color coded for infants. The Clinical & Laboratory Standards Institute (**CLSI**) made a change in the standard that applies to the depth of a heel stick for an infant. The depth should not exceed 2 mm to prevent infection caused by puncturing a bone. For adults, the average skin puncture depth should be 2 to 3 mm.

Automatic capillary puncture devices are used in home monitoring tests, but these usually do not result in a puncture sufficiently deep to collect the necessary amount of blood for POCT. Laser devices are also now available. They are used for glucose, hematocrit, and cholesterol screening. The laser concentrates on a small portion of the skin, makes an indentation 1 to 2 mm deep, and draws approximately 100 mcg/L of blood. All capillary puncture devices must be discarded in a biohazard sharps container.

POCT blood collection devices. Blood used in POCT tests is collected using a variety of devices. See Figure 4.6a–f. Figure 4.6a shows a slide that would receive a drop of blood directly from a finger stick. The drop of blood would then be smeared across the slide, stained, and observed under the microscope.

Capillary tubes. *Capillary tubes* are one type of device used to collect blood from a skin puncture site (see the two capillary tubes on the left of the circle in Figure 4.6b). Note: The capillary tubes must be plastic or plastic-covered glass for safety reasons. Blood moves freely into the capillary tubes during **microcollection** (collecting a small amount of blood). The blood is pulled into the tube by a process called **capillary action**. Red-marked capillary tubes contain **heparin**, a natural **anticoagulant**, which keeps the blood from clotting. Mixing these tubes by rolling them back and forth after collection is important. Blue-marked

capillary tubes do not contain anticoagulants, allowing the blood to clot naturally.

Capillary tubes may be sealed so that the specimen is less likely to be lost. Sealants may be clay, as seen in the on-line video, or the specimen may be contained in a self-sealing tube, as seen in Figures 4.7 and 4.8.

The following guidelines should be followed when using capillary tubes:

1. Air bubbles in a capillary tube may cause erroneous results. The best way to prevent bubbles is to start with a large drop of blood and then hold the capillary tube horizontally to the puncture site. Figure 4.7 shows the tube *incorrectly* held downward, which results in bubbles interspersed within the specimen.

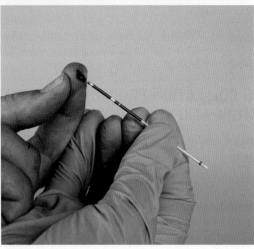

FIG. 4.7 The capillary tube was *improperly* held downward while collecting the sample resulting in air bubbles. (Photo by Zack Bent.)

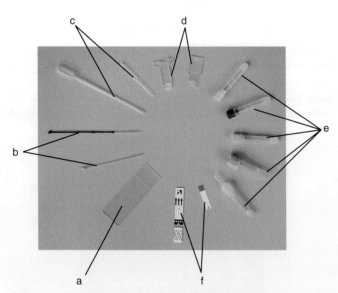

FIG. 4.6 Point-of-care testing (POCT) blood collection equipment. *(a)* glass slide for making blood smears; *(b)* capillary tubes that pull a blood sample inside by capillary action; *(c)* plastic pipettes provided in specific POCT kits; *(d)* cuvettes that fill with blood to be measured in hemoglobinometers; *(e)* microcontainers that receive the blood from a capillary puncture; *(f)* white strips to place in instruments that will record the patient's coagulation time (the large strip) and the patient's glucose (the small strip).

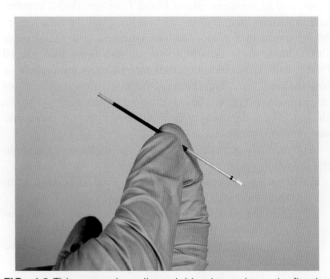

FIG. 4.8 This properly collected blood specimen is flowing down the tube and will connect with the self-sealing clay seen on the right end of the tube. Note: The tube must then be held vertically for 15 seconds so the self-sealing can take place. (Photo by Zack Bent.)

2. The blood specimen in self-sealing tubes must then be held downward, allowing the blood to flow down against the sealant (as seen in Figure 4.8). When it reaches the sealant, it then must be held vertical for 15 seconds, allowing the sealing to take place.

3. Capillary tubes are difficult to label. The recommended procedure is to place the sealed capillary tube into an empty vacuum tube and then label the vacuum tube. *Tip:* If the sealed capillary specimen is to be tested onsite, a sticky note with the patient's identification, technician's initials, and date may be used to hold the specimen against the adhesive portion while transporting the specimen from the collection area to the testing area. Another method is to thread the sealed capillary tube through two slits in a paper with the patient information written on it.

Plastic pipettes. The two pipettes seen in Figure 4.6c are used in two specific blood tests and are supplied by the manufacturer with instructions.

Microcollection tubes. *Microcollection tubes* hold more blood than capillary tubes. Some tubes have a lip that allows the drop of blood to flow into the tube (see the four color-coded microcollection tubes in Figure 4.6e. The lids on these tubes are coded with various colors corresponding to the anticoagulant present (or absent) in the container. Collect the specimen into the Microtainer tube by allowing the blood to run down the collection lip while holding the tube at a 30- to 45-degree angle. Do not scrape the tube across the blood specimen. Another type of collection tube consists of a plastic capillary tube inserted into the microtube receptacle. Blood flows into the container because of the same capillary action that takes place within the capillary tube.

Order of draw for capillary puncture tubes. Because of the different types of anticoagulants in microcollection tubes, the CLSI has recommended a specific order of draw for capillary punctures to prevent the transfer of substances among tubes and to allow for the clotting that takes place while collecting capillary specimens. The order of draw for capillary skin puncture is as follows (also see Table 4.2):

1. *Lavender*—Microtainer tubes used for hematology tests are filled first to avoid any microclots from forming, which distort the blood cells.

2. *Other tubes with anticoagulation additives* (i.e., green, mint green, and gray)—These microcontainers also prevent blood from clotting and produce "whole blood" samples.

3. Nonadditive tubes (*red* or *gold-topped* Microtainer tubes that contain no anticoagulants) are filled last because the capillary blood will clot in these tubes. Blood normally clots in 2 to 6 minutes. Nonadditive tubes are filled last because clotting always occurs in these tubes.

Appropriate Site Selection

The best site for capillary punctures is fleshy and vascular (pink not blue). A vascular site consists of a large capillary area without scars or calluses. Fleshiness helps protect against puncturing the bone. A bone puncture could lead to osteomyelitis, inflammation of the bone caused by bacterial infection. Sites that are swollen or callused should be avoided for skin puncture. Cyanotic sites, where the skin and mucous membrane are blue because of oxygen deficiency, should be warmed before use. A cyanotic site will not produce a good blood sample if it is not warmed or massaged.

In adults and children, the appropriate skin puncture site is the middle or ring finger (Figure 4.9). The little finger should be avoided because it is thinner and less fleshy than the other fingers. The index finger and thumb are also not recommended. The index finger could be more sensitive or callused, making it difficult to obtain blood, and the thumb has a pulse. With the middle or ring finger, the puncture should be made on the lateral part of the fingertip (slightly to the side of the center) and perpendicular to the whorls of the fingerprint. A puncture performed parallel to the fingerprint whorls will cause the blood to travel down the troughs of the fingerprint, preventing the blood from forming a drop.

The appropriate skin puncture site for newborns and infants who are not yet walking is the medial or lateral plantar surface of the heel of the foot (Figure 4.10). The puncture depth should be less than or equal to 2 mm to prevent puncturing the child's bone or connective tissue.

Site Preparation

Blood flow can be increased seven times by warming the site. This can be accomplished by massaging the area five or six times or by applying a warmed towel, an exam glove filled with warm water and tied at the wrist, a preemie diaper, or a commercially available device to the site for 3 to 5 minutes. The temperature of the warmed device should not be higher than 42°C. Microwave heating is not advisable because heating may be uneven.

The site should be cleaned with a 70% aqueous solution of isopropyl alcohol. Allow the cleaned site to dry thoroughly

TABLE 4.2	Order When Collecting More than One Microtainer by Capillary Puncture	
Order	**Microtainer Color**	**Rationale**
First	Lavender	EDTA specimen is drawn first to ensure adequate volume and accurate hematology test results (e.g., CBC). There cannot be a ny microclots in the specimen to interfere with the blood cell counts and blood smears.
Second	Green, gray	These "whole blood" tubes also prevent clotting using various anticoagulants.
Last	Gold, red	The clotted blood in these tubes is used to test the serum. Two gold tubes containing a gel barrier are needed to ensure that sufficient blood is collected to run the blood chemistry tests.

CBC, Complete blood count; *EDTA,* ethylenediaminetetraacetic acid.

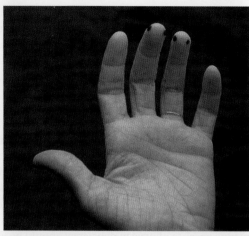

FIG. 4.9 Appropriate capillary puncture sites on the fingers. (From Proctor D, Adams A: *Kinn's the medical assistant: an applied learning approach,* ed 12, St. Louis, 2014, Saunders.)

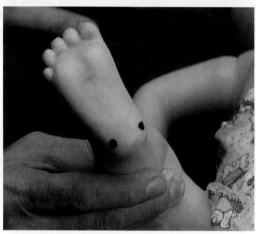

FIG. 4.10 Appropriate capillary puncture sites for infant. (From Proctor D, Adams A: *Kinn's the medical assistant: an applied learning approach,* ed 12, St. Louis, 2014, Saunders.)

because alcohol may cause hemolysis, contaminate glucose determinations, or prevent drops of blood from forming. Always follow the manufacturer's directions regarding how to cleanse the site before puncturing the site. Cleaning the site with povidone-iodine (Betadine) is not recommended because it may cause a false elevation of bilirubin, potassium, phosphorus, or uric acid measurements. After the site has been prepared, the skin puncture procedure can be performed.

Additional Information

When performing a capillary puncture, always remove the first drop of blood because it contains tissue fluid that could dilute the sample. (NOTE: Some tests do not require removal of the first drop; therefore, check the manufacturer's directions.)

If the blood has stopped flowing and insufficient blood was obtained, the entire procedure should be repeated at a new site with a new sterile puncture device. Never stick the same puncture site more than once.

Bandages are not recommended for small children because they can irritate the skin and cause choking if swallowed. If an adhesive bandage must be used to control bleeding, inform the parent that it should be removed as soon as the bleeding has stopped. Adhesive strips should not be used on infants because their skin is very delicate and could macerate when this type of bandage is used or be damaged when the bandage is removed. (See the Evolve capillary puncture video demonstration on-line and refer to Procedure 4.1 at the end of this section.)

Newborn Screening (Formerly PKU)

Neonatal (pertaining to a newborn) screening for two genetically transferred diseases, **PKU** (*phenylketonuria*) and *hypothyroidism,* is federally mandated in the United States for all newborns. These are conditions in which the newborn lacks the enzyme or hormone needed for certain metabolic reactions. If these conditions are not discovered and treated early, abnormalities as severe as mental retardation could develop. Some states require screening for other conditions as well, such as galactosemia, sickle cell anemia, cystic fibrosis, and human immunodeficiency virus (HIV). Each state determines a set core of tests that will be performed on all newborns born in the state and range anywhere from 24 to 65 plus tests. For more information, check out Baby's First Test: Conditions Screened by State at www.babysfirsttest.org/newborn-screening/states. More about these requirements can also be found at www.mchb.hrsa.gov, the website of the Maternal and Child Health Bureau of the Health Resources and Services Administration, and at www.aap.org, the website of the American Academy of Pediatrics.

The newborn screening blood collection must be performed between 24 and 72 hours after birth. If screening is done before the child is 24 hours old, it must be repeated before the child is 14 days old because many newborns have not yet had enough feedings to determine if a metabolic condition is present. The collection of blood for these tests is generally performed in the hospital, but sometimes the test samples are required in the outpatient setting. Be sure to read and follow the instructions for collecting these specimens properly and note the following guidelines.

1. After warming the newborn's heel, a capillary puncture (no deeper than 2 mm) is done on the medial or lateral plantar surface of the heel of the foot.
2. Remove the first drop of blood and then collect the blood in the appropriate microcontainer or on the screening card.
3. Apply a drop of blood to each circle on the screening filter paper form without touching baby's heel to the test circle, making sure to apply the blood to only one side of the paper (Figure 4.11).
4. All circles must be filled and completely saturated while the blood is extracted onto the circle (see Figure 4.11B). You may add a second drop to the same circle immediately if it soaks into the paper without sitting on top. Do not return to a circle that has started to dry.
5. Do not massage the foot of an infant with excessive force because this can cause bruising.
6. Allow the screening forms to dry in a horizontal position for a minimum of 3 hours.

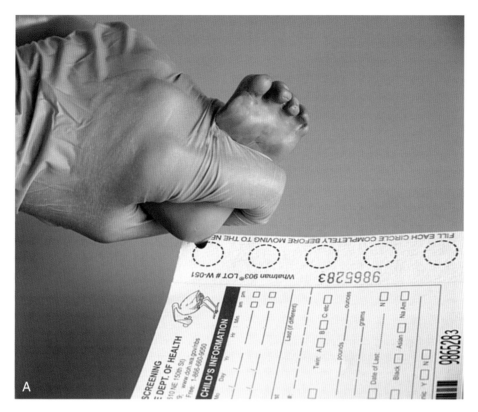

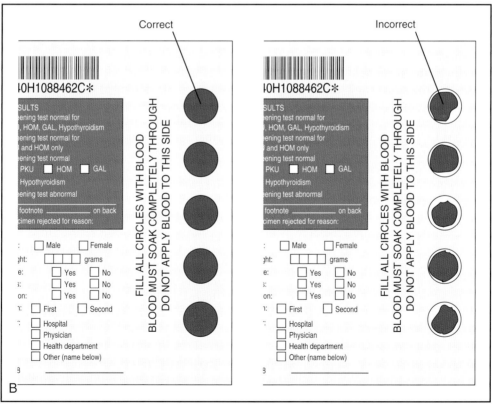

FIG. 4.11 A, Technique for placing a drop of blood from an infant's foot on the neonatal screening filter form. (Photo by Zack Bent.) **B,** Correct and incorrect completed screening forms. (Modified from Warekois R, Robinson R: *Phlebotomy: worktext and procedures manual,* ed 3, St. Louis, 2012, Saunders.)

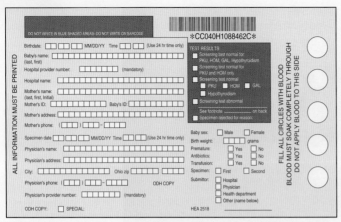

FIG. 4.12 Blank neonatal screening filter paper. (Modified from Warekois R, Robinson R: *Phlebotomy: worktext and procedures manual,* ed 3, St. Louis, 2012, Saunders.)

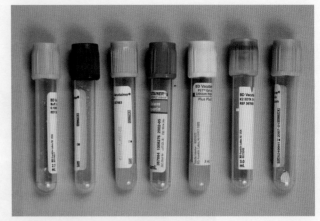

FIG. 4.13 Vacutainer Hemogard tubes in the proper order of draw. (Photo by Zack Bent.)

7. Do not stack wet forms.
8. Mail the forms to the testing center (the state health department) in the provided envelopes within 24 hours of collection. See sample form without blood collection in Figure 4.12.

Becoming Proficient at Capillary Puncture

Now that you have learned about the equipment, appropriate sites, site preparation, and the procedure for capillary punctures and neonatal screenings, you will want to reinforce your knowledge by doing the following:

1. Answer the capillary puncture questions in Chapter 4 of the workbook using your structured notes and text.
2. View Evolve videos online to see demonstrations of the following: Patient Identification, Capillary Collection Equipment, Pediatric Capillary Collection: Finger Stick, and Infant Capillary Collection: Heel Stick.
3. Perform the Evolve online Chapter 4 lessons designed to reinforce your knowledge of terminology and capillary puncture.
4. Review BEHAVIORAL Procedure 4-1 in workbook before your lab.
5. Study Procedure 4.1: Capillary Puncture Procedure at the end of this section before your lab.
6. Also study Procedure 4.2: Heel Stick for Neonatal Screening Test Procedure before your lab.

Venipuncture

Another method of collecting blood samples is venipuncture, which involves extracting blood from a vein. Venipuncture can be accomplished in three ways: by the evacuated tube (or vacuum tube) method, the syringe method, and the butterfly method.

Equipment Used in Venipuncture

Vacuum collection tubes. The collection containers for venipuncture are called *vacuum tubes* (Figure 4.13). These tubes are evacuated (the air has been removed to create a vacuum) so that a preset amount of blood will be collected. They are available in different sizes, ranging from 2 to 15 mL (5, 7, and 15 mL for adults and 2, 3, and 4 mL for children and adults). The tubes are available in glass or plastic, but OSHA recommends that plastic tubes be used for safety reasons. The manufacturer's label on each tube indicates the type of anticoagulant or additive that is present, the expiration date of the tube, and the amount of blood it will hold. Hemogard (Becton Dickinson, Franklin Lakes, NJ) plastic-covered tubes are designed with a special rubber stopper surrounded by a color-coded plastic closure that hangs over the outside of the tube and reduces the risk of blood splattering when the stopper is removed.

The expiration date on the tubes should always be checked and the tubes examined for cracks and other damage before use. If air enters the tube, the tube would be rendered useless because no blood would flow into it as a result of the lack of vacuum pressure.

Each tube has a colored stopper and a label that indicate whether anticoagulants or additives are present and, if so, what type. When blood is extracted from the body and nothing is added to the specimen, the cells automatically clot, yielding a liquid called serum and clotted cells. When anticoagulants are added to the collection tubes to prevent the blood from clotting, a "whole blood" sample is produced in which the cells are suspended in liquid that is referred to as plasma.

Figure 4.14A, shows a blood specimen collected in the left gold-topped tube that allows the blood to clot. The recommended time to allow blood to clot is 30 to 45 minutes, no longer than 1 hour, in an upright position at room temperature. NOTE: Tubes may also contain additives that accelerate clotting, such as silicone-coated interior, silica particles, or thrombin-based clot activators. If the appropriate amount of time is not allowed for clotting, insufficient liquid serum will be obtained. Also, fibrin clots could form in the serum if the clotting factors do not have time to settle into the clot. When the blood has clotted, the tube is then spun in a centrifuge for 15 to 20 minutes. The clot becomes compressed on the bottom of the tube with the serum on top (see Figure 4.14B, left tube). The polymer gel in the tube acts as a barrier between the *serum* and the clot.

Blood collected in an anticoagulant tube, as seen in the right lavender tube in Figure 4.14A, will not clot and can be used for testing when *whole blood* is needed. When whole blood is

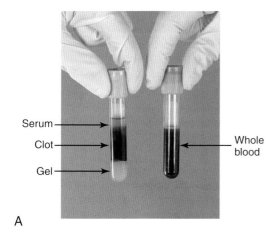

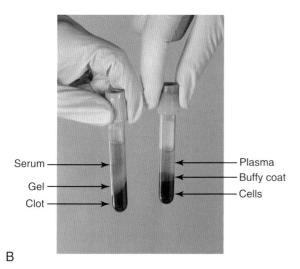

FIG. 4.14 A, Gold tube with clotted blood and lavender tube with whole blood before centrifuging. Note the composition of each. **B,** Clotted and whole blood after centrifuging. Note the layers in each tube.

centrifuged, the red cells pack into the bottom of the tube. The buffy coat is the narrow middle layer of white blood cells (WBCs) and platelets in the centrifuged whole blood specimen, and the liquid layer on top is referred to as *plasma* (see Figure 4.14B, right tube).

Anticoagulation occurs by using a variety of additives, such as oxalates, citrates, EDTA (ethylenediaminetetraacetic acid), and heparin. Oxalates, citrates, and EDTA bind with calcium, which is needed for clotting to occur. Heparin prevents clotting by inactivating thrombin and thromboplastin, the proteins needed in the blood-clotting mechanism.

Both serum and plasma are straw colored and contain essentially the same substances. The main difference between the two is that serum no longer has its clotting factors because they were used to form the fibrin clot.

Another common additive is the polymer gel that forms a barrier between the cells and the liquid (serum or plasma, depending on the tube) to stop further interaction between these layers. The gel has a lower density than that of the red blood cells (RBCs) or the clot and a higher density than that of the liquid part. After the blood

is centrifuged, the clot or RBCs will be on the bottom of the centrifuged tube, the gel in the middle, and the liquid portion on top. When this gel is in a "clot" tube, it is referred to as **SST**, which is "serum separator tube" or an RST "rapid serum tube." When the gel is in a whole blood tube with anticoagulant it is referred to as **PST**, or plasma separator tube. In both cases, the tubes must be centrifuged within 2 hours of the blood draw to prevent the living blood cells from metabolizing the chemicals in the serum or plasma.

Additives and color-coded vacuum tubes. The different types of anticoagulants and additives within the vacuum tubes are differentiated by the following color-coded plastic and rubber stoppers seen in Table 4.3 and described next:

1. Pale yellow—"Sterile" tubes contain preservatives or nutrients are used for growing bacteria from within the blood (e.g., blood cultures)
2. Light blue—"Coagulation" tubes contain liquid sodium citrate anticoagulant used for coagulation testing (e.g., prothrombin time). These tubes must be filled completely to maintain the ratio of one part liquid sodium citrate to nine parts of blood.
3. Red—"Clot" tubes contain no anticoagulants, which means the blood will automatically clot. (NOTE: *Red plastic* tubes contain a clot activator to accelerate the clotting process.)
4. Gold and tiger-topped (marbled red and gray)—"SST" *(serum separating tubes)* contain a silicone coating to accelerate clotting and a gel barrier to separate the serum from the cells (SST tube). They contain no anticoagulant. The serum is typically used for blood chemistry tests.
5. Green—"Heparin" tubes contain a heparin anticoagulant: sodium heparin, lithium heparin, or ammonium heparin; they are used for chemistry specimens, especially when a test is stat (needed immediately) because waiting for the blood to clot is not necessary as it is with serum tubes. It is important to note the type of anticoagulant substance that is in a heparin tube (e.g., a sodium heparin tube would not be used if sodium testing, and a lithium heparin tube would not be used for a lithium test because the sodium and lithium would falsely increase the patient's test results). Lithium heparin tubes are often used with the separating gel and are referred to as *PST (plasma separating tubes).* The *PST tubes* are distinguished from the non-gel heparin tubes by a lighter shade of green.
6. Lavender—EDTA tubes contain an anticoagulant and preservative for blood cells; they are used for hematology studies and molecular diagnostic testing. EDTA prevents platelet aggregation and allows preparation of blood smears with minimal distortion of WBCs.
7. Gray—"Glucose" tubes contain potassium oxalate, which removes calcium to prevent clotting, and sodium fluoride, which is used for glucose studies because the fluoride inhibits glycolysis (sugar breakdown).

Figure 4.15 shows additional tubes that might be ordered for the following special tests:
- Yellow topped with acid citrate dextrose (ACD) is used in blood banks, paternity testing, and genetic testing.
- Black is used for erythrocyte sedimentation rate (ESR).
- White Hemogard over blue is a non–liquid citrate–coated tube used for coagulation studies.

TABLE 4.3   List of Common Hemogard and Rubber Tube Stoppers

BD Hemogard Plastic Colors	Rubber Stopper Colors	Additive	Number of Inversions to Mix During Blood Draw and "Tube Descriptor"	Laboratory Use
Yellow, sterile	Yellow, sterile	Sodium polyanetholesulfonate (SPS)	8: "sterile tube"	Blood cultures
Light blue	Light blue	Sodium citrate	3–4: "citrate tube"	Coagulation studies
Red	Red	None or clot activator to produce clot and serum	0: "clot tube"	Chemistry, serology, blood bank
Gold	Marbled red and gray*	Thixotropic gel to separate serum from clot and clot activators	5: "SST tube"	Most chemistry; not suitable for blood bank testing
Light green	Marbled green and gray*	Thixotropic gel to separate plasma and cells and lithium Heparin	8: "PST tube"	Potassium determinations
Dark green	Dark green	Sodium heparin, lithium heparin, or ammonium heparin	8: "heparin tube"	Stat plasma chemistries, electrolytes
Lavender	Lavender	EDTA	8: "EDTA tube"	Whole blood hematology cell count, CBC
Gray	Gray	Sodium fluoride and potassium oxalate	8: "oxalate tube"	Glucose testing (usually), glucose tolerances

*Note the mixing requirements.
CBC, Complete blood count; EDTA, ethylenediaminetetraacetic acid; PST, plasma separator tube; SST, serum separator tube.
BD Hemogard plastic covers and rubber stopper colors from BD Diagnostics, Preanalytical Systems, 1 Becton Drive, Franklin Lakes, NJ, 07417, USA. www.bd.com/vacutainer. BD, BD Logo and all other trademarks are property of Becton, Dickinson, and Company. © 2014.

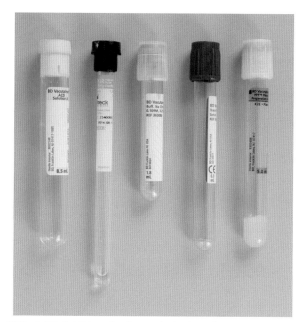

FIG. 4.15 Additional color-coded tubes for special tests.

- Royal blue is used for toxicology and detection of trace minerals in the blood (e.g., lead).
- White Hemogard over lavender is a PST tube for testing molecular diagnostics and viral load detection such as human immunodeficiency virus (HIV) and hepatitis C virus (HCV) levels.

Vacuum Tube Method Using the Vacutainer Collection System

The most commonly performed venipuncture method involves the use of vacuum tubes, which automatically fill with blood during the procedure. This method requires Vacutainer tubes, Vacutainer holders, and Safety Vacutainer needles, as seen in Figure 4.16.

Equipment used in the vacutainer method

Vacutainer needle. The *Vacutainer needle* is pointed at both ends (see Figures 4.16 and 4.17). When it is screwed into the plastic holder, the shorter end (with the rubber sleeve) punctures the vacuum tube, and the longer end, which has a beveled tip, is inserted into the vein. For a smoother and less painful puncture, the bevel end should always be turned upward. Safety needles are now required by law.

Most types of safety needles are activated by a one-hand thumb mechanism as seen in Figure 4.18.

The Vacutainer needle ranges in length from 1 to 1.5 inches. The space inside the needle is referred to as the lumen or *bore*. The diameter of the needle is called the *gauge*. The higher the gauge number, the smaller the diameter. The most frequently used gauges are 20 to 22. A high-gauge needle (e.g., 25) could cause hemolysis of the cells because the lumen is too small.

Butterfly Vacutainer needles have also become popular. See Figure 4.18C.

Vacutainer holder. The *Vacutainer holders,* seen in Figure 4.16, allow the Vacutainer needles on the right to connect to the vacuum tubes on the left. The Vacutainer double needles screw into one end of the holder. Then the needle is inserted into a patient's vein, and the vacuum tube is pushed all the way into the holder. The blood then starts to flow into the vacuum tubes seen on the left of Figure 4.16. The needle must be in the vein before pushing the vacuum tube all the way into the holder. NOTE: An indentation is present approximately ½ inch down from where the needle attaches to the holder. Pushing the vacuum tube into this ½-inch space *before* the needle is in the vein will result in the tube being filled with air.

Two types of Vacutainer holders are now available: one that will hold the Vacutainer multi-sample needle as described earlier and a new Vacutainer holder with the sleeved needle already attached inside as seen on the right in Figure 4.19. This new holder allows a butterfly needle or a sterile hypodermic needle, with the proper size lumen, to attach directly to the new holder containing the sleeved needle.

The plastic extension, or flange, is located at the large-opening end of all the holders (see Figure 4.16). The design of the flange prevents the holder from rolling and provides a ledge on which to position the fingers as the tube is inserted and removed.

OSHA recommends that Vacutainer needles not be removed from the holder after use but instead be disposed with the holder attached because the rubber-stoppered needle can expose health care workers to needle sticks.

Tourniquet. A tourniquet is a band placed above the venipuncture site to make the vein more prominent and easier to puncture. The average tourniquet is approximately 1 inch wide and 15 to 18 inches long and should be placed 3 to 4 inches above the venipuncture site. A tourniquet that is too tight is

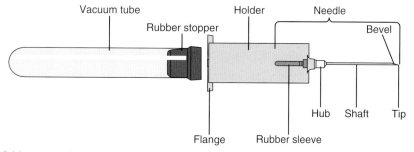

FIG. 4.16 Vacuum tube system. (From Hunt SA: *Saunders fundamentals of medical assisting,* Philadelphia, 2002, Saunders.)

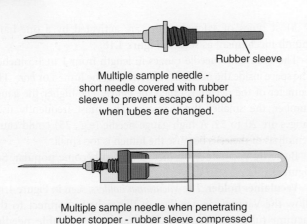

Multiple sample needle -
short needle covered with rubber
sleeve to prevent escape of blood
when tubes are changed.

Multiple sample needle when penetrating
rubber stopper - rubber sleeve compressed
between hub and stopper.

FIG. 4.17 Vacutainer multisample needles with rubber sleeves that allow blood to flow only when the sleeved needle is pushed into the vacuum tube. (From Hunt SA: *Saunders fundamentals of medical assisting*, Philadelphia, 2002, Saunders.)

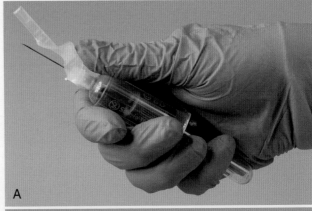

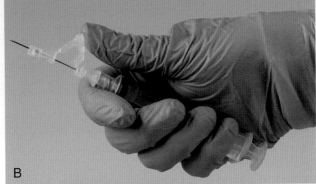

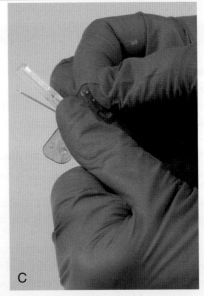

FIG. 4.18 A, One-hand thumb safety activation. **B,** One-hand spring device. **C,** Butterfly safety activation.

uncomfortable for the patient and can give inaccurate results. It should be tight enough to restrict venous flow but not so tight that it stops arterial flow. It should be looped so that it can be easily released with one hand. Do not place a tourniquet over sores or burned areas on the skin.

The recommended time to leave a tourniquet in place is 1 minute. If it is left on too long, results may be inaccurate because of hemoconcentration, a condition in which the blood concentration of large molecules (e.g., proteins, cells, and coagulation factors) increases. The recommended tourniquet procedure is to remove the tourniquet after a vein has been chosen, clean the site, prepare the equipment, and then reapply the tourniquet before making the incision. Tourniquets should be cleaned after use or discarded if they are disposable. See Procedure 4.3 steps A, B, and C for the proper application of the tourniquet.

Site preparation. Have the patient place his or her arm in a downward position to prevent reflux (backward flow of blood). For patients who do not want to feel the needle stick (e.g., children), a eutectic mixture of local anesthetics (EMLA) can be used to anesthetize the puncture area. EMLA is a topical cream that is a mixture of lidocaine and prilocaine. It is applied as a cream or patch and requires approximately 60 minutes for optimal anesthesia to occur. It may last as long as 2 or 3 hours. Some of the limitations to its use are the cost of the product, the need to wait 60 minutes, and the need to repeat the anesthetizing procedure if the venipuncture is not successful. Another topical anesthesia, IOMED "Numby Stuff" (IOMED, Inc., Salt Lake City, Utah), contains lidocaine hydrochloride 2% with epinephrine. It penetrates to a depth of 10 mm and takes 10 minutes to take effect.

See Procedure 4.3: Vacutainer Method at the end of this section for the pictorial sequence and step-by-step instructions on how to perform a successful venipuncture using the Vacutainer method.

Syringe Method

The syringe method is used on fragile veins that might collapse under the pressure of the Vacutainer method. The procedure is the same as the Vacutainer procedure, except that when the syringe needle is in the arm, the phlebotomist pulls *back* on the syringe plunger, creating back-pressure and drawing blood into the syringe. The syringe method allows control over the pressure exerted on the vein. This control helps keep the vein from collapsing, which makes the syringe method particularly useful for small, fragile veins.

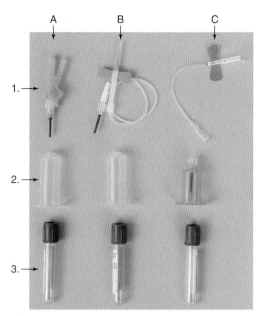

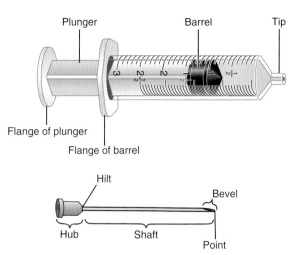

FIG. 4.20 Parts of a syringe and a hypodermic needle. (From Hunt SA: *Saunders fundamentals of medical assisting,* Philadelphia, 2002, Saunders.)

FIG. 4.19 Vacuum tube collection options:
Row 1. Needles: A, standard venipuncture needle; **B,** butterfly needle with sheathed needle attached, **C,** butterfly needle with luer-lok adapter to attach to a vacuum tube holder with a built-in sheathed needle (or to a syringe).
Row 2. Holders: A & B, standard vacuum tube holders **C,** vacuum tube holder with a built-in sheathed needle (used with IV butterfly needles that do not have a sheathed needle for venipuncture).
Row 3. Vacuum tubes.

Equipment used in the syringe method

Syringe. The *syringe* consists of a barrel and a plunger (Figure 4.20). The barrel is graduated into milliliters in sizes ranging from 2 to 20 mL and larger. The plunger should always be loosened by moving it back and forth several times before use and then pushed in before connecting the needle

(Figure 4.21). When the plunger is pulled back after the attached needle is in the vein, a backpressure is produced, and blood fills the syringe.

Syringe needle. A *syringe needle* is also called a *hypodermic needle.* Similar to a Vacutainer needle, it has a shaft and a hub, but the hub attaches directly to the syringe with no opposing sheathed needle. Blood can be seen entering the tip of the syringe as soon as the needle enters the vein. Syringe needles must have a safety section that allows the needle to be covered or blunted when the procedure is completed. The most commonly used needle gauge is 20 to 22, with a length of 1 to 1.5 inches. See Procedure 4.4: Syringe Method at the end of this section for a pictorial and written description of how to properly draw blood using a syringe. Blood drawn into a syringe must then be transferred to the appropriate evacuated tubes in the correct order using a safety transfer device.

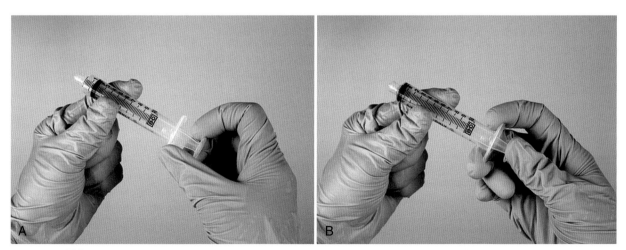

FIG. 4.21 A, The plunger should always be loosened by pulling it back *(a)* and pushing it in *(b)* several times before use. **B,** Make sure it is pushed in completely before connecting the needle and drawing blood from the patient. (Photos by Zack Bent.)

Butterfly Needle Method

The *butterfly needle method* of drawing blood has become popular. The phlebotomy equipment for this method consists of a uniquely designed needle with plastic wings used to grip the needle as it is inserted into the vein. When the needle enters the vein, the hub of the needle shows a "flash" of blood. The tubing then transports the blood to either a syringe or a Vacutainer collection system. Figure 4.22 shows three designs of butterfly needles, tubing, and their connecting devices that may be attached to the Vacutainer holder and vacuum tube or to a syringe.

Phlebotomists have found the butterfly needle system to be useful in drawing blood from very small veins, such as those in the hand of geriatric patients, and for pediatric draws. Hand veins tend to be very visible in all patients, so it is common to draw from a hand when having difficulty finding veins in the arm. However, veins in hands are also prone to collapse, roll, and bruise more easily because they have thin walls. More nerves are also present in this area, which makes a hand puncture more uncomfortable for the patient.

Butterfly needles may also be used in the antecubital space of the arm provided the lumen of the needle is the appropriate size (i.e., 21 gauge). When the needle is inserted into the vein, a "flash" can be seen, which gives the phlebotomist an assurance that the needle is "in" the vein.

When the Vacutainer method of collection is used, the small adapter device (Luer adapter) with the rubber-sheathed needle (located at the end of the butterfly tubing) is attached to a

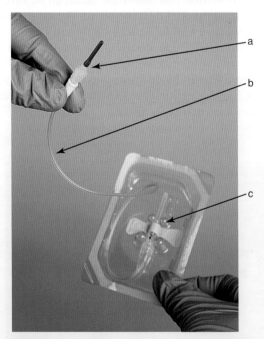

FIG. 4.22 The push-button butterfly needle consists of the sheathed needle *(a)* that will be attached to the Vacutainer holder and will penetrate the vacuum tube allowing the tubing *(b)* to transport the blood from the butterfly needle *(c)* after it enters the vein. Also note the black button just below the "wings." When pushed, the needle instantly retracts into the body of the butterfly. (Photo by Zack Bent.)

Vacutainer holder. When the syringe method of collection is used, the Luer adapter is removed, and the white end of the butterfly tubing fits directly onto the tip of the syringe. The syringe or butterfly method allows more control of the pressure, which is necessary when working with fragile veins.

In all three butterfly methods, a crucial safety issue arises when the needle is pulled out of the vein. Three recommended safety methods are described in Procedure 4.5. Laboratory professionals should stay informed of the most current safety devices and how they are safely activated. It is also wise to practice on a training model before using any new safety device on a patient. (The student workbook contains a form to evaluate and choose between various safety devices.)

See Procedure 4.5 to learn the steps for performing the butterfly method using both the Vacutainer method and the syringe method. Also, the safety activation techniques for three commonly used butterfly safety devices are presented.

Figure 4.23 displays all the supplies used in the three venipuncture procedures: Vacutainer, syringe, and butterfly methods. The vacuum tubes have also been placed in their correct order of draw from left to right.

Order of Draw for All Venipuncture Methods and Other Quality Assurance Considerations

When performing each of the aforementioned venipuncture methods, keep in mind that there is a recommended order of draw regarding which colored tube needs to be drawn up first, second, and so on. Based on the requisition order, the properly colored tubes will need to be set in their proper order of draw. The CLSI has recommended a specific order of draw for venipuncture. NOTE: The venipuncture order of the vacuum tubes is very different from the capillary order of Microtainers. This is because the sheathed needle that enters each Vacutainer tube is exposed to the additives in one tube that might affect the test result in a subsequent tube. Tests adversely affected by *additive contamination* from one tube to another are listed in Table 4.4.

The following pictures of the seven most common color-coded tubes in Figure 4.24 reflect the national recommendations on the order of drawing multiple tubes ("Order of Draw," CLSI). The following list of these colored tubes and their corresponding descriptions provides important quality assurance information:

1. The *yellow* "blood culture tube" is drawn first. The *SPS tubes* are used for blood culture specimen collection in microbiology, which are always drawn first to maintain sterility. NOTE: Chapter 8: Microbiology also discusses the drawing of both anaerobic and aerobic cultures. It is important to note that the anaerobic tube must always be drawn first, except when using the butterfly method. The aerobic tube is drawn first with butterfly needles because the air from the butterfly tubing should not enter the anaerobic bottle.

2. The *light blue* "coagulation tube" (sodium citrate) is drawn next because anticoagulants and additives from the other tubes will interfere with coagulation testing. This tube must be completely filled to achieve accurate clotting results. In the past, when a coagulation study (light blue tube) was ordered, a plain red glass tube with no additives was drawn first to absorb the tissue thromboplastin released from the traumatized

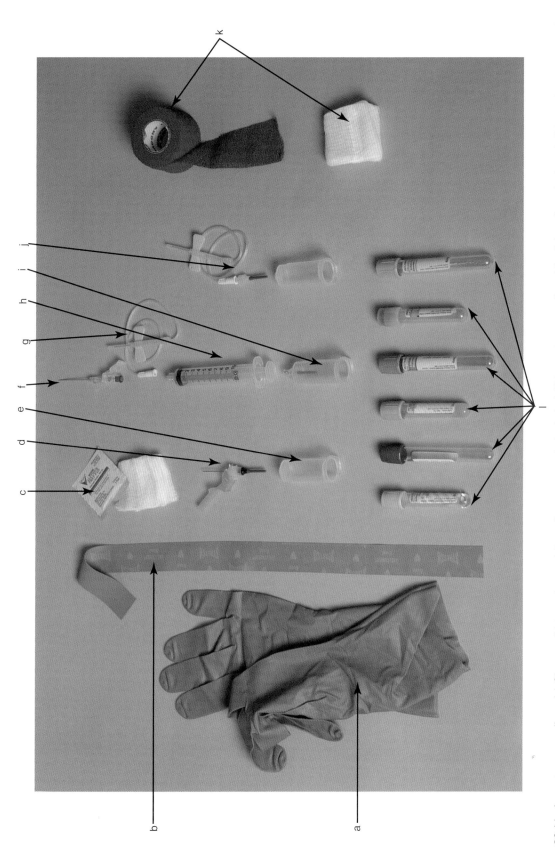

FIG. 4.23 Venipuncture supplies. *(a)* Gloves; *(b)* tourniquet; *(c)* sterile gauze and alcohol; *(d)* Vacutainer needle with pink safety device; *(e)* Vacutainer holder; *(f)* syringe needle with spring safety device; *(g)* butterfly needle assembled to connect directly to the tip of the syringe; *(h)* syringe; *(i)* safety transfer device for transferring blood from the syringe to the vacuum tube; *(j)* butterfly needle assembled to connect directly to the Vacutainer holder; *(k)* nonlatex (COFLEX) pressure bandage and gauze to control bleeding; *(l)* the six most commonly used Hemogard Vacutainer tubes in the recommended order of draw.

TABLE 4.4 **Tests Adversely Affected by Anticoagulant Additive Contamination from a Previously Drawn Tube**

	Additive	Tests Adversely Affected
Lavender stopper	EDTA	Chemistry: calcium, iron, sodium, potassium, Coagulation: APTT, PT
Green stopper	Heparin	Coagulation: PT, APTT, ACT
Gray stopper	Potassium oxalate	Chemistry: potassium, Coagulation: APTT, ACT

ACT, Activated clotting time; *APTT,* activated partial thromboplastin time; *EDTA,* ethylenediaminetetraacetic acid; *PT,* prothrombin time.

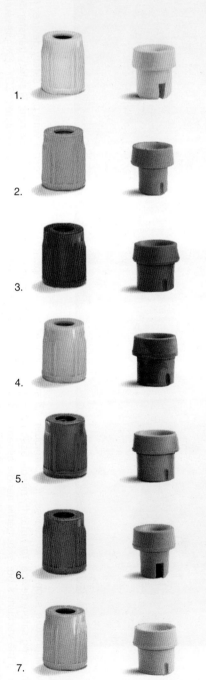

FIG. 4.24 The order of draw, according to Standard H3-A6. *(1)* Yellow, sterile; *(2)* light blue; *(3)* red; *(4)* gold Hemogard closure or red-gray rubber stopper; *(5)* green; *(6)* lavender; *(7)* gray. (From Warekois R, Robinson R: *Phlebotomy: worktext and procedures manual,* ed 3, St. Louis, 2012, Saunders.)

tissue that could interfere with coagulation testing. The red tube was referred to as the "waste tube" because its only purpose was to collect the tissue thromboplastin caused by the venipuncture. However, the new recommendations no longer require this. The new standard does, however, recommend that a plain red waste tube be drawn before a light blue tube when the butterfly method is being used. The tubing in the butterfly system has dead space in the line that reduces the volume of blood drawn, thereby resulting in an underfilled tube. An alternative, if a plain red tube is not available, is to use two blue tubes, with the first tube considered a waste tube whose only function is to clear the butterfly tubing of air. Neither the red nor the blue waste tubes need to be filled completely because they will not be sent to the laboratory. Their only purpose is to pull the blood through the tubing before connecting the blue tube that will then be filled accurately (with no air from the tubing) and sent to the laboratory.

3. The *red* "clot tube," with or without clot activators, yields a serum or clot specimen. A glass red top tube has nothing in it, but a plastic red top tube often contains a clot activator because blood does not clot well in plastic tubes.

4. The *gold* "SST tube" contains gel and clot activators and is also considered a "clot tube" that is able to separate the serum from the clotted cells. Some laboratories may also order a "tiger" rubber-topped tube that appears marbled with red and gray. This SST tube also contains gel and is similar to the Hemogard gold tube. In all three cases (red, gold, and tiger-topped tubes), it is important to follow the laboratory's designated serum tube choice based on the tests they will be running.

5. The *green* "heparin tube" (dark green plain and light green gel PST) must be drawn *before* the EDTA tubes because the EDTA interferes with some heparin tube chemistry tests, such as electrolyte testing. EDTA is usually bound to potassium or sodium. If an EDTA tube is drawn before a heparin tube for electrolyte testing, some of the EDTA potassium and sodium would be mixed in with the green tube's specimen and cause inaccurate electrolyte results (see Table 4.4).

6. The *lavender* "hematology tube" (EDTA) is drawn next and is most commonly used for hematology testing.

7. The *gray* "glucose tube" (potassium oxalate/sodium fluoride) is drawn last, after the EDTA tube, because the anticoagulant, potassium oxalate, also affects potassium results and RBC morphology. It is commonly used for glucose testing.

Table 4.5 Provides a helpful way to remember the order of drawing the seven most common plastic topped tubes. Visualize

TABLE 4.5　Order of Draw and Data for Seven Common Tubes

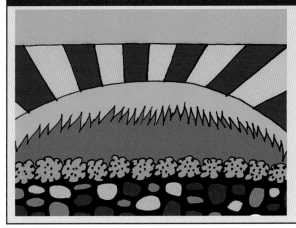

	a. Blue sky is usually the first plastic tube to draw for coagulation studies. (Do not forget the waste tube if using a butterfly needle and tubing.)
	b. The *red* and *gold* rays of the sun are on the horizon. Both of these "clot" tubes (along with the tiger topped tubes) must be drawn *after* the blue but *before* the remaining anticoagulant tubes.
	c. The *green* grassy hill is below the red and gold rays of the sunset. *Light green* is the PST heparin tube, and dark green is typically the lithium heparin tube.
	d. *Lavender* flowers are at the base of the hill below the green grass near the bottom of the picture.
	e. *Gray* rocks are at the bottom of the picture because the gray "glucose" tube is the last tube to draw.

PST, Plasma separator tube.
BD Hemogard plastic covers and rubber stopper colors from BD Diagnostics, Preanalytical Systems, 1 Becton Drive, Franklin Lakes, NJ, 07417, USA. www.bd.com/vacutainer. BD, BD Logo and all other trademarks are property of Becton, Dickinson, and Company. © 2014.

the picture in Table 4.5 with its descriptors on the right. The order of draw starts at the top of the picture with blue sky (citrate tube color). The colors then flow down in their proper order to the grey rocks (glucose tube), which is the last tube to draw.

Becoming Proficient at Venipuncture

Now that you have learned about the equipment, appropriate sites, site preparation, four methods of obtaining venous blood (Vacutainer, syringe, and two butterfly methods), and proper order of draw, you should reinforce your knowledge by doing the following:

1. Answer the venipuncture questions at the end of this chapter and in Chapter 4 of the workbook using your structured notes and text.

2. Perform the Chapter 4 Review Questions online to reinforce your terminology and venipuncture theory skills, and order of draw.

3. View the Evolve animated interactive venipuncture lesson and videos online to see Types and Applications of Tourniquets, Evacuated Collection Tubes, Locating a Vein, Routine Venipuncture: Evacuated Tube Method and Syringe Method, and Hand Collection Using a Winged Infusion Set (Butterfly).

4. Study the pictures and text in the following procedures before your lab:
   a. Procedure 4.3: Vacutainer Method.
   b. Procedure 4.4: Syringe Method.
   c. Procedure 4.5: Three Butterfly Needle Methods.

5. Review BEHAVIORAL Procedure 4-1 in your workbook before your lab.

PROCEDURE 4.1　Capillary Puncture Procedure

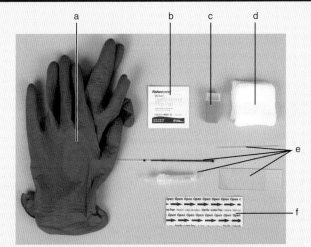

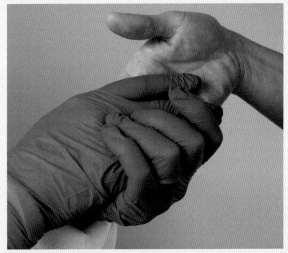

A, Capillary puncture setup (from *left* to *right* and *top* to *bottom*). *(a)* Nitrile gloves; *(b)* 70% isopropyl alcohol pads in sterile packages; *(c)* sterile, disposable, retractable, nonreusable lancet; *(d)* sterile gauze; *(e)* blood collecting devices: two capillary tubes, a microcontainer, and glass slide; *(f)* latex-free bandage, (and not pictured) a heel warmer if appropriate.

B, Warm the puncture site. NOTE: A nitrile glove half-filled with warm water and tied at the wrist also works well to warm the site.

Continued

PROCEDURE 4.1 Capillary Puncture Procedure—cont'd

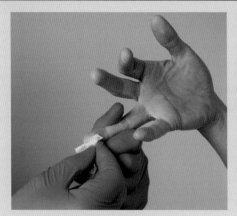

C, Disinfect with alcohol.

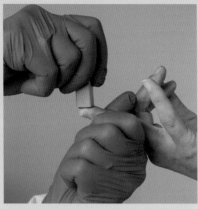

D, Perform the puncture with an incision-type safety lancet and then wipe away the first drop with gauze. Gently massage the finger to produce a large drop of blood.

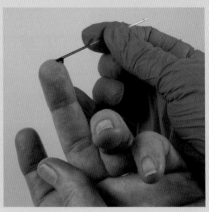

E, Collect the specimen in a capillary tube for testing.

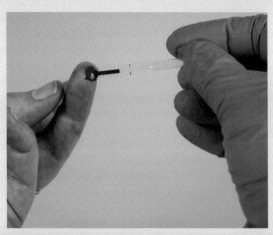

F, Alternatively, collect the specimen in a plastic pipette from a CLIA-waived test kit.

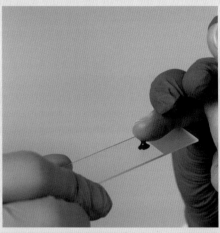

G, Alternatively, place 1 drop of blood on a slide for a blood smear.

Equipment and Supplies (Figure A)

- Nitrile gloves (NOTE: Latex gloves are no longer used due to possible allergic reactions)
- 70% isopropyl alcohol pads in sterile packages
- Sterile, disposable, retractable, nonreusable lancets (varying lengths for the appropriate depth)
- Sterile gauze
- Blood collection devices (based on test to be performed)
- Latex-free bandage (if age appropriate)

Additional supplies for collecting and processing specimens (not pictured): biohazard puncture-resistant sharps container, warming devices (optional), and a marking pen.

Preparation—Preanalytical

1. Wash the hands if they are visibly soiled. If not, use an alcohol-based rub for routine decontamination. Apply the hand rub to the palm of one hand and rub the hands together, covering all surfaces until dry.
2. Correctly identify the patient by using the three-way match. The patient should be sitting or lying.
3. Choose the appropriate site for a fingerstick according to the guidelines.

4. Put on gloves, first determining if the patient is allergic to latex. Nonlatex gloves should be worn if the patient is latex sensitive.
5. Warm the site, if needed, by massaging the area or applying a warming device to the site for 3 to 5 minutes (Figure B).
6. Clean the site with 70% isopropyl alcohol (Figure C). Allow the alcohol to dry and do not fan or blow on the cleansed site.

Blood Collection Procedure—Analytical

7. Determine the appropriate lancet device according to the age of the patient and the amount of blood needed.
8. Tell the patient, "You will feel a stick." Firmly hold the finger below the cleansed site and puncture the site in the appropriate place. When making the puncture, be sure to press hard to get a good blood flow so that the patient does not have to be stuck again (Figure D). Immediately after the puncture, discard the lancet into a biohazard sharps container placed nearby.
9. Wipe away the first drop of blood, which contains tissue fluid that could dilute the sample.
10. Gently massage the finger from the base of the finger to just below the puncture site to get a uniform drop of blood. Apply intermittent pressure and release below the site. You should be able to obtain an adequate drop to fill

---

PROCEDURE 4.1   Capillary Puncture Procedure—cont'd

at least a capillary tube (Figure E). NOTE: Do not squeeze excessively at the tip of the finger. Squeezing with too much force near the site could cause the blood sample to be contaminated with tissue fluid.

11. Collect the sample in the appropriate container based on the test ordered:
    a. Capillary tube for a hematocrit test (Figure E). NOTE: If a capillary tube is being filled, hold it horizontally to prevent air bubbles from getting into the tube
    b. A plastic pipette from a CLIA-waived test kit (Figure F)
    c. Slide for a blood smear (Figure G)
12. When collecting blood in a microcollection tube, do not scrape or scoop the container against the site because it could cause tissue fluid to contaminate the sample. Collect only free-flowing drops of blood. The microcollection tube should be collected in the color-coded order of draw for capillary puncture. Tubes with additives should be gently tapped or mixed during the collection procedure to prevent microclots from forming. Cap or seal the container when full. Invert the microtube 8 to 10 times to mix the specimen with any anticoagulants that may be present. Always follow the manufacturer's instructions.
13. Place gauze on the puncture site and ask the patient to apply pressure to it.

Follow-Up—Postanalytical

14. Recheck the puncture site. If the patient has stopped bleeding, apply an adhesive bandage to the puncture site as necessary. Make sure the patient is not allergic to the bandage material. If bleeding does not subside after 5 minutes, contact the physician.

15. Label the specimen(s) with the patient's name and identification number, the date and time the specimen was drawn, and your name (initials are sufficient in some facilities). When using capillary tubes, the recommended procedure is to place the filled tubes into unfilled vacuum tubes and label the vacuum tubes.
16. When the procedure is completed, discard blood-contaminated items in appropriate biohazard containers.
17. Remove gloves and discard in biohazard container. Sanitize hands.
18. Document the procedure on the specimen log sheet and in the patient's record, making sure to include the following six items:
    When: date and time of collection
    Where: location on the body where the blood was collected (e.g., right antecubital space, hand, finger) and where the specimen is being sent (e.g., reference lab, hospital, in office)
    What: types of tubes collected (e.g., gold and lavender)
    Why: what tests were ordered (e.g., blood chemistry profile, complete blood cell count)
    How: did the patient respond to the procedure (tolerated well? experienced pain? fasting state? difficult draw?)
    Who: person who collected the specimen (your name, credentials)
    Patient's name
    Date, time: Performed fingerstick and collected a lavender-topped microtainer of blood for hemoglobin testing in our lab. There were no complications.
    _____*First initial, last name, credentials*

PROCEDURE 4.2   Heel Stick for Neonatal Screening Test Procedure

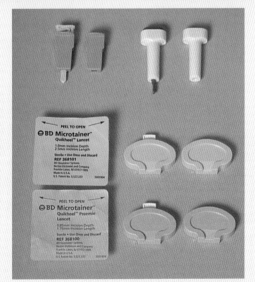

A, Neonatal safety lancets are the lower green and pink lancets designed to puncture the heel at a depth equal to or less than 2 mm.

Continued

PROCEDURE 4.2 Heel Stick for Neonatal Screening Test Procedure—cont'd

DO NOT WRITE IN BLUE SHADED AREAS–DO NOT WRITE ON BARCODE

ALL INFORMATION MUST BE PRINTED

CC040H1088462C

Birthdate: ☐☐ ☐☐ ☐☐ MM/DD/YY   Time ☐☐ ☐☐ (Use 24 hr time only)

Baby/s name: ☐☐☐☐☐☐☐☐☐☐☐☐☐☐☐☐☐☐☐☐☐☐
(last, first)

Hospital provider number: ☐☐☐☐☐☐ (mandatory)

Hospital name: ☐☐☐☐☐☐☐☐☐☐☐☐☐☐☐☐☐☐☐☐☐☐☐

Mother's name: ☐☐☐☐☐☐☐☐☐☐☐☐☐☐☐☐☐☐☐☐☐☐☐
(last, first, Initial)

Mother's ID: ☐☐☐☐☐☐☐☐☐   Baby's ID: ☐☐☐☐☐☐☐☐☐

Mother's address: ☐☐☐☐☐☐☐☐☐☐☐☐☐☐☐☐☐☐☐☐

Mother's phone: (☐☐☐) ☐☐☐–☐☐☐☐

Specimen date ☐☐ ☐☐ ☐☐ MM/DD/YY   Time ☐☐ ☐☐ (Use 24 hr time only)

Physician's name: ☐☐☐☐☐☐☐☐☐☐☐☐☐☐☐☐☐☐☐☐☐

Physician's address: ☐☐☐☐☐☐☐☐☐☐☐☐☐☐☐☐☐☐☐☐☐

City: ☐☐☐☐☐☐☐☐☐☐☐☐ Ohio zip ☐☐☐☐☐ ☐☐☐☐

Physician's phone: (☐☐☐) ☐☐☐–☐☐☐☐   ODH COPY

Physician's provider number: ☐☐☐☐☐☐☐ (mandatory)

ODH COPY: ☐ SPECIAL:

TEST RESULTS

☐ Screening test normal for
  PKU, HOM, GAL, Hypothyroidism

☐ Screening test normal for
  PKU and HOM only

☐ Screening test normal
  ☐ PKU ☐ HOM ☐ GAL
  ☐ Hypothyroidism

☐ Screening test abnormal
  _____
  See footnote _____ on back

☐ Specimen rejected for reason:

Baby sex: ☐ Male   ☐ Female

Birth weight: ☐☐☐☐ grams

Premature: ☐ Yes ☐ No

Antibiotics: ☐ Yes ☐ No

Transfusion: ☐ Yes ☐ No

Specimen: ☐ First   ☐ Second

Submittor: ☐ Hospital
         ☐ Physician
         ☐ Health department
         ☐ Other (name below)

HEA 2518 _____

FILL ALL CIRCLES WITH BLOOD
BLOOD MUST SOAK COMPLETELY THROUGH
DO NOT APPLY BLOOD TO THIS SIDE

B, Neonatal screening filter paper with five circles to saturate with the neonate's blood.

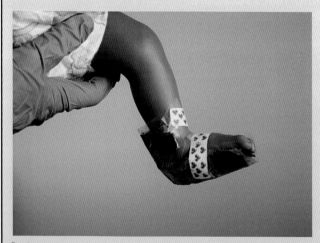

C, A commercial warming device designed for infant heels. After 3 to 5 minutes, the blood flow will increase 7 times. NOTE: A disposable glove half-filled with warm water and tied off at the wrist also works well to warm the heel.

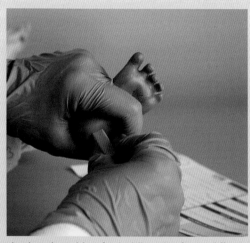

D, Note the hand position for holding the foot while the other hand performs the heel puncture on the lateral plantar portion of the heel.

PROCEDURE 4.2 Heel Stick for Neonatal Screening Test Procedure—cont'd

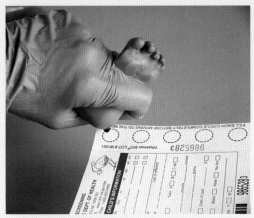

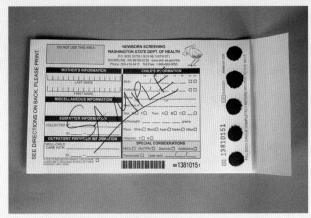

E, Apply gentle pressure with the thumb and forefinger and ease intermittently as drops of blood form.

F, Example of a thoroughly dried card with all five circles saturated.

Equipment and Supplies (see Figure A)
- Gloves (preferably nonlatex for latex-sensitive patients)
- Sterile gauze
- Warming device
- 70% isopropyl alcohol pads in sterile packages
- Sterile, disposable, retractable, nonreusable neonatal lancets with no more than 2 mm depth (Figure A)
- Neonatal screening filter paper (Figure B)

Preparation—Preanalytical
1. Wash the hands if they are visibly soiled. If not, use an alcohol-based rub for routine decontamination. Apply the hand rub to the palm of one hand and rub the hands together, covering all surfaces until dry.
2. Correctly identify the newborn by using the three-way match and fill out all the information required on the card.
3. Choose the appropriate site for the heel stick according to the guidelines.
4. Put on gloves.
5. Warm the site by applying a warming device to the site for 3 to 5 minutes (Figure C).

Blood Collection Procedure—Analytical
6. Clean the site with 70% isopropyl alcohol. Allow the alcohol to dry and do not fan or blow on the cleansed site.
7. With a gloved hand, place the lancet against the medial or lateral plantar surface of the heel of the foot.
8. Place the blade slot area securely against the heel and firmly and completely depress the lancet trigger (Figure D).
9. After triggering the lancet, remove the lancet and discard it into a biohazard sharps container.
10. Gently wipe away the first drop of blood with sterile gauze or a cotton ball.
11. Apply gentle pressure with the thumb and ease intermittently as drops of blood form. Be sure to apply pressure in such a way that the incision site remains open. Note the position of the hand in Figure E.
12. The filter paper should be touched gently against the large blood drop, and a sufficient quantity of blood should penetrate to completely fill a preprinted circle on the filter paper before going to the next circle. Do not go back and reapply additional drops in the same circle after you have left.
13. The paper should not be pressed or smeared against the puncture site of the heel. Simply hover the heel very close to the filter paper and allow the blood to fill the circle.

14. Blood should be applied only to one side of the filter paper, but both sides of the filter paper should be examined to ensure that the blood uniformly saturated the paper.
15. After all five circles of blood have been collected from the heel of the newborn, the foot should be elevated above the body. NOTE: A minimum of three successful circles is needed by the laboratory to test for multiple metabolic disorders.
16. A sterile gauze pad or cotton swab should be pressed against the puncture site until the bleeding stops.
17. It is not advisable to apply adhesive bandages over skin puncture sites on newborns.

Follow-Up—Postanalytical
18. Wash the hands.
19. Document the procedure on the specimen log sheet and in the patient's record, making sure to include the following six items:
    When: date and time of collection
    Where: location on the body where the blood was collected (e.g., right antecubital space, hand, finger) and where the specimen is being sent (e.g., reference lab, hospital, in office)
    What: types of tubes collected (e.g., gold and lavender)
    Why: what tests were ordered (e.g., blood chemistry profile, complete blood cell count)
    How: did the patient respond to the procedure (tolerated well? experienced pain? fasting state? difficult draw?)
    Who: person who collected the specimen (your name, credentials)
    Patient's name
    Date, time: Performed heel stick on a warmed right heel and collected five full samples of blood for neonatal screening. Specimen card was sent to the health department. There were no complications
    _____ *First initial, last name, credentials*
20. Allow filter paper to dry thoroughly on a horizontal, level, nonabsorbent open surface for 3 hours at ambient temperature and away from direct sunlight.
21. Do not touch or smear blood on the filter paper and do not contaminate the specimen card with cleaning chemicals or other substances.
22. Mail the thoroughly dried card (Figure F) in the envelope provided by the health department. (Photos C through F by Zack Bent.)

PROCEDURE 4.3 **Vacutainer Method**

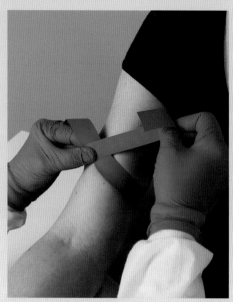

A, Apply the tourniquet. Pull the two ends of the tourniquet taut and then cross them in the front of the arm and grasp the center of the cross

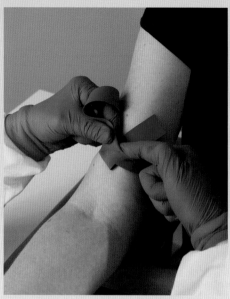

B, While holding the crossed area, pull up and tuck the top strap under the bottom strap from above so that the ends hang upward.

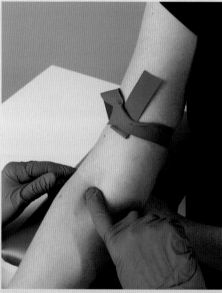

C, Palpate across the antecubital area and visualize the size, depth, and direction of the vein. If the location of the vein is not visible then make a mental note of its location by looking for "landmarks" such as a mole, freckle, crease in skin, nearby superficial veins, or other imperfections so that location can more readily be found after cleansing the site. An alternate method is to use a disinfected needle sheath and press down on the palpated location. It will leave an impression on the arm as a reference for cleansing and locating the vein in the next steps.

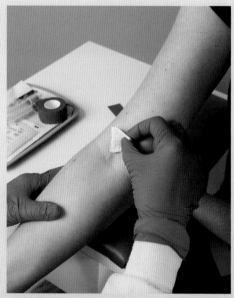

D, After removing the tourniquet, disinfect the area and assemble equipment on the appropriate side of the arm.

PROCEDURE 4.3 Vacutainer Method—cont'd

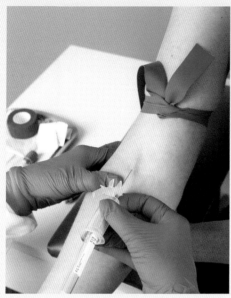

E, Reapply the tourniquet, remove the needle cover, and anchor the vein with the non-dominant hand.

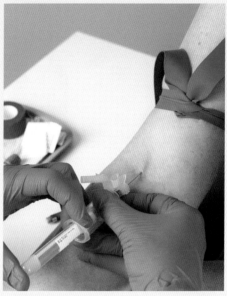

F, Insert the needle with the dominant hand. Then push the Vacutainer tube into the needle holder with the thumb of the nondominant hand while applying counterpressure on the flange of the Vacutainer holder.

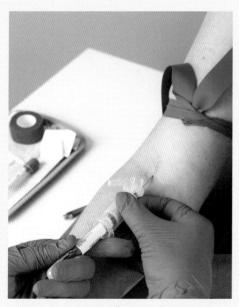

G, Pull out the tube with the fingers of the nondominant hand while applying counterpressure against the flange with the forefinger.

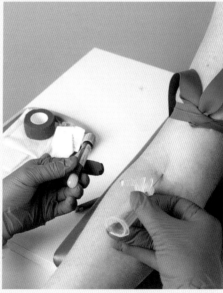

H, Mix the specimen by gently inverting the tube up and down allowing the blood to flow from one end of the tube to the other.

Continued

PROCEDURE 4.3 **Vacutainer Method—cont'd**

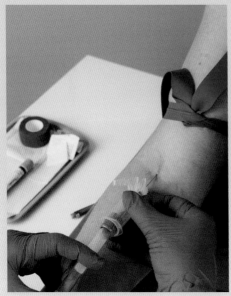

I, Insert the second tube with the nondominant hand.

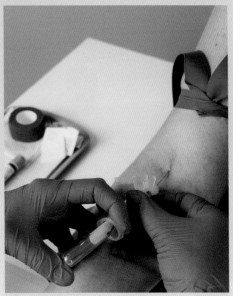

J, Push the vacuum tube into the holder.

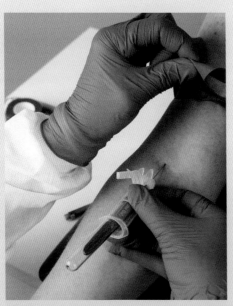

K, Remove the tourniquet as the last vacuum is filling, and have the patient relax her or his clenched fist.

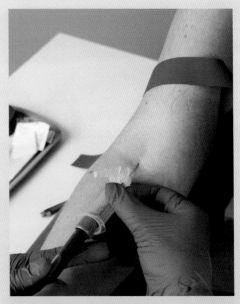

L, Remove the second tube from the holder.

PROCEDURE 4.3 Vacutainer Method—cont'd

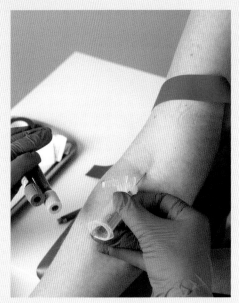

M, Mix both tubes while needle is still in the arm.

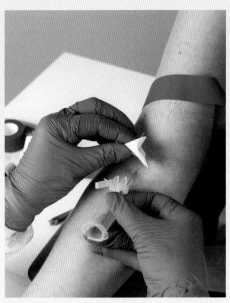

N, Hold sterile gauze over the site with the nondominant hand.

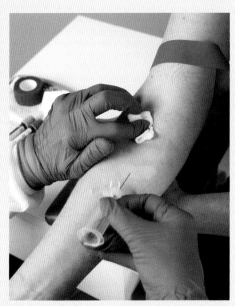

O, Remove the needle and immediately apply pressure on the site using the gauze.

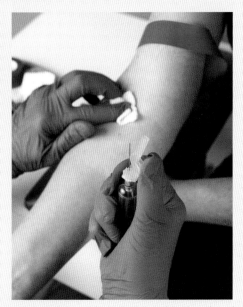

P, Activate the needle safety device with the thumb of the dominant hand.

Continued

PROCEDURE 4.3 Vacutainer Method—cont'd

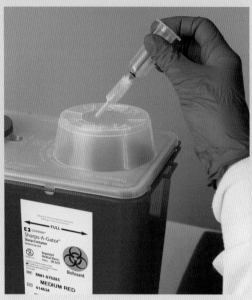

Q, Immediately dispose of the needle/holder assembly in a biohazard sharps container.

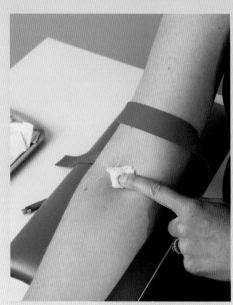

R, Label the tubes while the patient applies pressure to the puncture site.

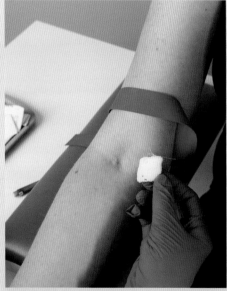

S, After 3 to 5 minutes, check for bleeding and apply an adhesive bandage or a nonlatex (COFLEX) Pressure bandage over the folded-over gauze.

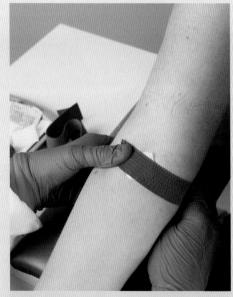

T, Apply a pressure bandage.

Equipment and Supplies
- Disposable gloves
- Tourniquet
- 70% isopropyl alcohol
- Vacutainer double-pointed needle
- Vacutainer holder
- Correct vacuum tubes for the requested tests
- Sterile gauze pads
- Adhesive bandages or non-latex (COFLEX) pressure bandage
- Test tube rack
- Biohazard sharps containers and bags

Preparation—Preanalytical
1. Wash the hands if they are visibly soiled. If not, use an alcohol-based hand rub. Apply the rub to the palm of one hand and rub the hands together, covering all surfaces until dry.
2. Correctly identify the patient by using the appropriate three-way match for your facility (spell name, date of birth, last four digits of their social security number, phone number, hospital identification number, or driver's license number).
3. Position the patient properly, such as in a semi reclining position or sitting in a chair with an arm support. Have the patient place his or her arm in a downward position to prevent reflux.

PROCEDURE 4.3 Vacutainer Method—cont'd

4. Determine if the patient is allergic to latex. Put on the appropriate type of gloves.
5. Apply the tourniquet and determine the appropriate site (Figures A and B). Have the patient make a fist and palpate the arm for a vein. NOTE: The patient should not open and close the fist and should avoid any vigorous pumping, which could result in muscle movement, making vein identification more difficult, and it may cause hemoconcentration.
6. Begin on one side of the antecubital space and palpate across to the other side with the index finger (Figure C). The vein will feel spongy. When the vein is found, determine its size and depth and follow it up and down to determine its direction.
7. Remove the tourniquet and have the patient release his or her fist.
8. Clean the arm with 70% isopropyl alcohol (Figure D). Rub the chosen site with the alcohol, working in concentric circles from the inside out, making sure not to backtrack. Allow the alcohol to dry for a minimum of 30 seconds to 1 minute without fanning or blowing on the cleansed site.
9. While the site is drying, assemble the equipment. Take the sheath off the holder end of the Vacutainer needle and screw it into the holder (while leaving the puncturing needle covered). Determine which vacuum tubes are needed for the testing and place them in a rack in the order of draw. Check the expiration date of the tubes and look for cracks. Be sure to tap the tubes that contain additives to release any additives that may be on the lids. Place the gauze, tubes, and all equipment close to the drawing station on the side of your free hand so they can be easily reached during the procedure.

Blood Collection Procedure—Analytical

10. The collection process begins after the alcohol has dried. Reapply the tourniquet, being careful not to contaminate the cleansed site. Have the patient make a fist again.
11. Remove the needle sheath, exposing the needle.
12. Anchor the vein with the nondominant thumb, placing it approximately 1 to 2 inches below and to the side of the puncture site so that it is not in the way of the entry of the needle into the vein (Figure E). Make the skin over the vein taut by pulling toward the patient's hand. This will help keep the vein from moving and allow the needle to enter more easily.
13. Approximately ¼ to ½ inch below the site, note any "landmarks" previously identified and with the bevel up, insert the needle at a 15-degree angle with one swift yet gentle, continuous motion to prevent tissue damage. It should *not* be a jab. The phlebotomist and needle should be positioned in the same direction as the vein. The correct angle will vary depending on the depth of the palpated vein. The common angle is 15 degrees. If the angle is less than 15 degrees, the needle may go above the vein; conversely, if the angle is greater than 15 degrees, the needle may go through the vein. Never stick unless a vein has been determined. The holder should be held steady with the dominant hand during the procedure so that the needle does not move through the vein or pull out.
14. Push the tube into the needle holder (Figure F). Put the index and middle fingers of the nondominant hand on both sides of the flange of the holder and push the tube into the Vacutainer needle with the thumb of the same hand.
15. Follow the order of draw for vacuum tubes when filling the tubes. If possible, fill the tubes from the bottom up so that the sheathed needle inside of the collecting tube does not make contact with additives in one tube and cross-contaminate the next tube. To remove a tube from the holder, put the forefinger of the nondominant hand against the flange of the holder and pull the tube out with the fingers of the nondominant hand (Figure G). Gently invert the tube a few times to start mixing the blood with the additives (Figure H).
16. Insert the next tube into the holder and use the same method of pushing the tube into the holder (Figure I). (NOTE: When the second tube is

filling, you may invert the previous tube to reach the required five to eight times.)
17. While the *last* tube is filling, remove the tourniquet (Figure K) and make sure the patient's hand is relaxed. NOTE: The tourniquet is removed *before* you take the needle out of the arm. If this is not done, blood may leak into the tissues from the venous puncture site, causing a hematoma (literally, a tumor or swelling of blood in the tissues).
18. When the last tube is filled, remove it (Figure L) and mix it and all other tubes by inverting (Figure M). NOTE: The last tube must be removed *before* removing the needle from the arm to prevent blood from dripping out of the needle.
19. Hold a sterile gauze or cotton ball over the needle (Figure N). Then swiftly pull out the needle and press down on the gauze immediately after the needle has been removed (Figure O). Pressure on the needle is painful for the patient.
20. After exiting the vein, activate the one-handed needle safety device (Figure P) and discard the entire Vacutainer device (holder with attached needle) into a biohazard sharps container (Figure Q).

Follow-Up—Post Analytical

21. With the gauze over the site, ask the patient to apply pressure for 3 to 5 minutes with the arm straight (Figure R). This pressure will help prevent a hematoma from forming. Bending the arm at the elbow can cause blood flow from the puncture site to increase.
22. While the patient is applying pressure, gently continue to invert the tubes 5 to 8 times. Label them with the patient's name, identification number, the date and time that the specimen was drawn, and your initials, if appropriate NOTE: Never prelabel tubes before the actual specimen is obtained; a prelabeled tube may end up with someone else's specimen!
23. During the entire process, assess the patient for signs of fainting. Check the site for bleeding after 3 to 5 minutes (Figure S). If bleeding has subsided, first determine if the patient is allergic to any type of bandage; then apply a pressure bandage (Figure T). Tell the patient not to lift any heavy objects for approximately 1 hour. If the site is still bleeding, continue to apply pressure. If bleeding has not stopped after 5 minutes, contact the physician. During the entire process, make sure that the patient is feeling well.
24. Discard all materials in the appropriate containers.
25. Remove gloves in the appropriate manner discussed in Chapter 1 and discard them in a biohazard bag.
26. Wash the hands.
27. Document the procedure on the specimen log sheet and in the patient's record, making sure to include the following six items:
    When: date and time of collection
    Where: location on the body where the blood was collected (e.g., right antecubital space, hand, finger) and where the specimen is being sent (e.g., reference lab, hospital, in office)
    What: types of tubes collected (e.g., gold and lavender)
    Why: what tests were ordered (e.g., blood chemistry profile, complete blood cell count)
    How: did the patient respond to the procedure (tolerated well? experienced pain? fasting state? difficult draw?)
    Who: person who collected the specimen (your name, credentials)
    Patient's name
    Date, time: Performed venipuncture on the left arm and collected a lavender tube for CBC and a gold tube for a Chemistry Profile. Tubes were processed and picked up by the ABC lab. There were no complications.
    _____ *First initial, last name, credentials*

PROCEDURE 4.4   Syringe Method

Deep clean kitchen or baths.

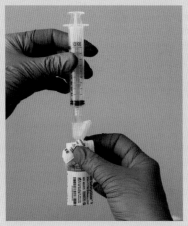

A, Assemble the sterile syringe and safety needle. NOTE: Pull and push the plunger back and forth in the barrel, and then make sure the plunger is pushed all the way into the barrel to remove all air.

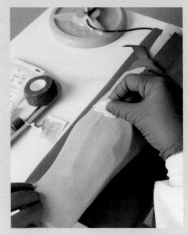

B, Apply the tourniquet as in the Vacutainer method, disinfect the site, and have supplies ready.

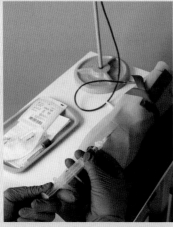

C, After anchoring the vein with the nondominant hand and inserting the needle with the dominant hand, withdraw blood by pulling back on the plunger. Note the thumb or forefinger is placed against the flange to provide counter-pressure while the other fingers pull back the plunger.

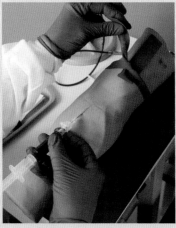

D, Instruct the patient to unclench the fist and remove the tourniquet before collecting the last portion of the blood specimen.

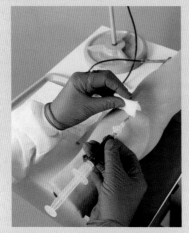

E, Hold the sterile gauze over the puncture site while removing the needle.

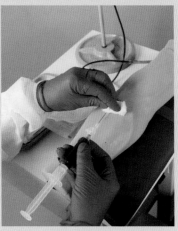

F, After the needle is removed, immediately apply pressure.

PROCEDURE 4.4 **Syringe Method—cont'd**

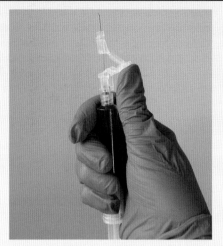

G, Immediately activate the one-handed spring needle safety device.

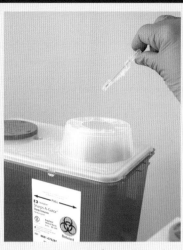

H, Remove the protected needle from the syringe and discard the needle in a biohazard sharps container.

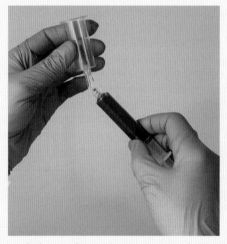

I, Attach the safety transfer device to the tip of the syringe.

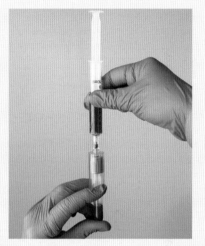

J, Invert the syringe above the device and connect the vacuum tubes in their proper order of draw by pushing them into the transfer device from below. Make sure the blood runs down the side of the tube to prevent rupture of the red blood cells. Invert each tube after it is filled.

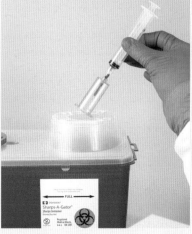

K, When the transfer is finished, discard the entire syringe and transfer device assembly in the biohazard sharps container.

Continued

PROCEDURE 4.4   Syringe Method—cont'd

Equipment and Supplies

- Disposable gloves
- Tourniquet
- 70% isopropyl alcohol
- Syringe and needle in correct sizes
- Correct vacuum tubes for the requested tests
- Safety transfer device
- Sterile gauze pads
- Adhesive bandages
- Test tube rack
- Biohazard sharps containers and bags

Preparation—Preanalytical

1. Follow steps 1 through 8 of Procedure 4.3.
2. While the site is drying, assemble the equipment. Remove the sterile syringe and needle from their packages, keeping them sterile (Figure A). Move the plunger back and forth several times to break the seal on the syringe. Make sure the plunger is fully pushed into the barrel to remove all air. Screw the hub of the needle tightly onto the syringe. Determine which vacuum tubes are needed for the testing and place them in a rack in the order of draw for vacuum tubes. Check the expiration date of the tubes, look for cracks, and tap the tubes that contain additives to release any additives that may be on the lids. Place all equipment close to the draw station on the side of your free hand so it is easily reached during the procedure.

Blood Collection Procedure—Analytical

3. Follow steps 10 through 12 of Procedure 4.3, including applying the tourniquet, disinfecting the site (Figure B), and anchoring the vein while inserting the needle.
4. When the needle is in the vein, blood may be seen in the hub of the syringe. Gently pull back on the plunger to pull blood into the syringe (Figure C). If the plunger is moved too fast, the blood may be hemolyzed or the vein may collapse. Be careful not to move the needle while it is in the vein, which could be painful for the patient. Also, do not withdraw the needle out of the patient's arm while pulling back on the plunger.

5. When the syringe has filled with the required amount of blood, have the patient unclench his or her fist and release the tourniquet (Figure D). Place sterile gauze over the puncture site as you remove the needle (Figure E). Be careful to remove the needle in the same path it was inserted. Then apply pressure to the site (Figure F). Do not press down on the gauze until the needle has been removed; such pressure would be painful for the patient.
6. Activate the syringe needle safety device after the needle has been removed from the arm (Figure G). Detach the needle from the syringe and discard the protected needle in the sharps biohazard container (Figure H).

Follow-Up—Postanalytical

7. With the gauze on the site, ask the patient to apply pressure for 3 to 5 minutes with the arm straight.
8. The blood must be transferred into the vacuum tubes as quickly as possible so that it does not clot in the syringe. While the patient applies pressure to the puncture site, transfer the blood from syringe to vacuum tubes with a *safety transfer device*. This device looks like a Vacutainer holder with only the inner sheathed needle in the holder. One end of the safety transfer device attaches to the end of the syringe (Figure I). The inside of the holder containing the rubber-sheathed needle then pierces the Vacutainer tube when the syringe and holder are inverted (Figure J). The blood in the syringe is drawn automatically into the tubes because of the vacuum in these tubes. To keep from hemolyzing the red blood cells, hold tube so that the flow of blood runs down the side of the tube and never push on the syringe plunger while transferring blood with this device.
9. Invert the tubes 8 to 10 times and label them with the patient's name and identification number, the date and time that the specimen was drawn, and your name (or initials, if appropriate).
10. Discard the entire connected syringe and transfer device into the sharps container (Figure K). Discard all other potential biohazard materials in a biohazard bag.
11. Follow steps 20 through 24 of Procedure 4.3.

PROCEDURE 4.5   Two Butterfly Needle Methods

Butterfly Safety Lock and Push-Button
Butterfly Safety Lock Needle Using a Vacutainer Tube System

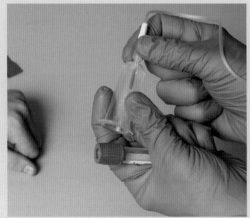

A, Firmly attach the Vacutainer adapter to the butterfly tubing and then screw the rubber sheathed needle into the Vacutainer holder. Reaffirm that the adapter is firmly attached to avoid air leaks during the blood draw.

Equipment and Supplies

- Tourniquet
- Sterile gauze pads
- 70% isopropyl alcohol
- Disposable gloves
- Vacutainer holder
- Vacutainer tubes
- Winged butterfly with safety lock needle and Vacutainer adapter to connect to Vacutainer holder
- Biohazard sharps containers and bags

Preparation—Preanalytical

1. Follow steps 1 through 4 of Procedure 4.3. The procedure for entering a vein in the arm is the same as those for the syringe and vacuum tube methods. If blood is being drawn from the hand, apply the tourniquet above the wrist and have the patient make a half fist.
2. Beginning on one side of the puncture area, palpate across to the other side with the index finger. The vein will feel spongy. When the vein is found, determine its size and depth and follow it up and down to determine its direction.
3. Remove the tourniquet.

PROCEDURE 4.5 **Two Butterfly Needle Methods—cont'd**

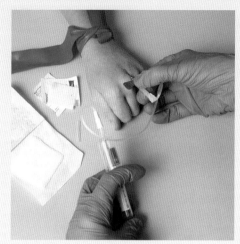

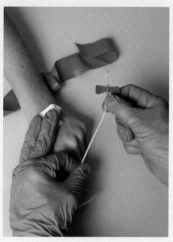

B, After disinfecting the hands, apply the tourniquet and anchor the vein. Insert the butterfly needle into the vein. Push the vacuum tubes into the holder, which will draw the blood through the tubing into the tubes. Note: When possible, angle the Vacutainer tube with the stopper up allowing the blood to flow to the bottom of the tube.

C, Remove the needle after the last tube has been collected and mixed. Activate the safety device using the "OK" method, making sure both hands are behind the exposed needle.

4. Clean the hand with 70% isopropyl alcohol. Allow the alcohol to dry without fanning or blowing on the cleansed site.
5. While the site is drying, assemble the equipment. Remove the winged infusion set from the package and stretch the tubing to straighten it. If you are using the Vacutainer method, attach a Luer adapter to the end of the tubing of the winged infusion and then screw the other end into a Vacutainer holder. Double check to affirm there is a tight seal where the Luer adapter fits onto the sheathed needle to prevent air from entering the Vacutainer tubes (Figure A).
6. Determine which vacuum tubes are needed for the testing and place them in a rack in the order of draw. Note: If a blue top is ordered, it is necessary to draw a waste tube first to remove the dead space in the tubing. A red tube with no additives or an additional blue top may be used to clear the air in the tubing with blood. The waste tubes do not need to be filled because they will be discarded after the procedure. Check the expiration date of the tubes, look for cracks, and tap the tubes that contain additives. Place all equipment close to the draw station so it can be easily reached during the procedure.

Blood Collection Procedure—Analytical
7. When the alcohol has dried, reapply the tourniquet. Remove the needle sheath from the needle.
8. Anchor the vein by placing the nondominant thumb 1 to 2 inches below and to the side of the puncture site. Make the skin over the vein taut by pulling toward the patient's knuckles.
9. Grip the folded plastic wings to guide the needle into the vein (Figure B). At approximately ¼ to ½ inch below the site, note the landmarks previously identified, and with the bevel up, quickly and gently insert the bevel of the needle into the vein at a 15-degree angle or less when drawing from a hand. Continue to "thread" the needle with one continuous, swift motion to keep the needle from twisting out of the vein.

10. If you are using the Vacutainer holder or system, push the vacuum tubes into the holder (Figure B). After each tube has filled with blood, remove it and gently invert it back and forth.
11. After the required amount of blood has been obtained, have the patient unclench his or her fist and release the tourniquet. Place a piece of sterile gauze over the puncture site and remove the needle by holding the tail of the needle device with the thumb and forefinger of the dominant hand forming the "OK" sign. Swiftly pull the needle out and to the side. Note: Do not press down on the gauze until the needle has been removed.
12. Immediately activate the safety device by using the nondominant hand to grab the tubing with its thumb and forefinger forming the "OK" sign and then pull on the tubing. The needle will retract into the butterfly body. Use the remaining fingers to apply pressure to the site as seen in (Figure C). (Note: Always keep both hands behind the needle tip to prevent an accidental stick.) After the safety device has been activated with the butterfly or Vacutainer method, the entire Vacutainer holder and butterfly apparatus should be discarded in a biohazard sharps container.
13. With the gauze on the site, ask the patient to apply pressure for 3 to 5 minutes with the arm straight or elevated above the heart.

Follow-Up—Postanalytical
14. Follow steps 20 through 26 of Procedure 4.3.

Butterfly Push-Button Needle Using a Syringe
This procedure is basically the same as the previously described safety lock butterfly procedure, with a few changes. The push-button butterfly needle is considered safer than the safety lock needle when used properly. The best way to learn any new safety device is to practice first on a training model. Figures D through L demonstrate the ways in which this method differs from the previous procedure.

Continued

PROCEDURE 4.5   **Two Butterfly Needle Methods—cont'd**

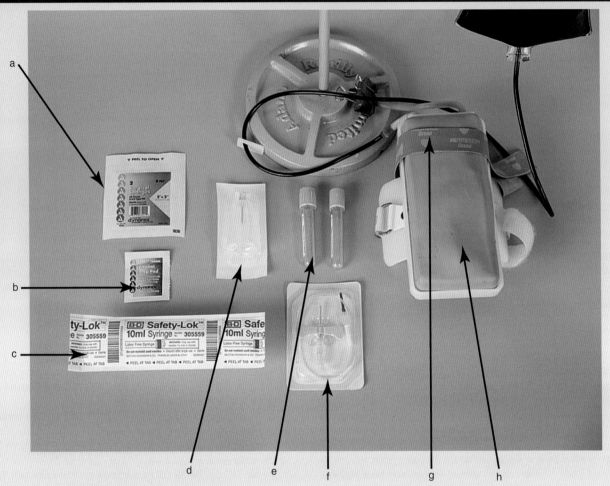

D, Equipment and supplies for push-button method using a syringe: *(a)* Sterile gauze pads; *(b)* 70% isopropyl alcohol; *(c)* sterile syringe; *(d)* transfer device; *(e)* Vacutainer tubes; *(f)* butterfly with push-button safety needle; *(g)* tourniquet; *(h)* training model with artificial blood for practicing.

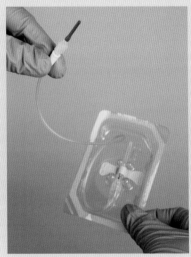

E, Proper removal of the butterfly from its container consists of pulling out the entire assembly using the adapter end of the tubing to prevent accidental activation of the black push button located just under the blue "wings."

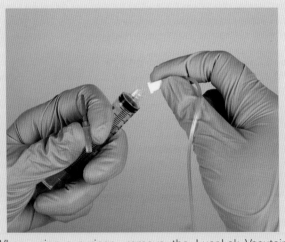

F, When using a syringe, remove the Luer-Lok Vacutainer holder adapter (seen in the left hand) and place the syringe adapter tightly onto the tip of the syringe. Also, remember to move the plunger back and forth several times to break the seal on the syringe and then push the plunger all the way in to remove all air from the syringe.

PROCEDURE 4.5   Two Butterfly Needle Methods—cont'd

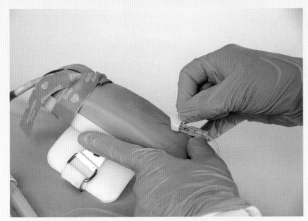

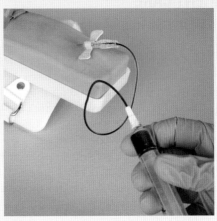

G, While anchoring the vein with the nondominant hand, quickly insert the bevel of the butterfly needle at a 15-degree angle (or less if drawing from a hand) and observe the flash of blood entering the tail of the butterfly. Continue to thread the needle along the lumen of the vein to anchor the needle.

H, With the needle in place, both hands may be used to slowly pull the blood into the syringe. It may be necessary to pull back the plunger a little at a time to keep the vein from collapsing.

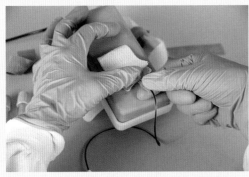

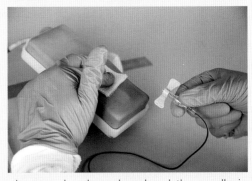

I, After you have collected enough blood in the syringe, grasp the body of the butterfly using the thumb and forefinger of the dominant hand to stabilize the needle. Place gauze over the needle to safely prevent splattering of the blood during the retraction of the needle. NOTE: Tell the patient to expect a snapping sound that will indicate the procedure is over. The nondominant hand uses the side of the thumb to push down the black button located just below the wings. The needle then instantly retracts inward and juts out the back end of the butterfly body.

J, After the snap has been heard and the needle is safely tucked into the body of the butterfly, the nondominant hand immediately applies pressure to the site.

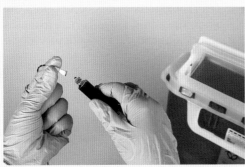

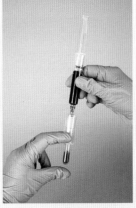

K, Remove the hub of the butterfly from the syringe and throw the tubing into the sharps container.

L, Using the transfer device, transfer the blood into the appropriate tubes in their correct order of draw. Hold the syringe above and the vacuum tubes below in an upright position, allowing the blood to run down the side of the tube. Also, keep pushing on the tubes as they are filling so they do not slip off the sheathed needle in the transfer device, causing an incomplete fill.

❖ ADVANCED CONCEPTS: SPECIMEN AND PATIENT CARE

Preparing Blood Specimens for Laboratory Pickup

The last step in blood collection is the processing of the blood before the laboratory retrieves the specimen for testing. Each laboratory or CLIA-waived test procedure has a specific protocol regarding how to process the blood for the test they will be performing. Therefore, it is important to check the lab manual provided by the laboratories that will be picking up the specimens and to perform the following steps:

- Log each collection on the laboratory log sheet, indicating the date, time, patient identification, tubes drawn, tests ordered, lab where tests will be performed, and the phlebotomist's initials. (See the Workbook Appendix—Chapter 4 "Specimen Log Sheet" for logging lab specimens.)
- Allow 30 minutes for gold, red, and tiger rubber-topped tubes to clot in an upright position in a test tube rack. They should then be centrifuged within 2 hours of collection to separate the serum from the clotted cells (Figure 4.25).
- Place the closed tubes in the centrifuge, creating a balanced load. Opposing centrifuge holders must be equally weighted with loaded samples that are the same size and equal in fill.
- Fill a tube with water to match the weight of any unpaired sample and place it across from the sample.
- The tubes should remain closed with their tops on at all times during the centrifugation process.
- Centrifuge the clotted specimens for 15 to 20 minutes depending on centrifuge speed (usually 3000 rpm) and laboratory recommendations (Figure 4.26).
- PSTs should also be centrifuged for 15 to 20 minutes within 2 hours of collection, according to laboratory protocol.
- Store all specimens at room temperature or refrigerate, according to laboratory guidelines.
- Place specimens in a biohazard specimen bag with their corresponding requisition placed in the front pocket of the bag.

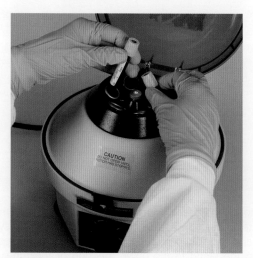

FIG. 4.25 Place the capped tubes in the centrifuge, creating a balanced load. Opposing centrifuge holders must be equally weighted with loaded samples that are the same size and equal in fill. (Photo by Zack Bent.)

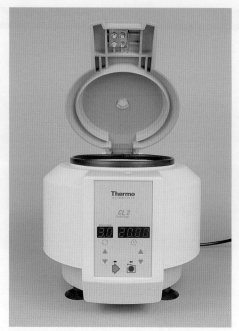

FIG. 4.26 Observe the settings for spinning a clotted blood specimen: $3.0 \times 1000 = 3000$ rpm for 20 minutes. (Photo by Zack Bent.)

Centrifuge Safety

- Do not spin uncovered specimen tubes and always have the centrifuge lid cover closed when the centrifuge is running to prevent the vaporization of hazardous droplets.
- If an abnormal noise, vibration, or sound is noted while the centrifuge is in operation, immediately stop the unit by turning off the switch and check for a possible load imbalance.
- Centrifuges must never be slowed or stopped by grasping any part of the device with your hand or applying another object against the rotating equipment.
- Broken tubes or liquid spills must be cleaned according to OSHA standards. Clean the centrifuge daily with a disinfectant and paper towel.

NOTE: Watch the online Evolve video: Preparing a Serum Specimen Using a Serum Separator Tube.

Patient Issues When Locating a Suitable Vein

Patient issues and complications may occur before, during, and after a phlebotomy procedure. It is important to understand the following complications and learn ways to prevent them when possible.

Obesity

The veins on obese patients may be difficult to visualize and palpate, making them a challenge to find and penetrate. The following are some possible solutions to this challenge:

- Ask the patient if he or she has had blood drawn previously and if there is a "favorite" vein of choice.
- Have the patient warm the antecubital space for several minutes and then use a blood pressure cuff as a tourniquet and

inflate to about 30 to 40 mm Hg on the patient's downward extended arm.

- First palpate for the median vein by feeling between the creases in the antecubital space while the patient makes a fist.
- If the median vein is not palpable, then have the patient turn his or her extended lower arm with the thumb up, which may then expose the cephalic vein when a fist is made.
- If the cephalic vein is not palpable, apply the tourniquet above the wrist and check the hand for visible or palpable veins on the back of the hand (Figure 4.27) or on the thumb side of the hand.
- Currently, there is an instrument that trans illuminates the surface of the skin with infrared light to assist in locating difficult to find veins (Figures 4.28 and 4.29).
- Caution must be taken not to probe the area excessively if a vein is missed.

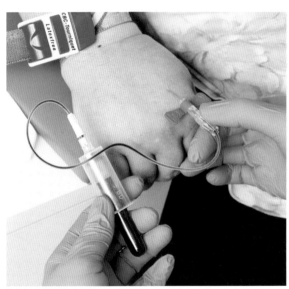

FIG. 4.27 Drawing blood from a hand when veins are difficult to find in the antecubital space. Note how the vacuum tube is held to allow the blood to flow down to the bottom of the tube. Also note the specialized tourniquet at the wrist, which improves patient comfort. (Photo by Zack Bent.)

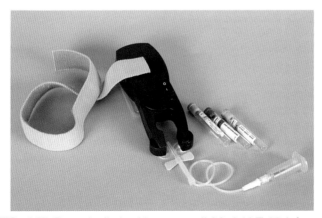

FIG. 4.28 The vein finder. Venoscope II Model VT 03 infrared light source displays vein. (Photo by Zack Bent.)

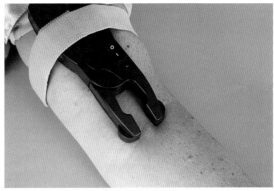

FIG. 4.29 Attaching Venoscope to arm for assisting in blood draw. (Photo by Zack Bent.)

Complications During Blood Collection

Hematomas

A hematoma is a swelling or tumor of blood under the skin causing a bruise. It results from an open break in a blood vessel. It can occur around a puncture site when blood leaks from the vein into the surrounding tissue. A hematoma may result when any of the following occurs:

- The needle penetrates the vein.
- The needle is only partially in the vein (Figure 4.30A).
- Insufficient pressure was applied to the puncture site after the procedure was completed.
- The patient has lifted heavy objects with the arm too soon after the draw, causing the puncture site to reopen.

If a hematoma occurs during the procedure, remove the tourniquet and needle immediately followed by applying direct pressure for 3 to 5 minutes. If the bleeding continues, call for assistance.

Failure to Obtain Blood When Needle Is in the Arm

If blood is not seen after connecting the vacuum tube, one of the following problems may have occurred as seen in Figure 4.30B–E:

- The bevel is against the upper wall of the vein and the vein has collapsed (see Figure 4.30B). Adjust by slightly tipping the needle downward.
- The needle pierced all the way through the vein (see Figure 4.30C). Insertion of the needle at an angle greater than 15 degrees is a likely cause. Adjust by slightly pulling back and correcting the angle.
- The needle is inserted above the vein, possibly because the needle is inserted at less than a 15-degree angle (see Figure 4.30D). Adjust by slightly correcting the angle and pushing forward.
- The needle has missed the vein entirely (see Figure 4.30E). Do not probe if the vein is missed because this bruises the arm and could hemolyze the RBCs. Slight repositioning of the needle may result in blood flow. If not, remove needle and begin the process on a new site.
- A defective vacuum tube has been used. Always inspect tubes before using them and never reuse a tube from a failed blood draw. It must be discarded.

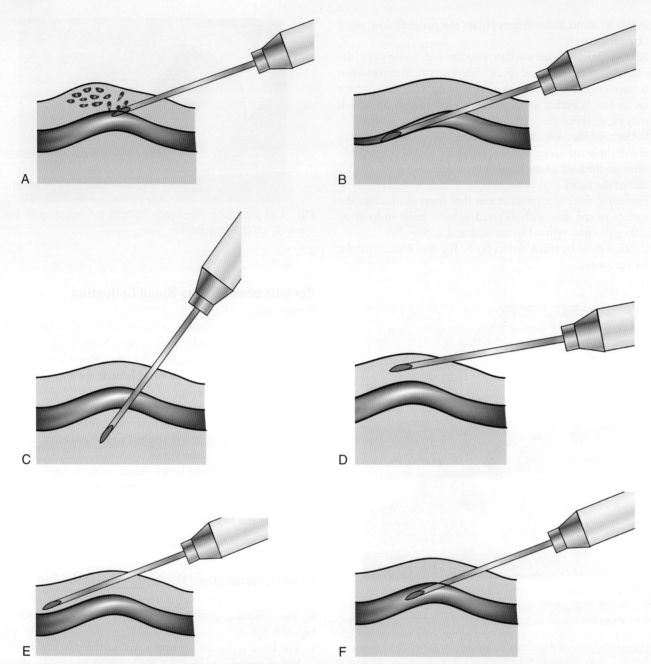

FIG. 4.30 Complications when searching for a vein. **A,** Hematoma caused by blood escaping into the tissue from partially inserted needle. **B,** The needle bevel is on the wall of a collapsed vein. **C,** The needle bevel has gone entirely through the vein. **D,** The needle is above the vein because of an incorrect angle. **E,** The needle has completely missed the vein. **F,** A successful insertion at the correct angle and the proper depth. (Art provided by Gala Bent.)

If none of these issues are resolved, remove the tourniquet and needle, observing the same safety techniques as a successful draw and repeat the procedure on the other arm. A patient should never be stuck more than two times by the same phlebotomist. See Evolve on-line Lessons with 6 scenarios of missed veins.

Mastectomy

Do not perform a venipuncture on the arm adjacent to a **mastectomy** (removal of the breast) site. A patient who has undergone a mastectomy may have no lymph flow to that arm because the axillary lymph nodes on the mastectomy side may have been removed. This condition carries a potential risk for infection, along with alterations in the levels of body fluids and blood analytes in that arm. In addition, the tourniquet may injure the patient's arm.

Intravenous Therapy

Drawing blood from a patient's arm in which there is an intravenous (IV) fluid running is not recommended because the fluid could dilute or influence the results of the tests. A glucose drip, for example, could falsely increase glucose values. If an arm with an IV tube must be used, always draw on the arm *below* the IV insertion area (e.g., from the hand). The nurse should turn off the IV drip for 2 minutes before the venipuncture, and a discard volume of 5 mL should be drawn first.

Edema

Areas affected by *edema* (abnormal accumulation of fluid in interstitial spaces) should not be used for venipuncture because the extra tissue fluid may contaminate and dilute the test results. An example of an edematous arm would be one that is in a cast.

Areas to Avoid

Veins that are obstructed in some way—such as when the skin is sclerosed (hardened), psoriatic with plaque, or scarred—should not be used. Sites with open wounds or that are burned and susceptible to infection should also be avoided.

Hemolysis

Hemolysis is the breaking open or rupture of RBCs and the release of their hemoglobin. Hemoglobin turns serum or plasma pink or red. Hemolysis can be caused by one of the following actions:

- Using a needle that is too small
- Collapsing the vein by putting too much pressure on it, either by using the Vacutainer method on a small vein or by pulling back the plunger too quickly with the syringe method
- Vigorously shaking the filled tubes
- Allowing hemolyzed blood to release chemicals into the plasma and serum that adversely affect the test results for the following analytes:
  - Potassium
  - Magnesium
  - Iron
  - Lactate dehydrogenase
  - Phosphorus
  - Ammonia
  - Total protein

Excessive Bleeding

A patient typically stops bleeding in 2 to 6 minutes after applying pressure to the site. However, patients who take medications such as blood thinners and arthritis medications may bleed for a longer time. Even aspirin can act as a blood thinner. Patients may also have coagulation abnormalities such as platelet defects. In this case, petechiae (small red or purple spots) may appear on the patient's skin. Petechiae are caused by small amounts of bleeding under the skin. Let the physician know if bleeding does not stop.

Neurologic Problems

Syncope, or fainting, is common for some patients to experience during or after phlebotomy procedures. Signs of fainting include pallor, sweating, and hyperventilation. If a patient expresses concern about fainting, place him or her in a reclining position before starting the procedure.

If a patient feels faint during the procedure, release the tourniquet and remove the needle and apply pressure. Be sure to activate the safety device. Have the patient lower his or her head and breathe deeply. Place a cold or wet towel on the forehead and back of the neck. Do not attempt to put anything in the patient's mouth. If possible, place the patient in a reclining position and stay with the patient for at least 15 minutes after the patient has recovered. Instruct the patient not to drive for at least 30 minutes. Giving the patient a glass of juice may be helpful. An incident report from your health care facility should be completed describing the fainting incident and any follow-up action taken.

Seizure is another neurologic problem that could occur during a phlebotomy procedure. If a patient has a seizure, remove the tourniquet and needle immediately and apply pressure to the puncture site. Call for help and do not attempt to put anything in the patient's mouth unless authorized to do so.

Hitting a nerve during venipuncture is rare but serious. The patient will probably experience a tingling sensation, electric-like shock or sharp pain radiating down the affected nerve. The patient may suddenly jerk. Immediately remove the tourniquet and needle and apply pressure to the site. Notify an authorized person and file an incident report.

Risk Management

OSHA regulates the Bloodborne Pathogens Standard by requiring all health care facilities to have an exposure control plan in place to help reduce employee exposure. The most common exposure to bloodborne pathogens in health care results from accidental puncture wounds with contaminated needles, glass, or other sharp items. In an effort to reduce these percutaneous incidents in the workplace, the Bloodborne Pathogens Standard requires documentation of the selection and evaluation of any new safety technology used by employees. The goal is to determine the effectiveness of new safety devices in the following areas:

- Decreased risk of injuries
- Acceptance of the device by users
- Ability of the device to not affect patient care adversely

Two sample safety device evaluation forms from OSHA are included in the workbook appendix Chapter 4 forms: "Sample Device Preselection Worksheet" and "Sample Device Evaluation Form." All employees who are at risk of exposure must be alert and involved in finding ways to eliminate exposure to bloodborne pathogens. Be sure to take the time to complete the forms and answer the questions during the blood-collecting laboratory practice sessions.

REVIEW QUESTIONS*

1. What is the *most serious* error a phlebotomist can make before collecting a specimen?
   a. Not collecting enough blood
   b. Not releasing the tourniquet before removing the needle
   c. Misidentifying the patient
   d. Collecting the blood in the wrong tube

2. A certified medical assistant is in the process of collecting a blood sample by the Vacutainer method. During the procedure, a hematoma begins to form. Which of the following scenarios could explain why this occurred?
   a. The bevel is against the wall of the vein.
   b. The bevel is in the middle of the vein.
   c. The bevel was inserted above the vein.
   d. The bevel is only partially inserted in the vein.

3. Which of the following tubes is used for coagulation studies?
   a. Lavender
   b. Light blue
   c. Green
   d. Gray

4. A capillary puncture is performed on a newborn. All the following steps are correct *except*
   a. the puncture site is warmed before the puncture is made.
   b. the medial or lateral section of the plantar surface of the foot is the site of the puncture.
   c. a 3-mm lancet is used for the puncture.
   d. the first drop of blood is wiped away.

5. A certified medical assistant is performing a Vacutainer blood collection. Which of the following techniques is *incorrect?*
   a. The tourniquet is placed 3 inches above the puncture site.
   b. The puncture site is cleaned using friction with 70% isopropyl alcohol.
   c. The tourniquet is removed after the last tube and the needle are removed.
   d. The tubes are mixed 8 to 10 times after being filled with blood.

6. If the angle of needle insertion is lower than 15 degrees during a venipuncture procedure, which of the following may occur?
   a. The needle may end up above the vein.
   b. The needle may pierce completely through the vein.
   c. The vein may collapse.
   d. The needle bevel may stick to the bottom of the vein wall.

7. You are in the process of drawing blood when you notice that the patient is looking pale and sweating. Which of the following steps should you *not* do?
   a. Continue with the procedure until all the required blood is drawn.
   b. Call for help.
   c. Try to get the patient into a reclining position.
   d. Apply cold compresses to the patient's head and back of the neck.

8. What is the recommended maximum time to apply a tourniquet?
   a. 4 minutes
   b. 3 minutes
   c. 2 minutes
   d. 1 minute

9. Which of the following tests should *not* be done by the capillary puncture method?
   a. Glucose
   b. Complete blood count
   c. Blood cultures
   d. Cholesterol

10. The following tubes are being used in a Vacutainer venipuncture procedure: green, lavender, red (plastic), and light blue. Place them in the correct order of draw.

*Answers to these Review Questions are located in the Appendix on p. 278.

WEBSITES

Newborn screening:
www.nlm.nih.gov/medlineplus/newbornscreening.html
http://kidshealth.org/parent/medical/genetic/newborn_screening_tests.html
www.marchofdimes.com/pnhec/298_834.asp
Baby's First Test: Conditions Screened by State:
www.babysfirsttest.org/newborn-screening/states
American Academy of Pediatrics:
www.aap.org
Clinical and Laboratory Standards Institute (formerly NCCLS):
www.clsi.org/

Occupational Safety and Health Administration:
www.osha.gov
Phlebotomy:
www.phlebotomypages.com/phlebotomist_skills.htm
www.phlebotomy.com/index.html
www.bd.com/safety/products/b_collect/index.asp#b3
Maternal and Child Health Bureau of the Health Resources and Services Administration:
www.mchb.hrsa.gov
Website for vein finder:
www.venoscope.com

Hematology

OBJECTIVES

After completing this chapter, you should be able to do the following:

1. Define and match terms and abbreviations in this chapter.

Fundamental Concepts

2. Identify the proper specimen collection for hematology testing.
3. Identify the blood components found in bone marrow and peripheral blood. Describe their functions, their characteristics, and their basic formation in the bone marrow.
4. Perform a blood smear and stain and identify typical blood cells from the smear.
5. Observe selected abnormal cells from visual aids.
6. Describe the basic principles of hemostasis (including the involvement of blood vessels, platelets, clotting factors, and anticoagulants).

CLIA-Waived Procedures

7. Identify equipment and supplies used in waived hematology and coagulation tests.

8. Follow the most current Occupational Safety and Health Administration safety guidelines when performing hematology and coagulation tests and apply the correct quality control for the CLIA-waived hematology tests.
9. Perform the following Food and Drug Administration–approved waived tests according to the stated task, conditions, and standards listed in the Learning Outcome Procedure Sheets in the student workbook: hemoglobin, hematocrit, erythrocyte sedimentation rate, and prothrombin time.
10. Describe the role of prothrombin in blood coagulation and explain the major use of the prothrombin time test.

Advanced Concepts

11. Describe the seven tests involved in the complete blood count.
12. Identify the red blood cell indices and explain their significance in determining anemia.
13. Explain the significance of the white blood cell count and differential.

KEY TERMS

agranulocytes: white blood cells that do not contain granules in their cytoplasm: monocytes and lymphocytes

anemia: condition in which the red blood cell count or hemoglobin level is below normal

anisocytosis: abnormal variances in red blood cell size

band: an immature neutrophil whose nucleus has not segmented (also called stab)

baso-: prefix meaning blue or basic

basophils: white blood cells with large granules that stain dark blue

cytoplasm: fluid within the cell containing the nucleus and other organelles

differential count: procedure for determining the percentage of the various types of leukocytes based on their staining characteristics, shapes, and sizes

eosino-: prefix meaning red

eosinophils: white blood cells with large red granules

erythroblasts: immature red blood cells

erythrocyte sedimentation rate (ESR): the distance red blood cells fall or settle out of an anticoagulated blood specimen after 60 minutes

fibrinogen (factor I): one of plasma proteins involved in clotting

formed elements: cells and cell fragments that can be viewed under a microscope

granulocytes: white blood cells that contain granules in their cytoplasm: neutrophils, basophils, and eosinophils

hematocrit (Hct): test that measures percentage of packed red blood cells compared with total blood volume

hematologists: specialists who studies blood, blood-forming organs, and blood diseases

hematology: the study of blood and blood-forming organs in health and in disease

hematopoiesis: blood production

hemocytoblast: a stem cell that differentiates (changes) and becomes any of the seven visible blood elements found in circulating blood

hemoglobin (Hgb): oxygen-carrying reddish pigment in red blood cells

hemolysis (hemolyzing): destruction of the red blood cells

hemostasis: body's ability to initiate a clotting response to stop bleeding and at the same time prevent the blood from forming an unwanted stationary clot

hypochromic: decrease in color caused by a decrease of hemoglobin in red blood cells

hypoxemia: lack of oxygen in the blood

immunoglobulins: antibodies that destroy or render harmless foreign invaders containing antigens

leukemia: cancer of the blood-forming tissues in bone marrow, lymphatic system, or both

leukocytosis: abnormal increase in number of white blood cells

leukopenia: abnormal decrease in number of white blood cells

lymphocytes: small, nongranular white blood cells

macrophages: large, engulfing monocytes when they enter the tissues

megakaryocyte: large nuclear cell in the bone marrow that fragments its cytoplasm to become platelets

monocytes: large, nongranular white blood cells that develop in bone marrow

myeloblasts: bone marrow cells that differentiate into the three kinds of granulocytes

neutro-: prefix meaning neither acidic nor alkaline

neutrophil: white blood cells with fine granules that stain lavender or pink

nongranulocytes: white blood cells that do not contain granules in their cytoplasm: monocytes and lymphocytes

normocytes: mature red blood cells with normal size, shape, and color

nuclei: central controlling structures in cells

-phil: suffix meaning attraction

poikilocytosis: abnormal shapes in red blood cells

polycythemia: abnormal condition of increased number of red blood cells

polymorphonuclear (PMN): having a multishaped, segmented nucleus; sometimes abbreviated as PMN or seg

prothrombin (factor II): one of 21 plasma proteins involved in clotting

protime test: test for monitoring coagulation times for patients taking anticoagulants such as coumadin

RBC indices: mathematical ratios of the three red blood cell tests (hemoglobin, hematocrit, and red blood cell count)

reticulocytes: newly released red blood cells in the blood that still contain some nuclear RNA

rouleaux formation: arrangement of red blood cells resembling stacked chips caused by an increase in serum proteins

thrombocytes: platelets; cellular fragments that gather at the site of a damaged blood vessel and release clotting chemicals to form a clot

thrombosis: formation of clots inside blood vessels

vitamin K: critical element in the production of coagulation factors

ABBREVIATIONS

ALL: acute lymphocytic leukemia
AML: acute myelocytic leukemia
CBC: complete blood count
CLL: chronic lymphocytic leukemia
CML: chronic myelocytic leukemia
ESR: erythrocyte sedimentation rate
g/dL: grams per deciliter, which represents the weight of a substance (g) per volume (dL)
Hct: hematocrit

Hgb: hemoglobin
INR: international normalized ratio (for prothrombin time test results)
MCH: mean cell hemoglobin
MCHC: mean (average) cell hemoglobin concentration
MCV: mean cell volume
PMN: polymorphonuclear
PT: prothrombin time (protime)

❖ FUNDAMENTAL CONCEPTS

Overview of Hematology and Blood

Hematology is the study of blood and blood-forming organs in health and in disease. The complete blood count (CBC) is one of the most commonly ordered "routine" tests for evaluating a person's internal health status. Hematologists are physicians who may work in the hematology departments of hospitals, reference labs, and private practices, where they evaluate the blood's cellular elements microscopically and analytically by using a variety of test methods. Hematologists may also evaluate hemostasis, the body's ability to initiate a clotting response to stop bleeding and at the same time prevent the blood from forming an unwanted stationary clot.

In the ambulatory setting, basic CLIA-waived hematology tests and coagulation (clotting) tests are performed on capillary blood. If a reference laboratory does the testing, the requisition and laboratory protocol must be checked to ensure the proper tubes are drawn and correctly processed. The blood for hematology tests is usually collected in lavender-topped vacuum tubes containing the anticoagulant ethylenediaminetetraacetic acid (EDTA), which also preserves cellular elements in their natural state.

The blood for coagulation studies is usually collected in blue-topped vacuum tubes that must be allowed to fill accurately because the blood and the liquid anticoagulant in the tube must be in the proper ratio. This is why a "waste" tube is needed when using the butterfly needle and tubing.

Blood is a complex liquid connective tissue that is constantly circulating through the blood vessels. The formed elements within blood can be viewed under a microscope as cells and cell fragments (Figure 5.1, left). These formed elements (erythrocytes, or red blood cells [RBCs]; thrombocytes, or platelets; and leukocytes, or white blood cells [WBCs]) are suspended in the watery liquid called plasma, which contains hundreds of dissolved biochemical substances (Figure 5.1, right).

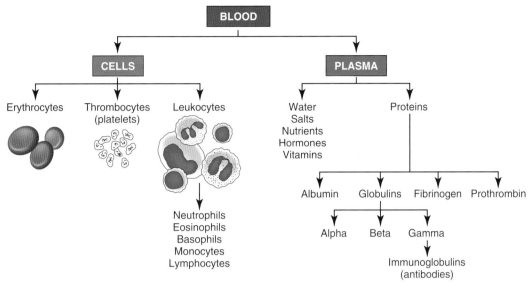

FIG. 5.1 Blood components. *Left,* Formed cellular elements; *right,* liquid plasma and its chemical divisions. (From Chabner D: *The language of medicine,* ed 10, St. Louis, 2014, Saunders.)

(NOTE: Chapters 6 and 7 focus on the biochemical substances located in the plasma.)

Blood cells are produced in the red bone marrow found in flat bones and at the ends of long bones (Figure 5.2). All the cells originate from a stem cell, or hemocytoblast, that differentiates (changes) and becomes any of the following seven formed elements that are seen in circulating blood:

- Red blood cells (RBCs, also called *erythrocytes*)
- Five types of white blood cells (WBCs, also called *leukocytes*):
  - Basophils
  - Neutrophils
  - Eosinophils
  - Monocytes
  - Lymphocytes
  - Platelets (also called *thrombocytes*)

Figure 5.3 is a simplified flow chart illustrating blood production, or hematopoiesis. Each of the seven formed elements is viewed and discussed as it is developed in the bone marrow and then released into the bloodstream or tissue, where it fulfills its function.

Red Blood Cells (Erythrocytes)

The bone marrow is constantly producing new RBCs. The beginning stages of RBC production in the bone marrow are shown in the upper left of Figure 5.3. Erythroblasts (immature RBCs) become normocytes that shed their nuclei before entering the bloodstream. In the bloodstream, the young RBCs, which still contain some nuclear remnants, are called reticulocytes (Figure 5.4). The average number of reticulocytes found in peripheral blood is approximately 1%. A percentage higher than 3% indicates that the individual is actively producing new RBCs because of a loss of RBCs, such as when hemorrhaging occurs. As the reticulocytes continue to mature, they shed their remaining intracellular

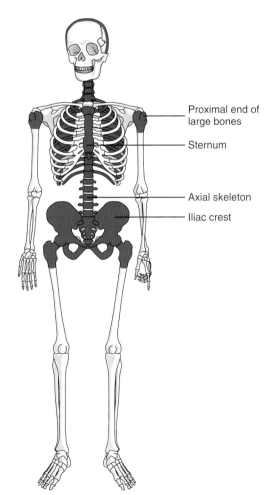

FIG. 5.2 Red bone marrow sites of hematopoiesis. (From Rodak BF: *Hematology: clinical principles and applications,* ed 4, St. Louis, 2012, Saunders.)

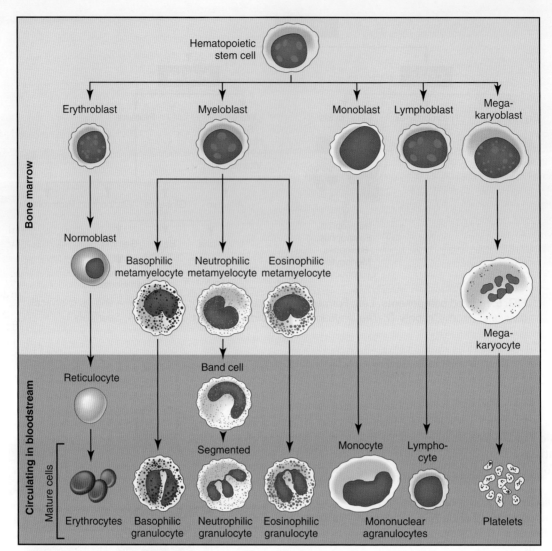

FIG. 5.3 Hematopoiesis. Note the stem cell's differentiation in the bone marrow *(top yellow area)* and immature and mature cellular elements in the peripheral bloodstream *(bottom tan area).* (From Chabner D: *The language of medicine,* ed 10, St. Louis, 2014, Saunders.)

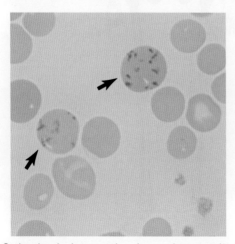

FIG. 5.4 Stained reticulocytes showing nuclear remains *(arrows).* (From Rodak BF: *Hematology: clinical principles and applications,* ed 4, St. Louis, 2012, Saunders.)

nuclear material while retaining millions of hemoglobin (Hgb) molecules (reddish pigment capable of carrying oxygen).

Mature RBCs are biconcave disks filled with a reddish pigment called *hemoglobin.* Hgb consists of an iron (heme) and a protein (globin) molecule. Hgb has a strong affinity for oxygen that it picks up and carries from the lungs to the cells of the body. This oxygen-carrying capacity of RBCs is critical to sustaining life energy throughout the body. Because of their critical role, RBCs account for almost half of the blood volume. After 80 to 120 days, RBCs disintegrate, releasing heme and globin. The iron from the heme portion goes back to the bone marrow to make new RBCs (Figure 5.5). The remaining elements from the heme convert to bilirubin, which is further processed through various stages in the liver, intestines, and kidneys (Figure 5.6).

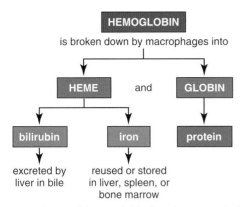

FIG. 5.5 Breakdown of hemoglobin into heme and globin and their further breakdown into bilirubin, iron, and protein. (From Chabner D: *The language of medicine,* ed 10, St. Louis, 2014, Saunders.)

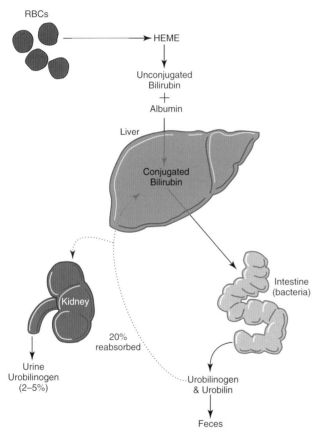

FIG. 5.6 Bilirubin metabolism in the liver, intestines, and kidney. (From Rodak BF: *Hematology: clinical principles and applications,* ed 4, St. Louis, 2012, Saunders.)

White Blood Cells

White blood cells fall into two general categories: granulocytes, consisting of neutrophils, basophils, and eosinophils; and nongranulocytes, consisting of lymphocytes and monocytes.

Granulocytes. Myeloblasts are the most primitive and first identifiable cell in the granulocytic cell line in the bone marrow (see Figure 5.3). The myeloblasts develop into the three kinds of granulocytes: neutrophils, eosinophils, and basophils. Unlike the erythrocyte, the granulocytes enter the bloodstream with their nuclei (the central controlling structure in the cell) in an elongated "band" shape, or in a "segmented" shape. The maturing nuclei of the eosinophils and basophils become segmented into two lobes. The mature neutrophil's multisegmented nucleus is referred to as polymorphonuclear (PMN) or as a *seg.* Compare the shapes for the three mature granulocytes at the bottom of Figure 5.3.

The three mature granulocytes in the bloodstream are distinguished from one another by the staining characteristics of the granules located in their cytoplasm (fluid within cells between the nucleus and the outer cell membrane). When a drop of whole blood is smeared onto a slide and then stained, the three different granulocytic WBCs show an affinity, or attraction, to the *red* acid dye (eosino-), the *blue* alkaline dye (baso-), or *both* colors (neutro-). The WBCs are named on the basis of their *attraction* to the dyes (indicated by the suffix -phil) and have distinct purposes in aiding the body during infection and inflammation.

Neutrophils. Neutrophils have small granules that stain lavender or pink. They are usually the most numerous WBCs seen in the blood because of their constant need to engulf and digest foreign matter, especially pathogenic bacteria.

Eosinophils. Eosinophils have large granules that stain reddish-orange. They increase in number during allergic reactions and parasitic infestations.

Basophils. Basophils have large granules that stain dark blue. Basophils synthesize and store histamine, which helps the inflammatory response. These cells also contain other inflammatory chemicals such as heparin, serotonin, and leukotrienes.

Nongranulocytes (Agranulocytes). Bone marrow also produces the following two nongranulocytes, or agranulocytes, which may have a few or no granules in their gray and sky-blue cytoplasm (refer to the third and fourth column coming from the stem cell in Figure 5.3):

1. Monocytes in the blood develop from monoblasts (immature monocytes) in the bone marrow. They are the largest WBCs and can leave the bloodstream to enter the tissues as macrophages (large, engulfing cells). Their numbers increase during the recovery stage of infection and during the healing of traumatized tissue when debris needs to be cleared.
2. Lymphocytes are the smallest, nongranular WBCs that develop from lymphoblasts (immature lymphocytes) in the bone marrow. They further differentiate into B and T cells, as seen in Figure 5.7.
   - *T lymphocytes* are stimulated by the thymus gland to develop a variety of immune responses toward invaders.
   - *B lymphocytes* become plasma cells capable of producing specific antibodies (immunoglobulins) that destroy or render harmless foreign invaders, especially viruses. (NOTE: The immune response involving T and B lymphocytes is covered in Chapter 7.)

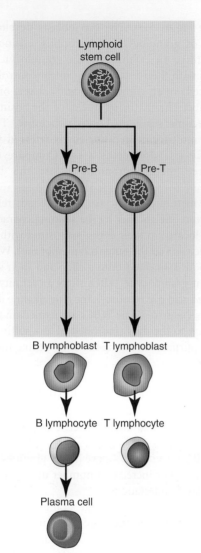

FIG. 5.7 Lymphocytic flow chart showing the lymphoblast differentiating into B and T lymphoblasts and cells. The B cells become plasma cells when they leave the bloodstream and enter body tissues. (From Rodak BF, Carr JH: *Clinical hematology atlas,* ed 4, St. Louis, 2013, Saunders.)

Lymphocytes are the smallest WBCs in the bloodstream. They move freely among the blood vessels, lymph vessels, and tissues as they constantly survey for and respond to foreign invaders.

Platelets (Thrombocytes)

The seventh formed element also comes from the stem cell (hemocytoblast) after it differentiates into a megakaryoblast and then into a **megakaryocyte** (large nuclear cell) in the bone marrow. (Refer to the last column on the right in Figure 5.3.) This very large cell releases fragments of its cytoplasm into the bloodstream, which are seen as small **thrombocytes**, or platelets.

Platelets also release clotting chemicals that activate the formation of sticky fibrin strands that entangle the blood cells and form a clot (Figure 5.8). They gather around the

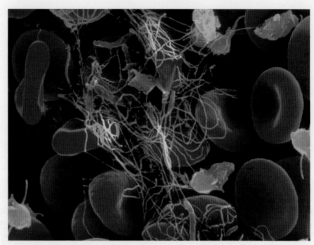

FIG. 5.8 Fibrin strands enmesh the cells and form a clot that plugs the bleeding vessel. (From Chabner D: *The language of medicine,* ed 10, St. Louis, 2014, Saunders. Originally from Page J, et al: *Blood: the river of life,* Washington, DC, 1981, New Books.)

site of a damaged blood vessel in an effort to "plug" the leak (Figure 5.9).

Preparing a Blood Smear to Be Viewed by the Physician or Laboratory Technician

A blood smear can be made by using fresh blood from a gently mixed lavender-topped EDTA Vacutainer tube (Becton Dickinson, Franklin Lakes, NJ) or from a fresh capillary puncture. A drop of blood is placed on the end of a clean slide with a Diff safety device (Becton Dickinson) inserted into the lavender EDTA tube. This device is a convenient and safe way to obtain a drop of blood from the Vacutainer tube without removing the sealed top of the tube. Push the white device into the top of the EDTA lavender tube; then invert the tube and press the device against the slide (Figure 5.10). The pressure on the slide causes a drop of blood to flow onto the slide. A drop of blood can also be obtained from a finger capillary puncture. Next, the drop of blood is spread across the slide by bringing a clean "pusher" slide back into the drop at a 30- to 35-degree angle. As soon as the blood spreads approximately three fourths along the edge, quickly move the pusher slide forward (Figure 5.11). Allow the slide to air dry.

A properly performed smear will look like the one illustrated in Figure 5.12. Improper, unacceptable smears resemble those depicted in Figure 5.13.

Evaluate the smear to see if the following are present:
1. A feathered edge
2. A well-distributed "body" with margins on each side
3. Smooth, thick-to-thin spreading of the smear with no ridges or tails

The smeared blood slide is then stained with either Wright's stain or a Diff-Quick (Becton Dickinson) stain. Both of these staining methods use three ingredients: a methanol fixative, a red acid dye, and a blue alkaline dye. The Wright's stain also uses a buffer solution to change the pH. Refer

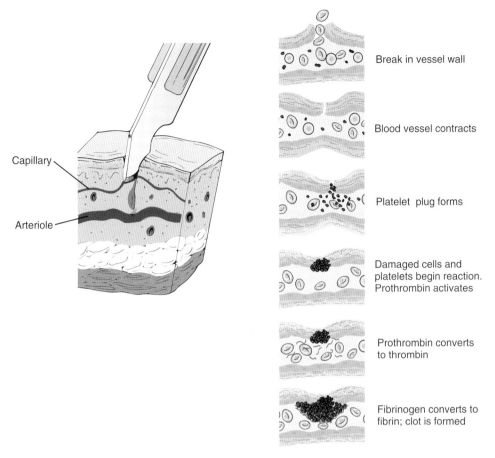

Capillary

Arteriole

Break in vessel wall

Blood vessel contracts

Platelet plug forms

Damaged cells and platelets begin reaction. Prothrombin activates

Prothrombin converts to thrombin

Fibrinogen converts to fibrin; clot is formed

FIG. 5.9 Hemostasis. The damaged blood vessel constricts, platelets congregate, and a fibrin clot is formed. (From Stepp CA, Woods M: *Laboratory procedures for medical office personnel*, Philadelphia, 1998, Saunders.)

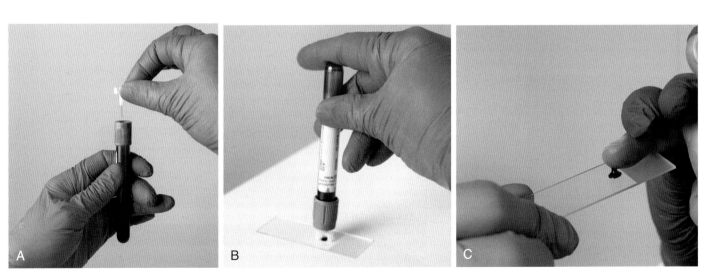

FIG. 5.10 A, One way to apply a drop of blood to a slide for smearing is to push a Safety Diff device into a lavender-topped Vacutainer tube. **B,** Press the device against the slide to deliver a drop of blood. **C,** Another method is to apply the drop of blood directly from a finger stick.

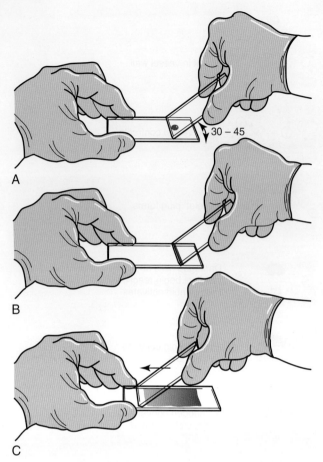

FIG. 5.11 Proper blood smear technique. **A,** Pull the upper slide back into the drop of blood. **B,** Allow blood to spread along the edge of the slide. **C,** Then, with downward pressure, quickly push the slide to the other end until stopped by the fingers. (From Rodak BF: *Hematology: clinical principles and applications,* ed 4, St. Louis, 2012, Saunders.)

to the safety data sheets (SDS) in the workbook and the labels on the bottles when working with stains and take appropriate precautions. The simple Diff-Quick staining procedure used in ambulatory settings is provided in the workbook and is demonstrated in Procedure 5.1 at the end of this section.

Stained blood smears must be observed by the physician, a trained hematologist, or a medical laboratory technician.

White Blood Cell Identification and Differential

The hematologist scans stained blood smears to identify the distribution of the five types of leukocytes on the basis of their staining characteristics, shapes, and sizes. This procedure is called a differential count. See the WBC Atlas, which lists and shows the distinguishing characteristics that are observed for each of the leukocytes. The WBC Atlas is presented on pp. 122 to 123.

Note the following facts found in the atlas for each of the following:

- Segmented neutrophil—most prevalent WBC; fine lavender or pink granules in the cytoplasm and a segmented nucleus (A)
- Banded neutrophil; nucleus has a banded shape (B)
- Small (mature) lymphocyte—second most prevalent WBC: dense circular nucleus and scant blue cytoplasm (C)
- Monocyte—largest of the leukocytes; has large, lacy nucleus (D)
- Eosinophil—has large red granules (E)
- Basophil—least numerous; has large, dark-blue or black granules (F)

Each time a leukocyte is found, the hematologist identifies it and presses the corresponding key on a differential counter (Figure 5.14). After identifying 100 leukocytes, the counter sounds a bell. Each of the five leukocytes is then displayed as a percentage of the total 100 cells identified.

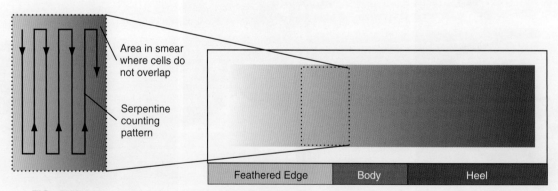

FIG. 5.12 Ideal smear, showing the thinning out of the "feathered edge" on the left with the "body" of the slide for viewing the cells. The "heel" is the thick area of blood cells that were pulled from the drop of blood. Note the serpentine pattern of moving the slide up and over and down and over the body of the smear to observe many different fields without duplicating an area. (From Stepp CA, Woods M: *Laboratory procedures for medical office personnel,* Philadelphia, 1998, Saunders.)

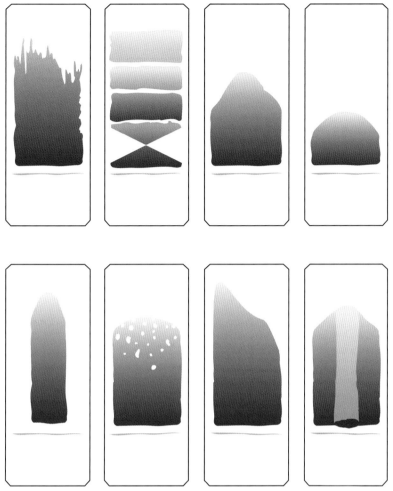

FIG. 5.13 Improper smears resulting from dirty slides and improper pushing techniques. (From Rodak BF: *Hematology: clinical principles and applications,* ed 4, St. Louis, 2012, Saunders.)

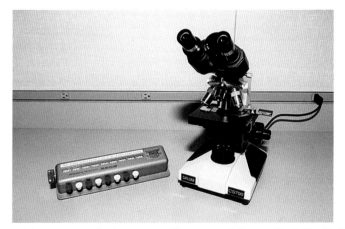

FIG. 5.14 Differential counter and microscope. (Courtesy of Cymar, Carliville, IL. From Proctor D, Adams A: *Kinn's the medical assistant: an applied learning approach,* ed 13, St. Louis, 2017, Elsevier Inc.)

WHITE BLOOD CELL ATLAS

	Cell Type	Cell Size (µm)	Nucleus	Chromatin in Nucleus	Cytoplasm
A	Polymorphonuclear neutrophil (poly, PMN), segmented neutrophil (seg)	10–15	Two to five lobes connected by thin filaments	Coarsely clumped	Pale blue to pink
B	Band neutrophil (band)	10–15	C or S shaped; constricted but no threadlike filaments	Coarsely clumped	Pale blue to pink
C	Lymphocyte (lymph)	7–18	Round to oval; may be slightly indented; occasional nucleoli	Condensed to deeply condensed	Scant to moderate; sky blue; vacuoles may be present
D	Monocyte (mono)	12–20	Variable; may be round or horseshoe or kidney shaped; often has folds producing "brainlike" convolutions	Lacy	Blue-gray; may have pseudo-pods; vacuoles may be absent or numerous
E	Eosinophil (eos)	12–17	Two to three lobes connected by filaments	Coarsely clumped	Pink; may have irregular borders
F	Basophil (baso)	10–14	Usually two lobes connected by thin filaments	Coarsely clumped	Lavender to colorless

A, **Segmented neutrophils**, the most prevalent white blood cell, have fine lavender or pink granules throughout the cytoplasm.
B, **Banded neutrophils** show immature nonsegmented nuclei.
C, **Lymphocytes** are typically the second most frequently seen white blood cell. Note the dense nucleus with scanty cytoplasm.
D, **Monocytes** contain a convoluted nucleus and abundant cytoplasm. They are the largest white blood cell.
E, **Eosinophils** have large, red granules.
F, **Basophils** have large, dark-blue granules.
(Illustrations modified from Carr JH, Rodak BF: *Clinical hematology atlas*, ed 4, St. Louis, 2013, Saunders.)

Granules	Reference Range (%)	Microscopic View
Abundant lavender or pink granules	50–70	
Abundant lavender or pink granules	0–5	
±Few	20–40	
Many fine granules frequently giving the appearance of ground glass	3–11	
Granules are large red to orange, round	0–5	
Large dark blue/black; variable in number with uneven distribution	0–1	

Red Blood Cell Identification and Description

Next, the hematologist observes and reports the appearance of the RBCs. Normal RBC appearance and distribution are shown at the top of the RBC Atlas Figure 5.15.

In a diseased state, the RBCs may become altered in appearance. The three columns in the flow chart (see Figure 5.15) show how RBCs can vary in size (**anisocytosis**), shape (**poikilocytosis**), and color (*hypochromic*, basophilic stippling, and *polychromatic*). The hematologist reports the degree of these variances by using +1, +2, and so on. The following descriptive terms are used for abnormal RBC sizes, shapes, and colors shown in the RBC Atlas (see Figure 5.15).

Red blood cell atlas. Abnormal sizes:
- Macrocytes (large RBCs)
- Microcytes (small RBCs)
- Anisocytosis (varying sizes of RBCs)

Abnormal shapes:
- Target cells
- Spherocytes (ball-shaped round cells, rather than disc shaped)
- Ovalocytes (elliptical-shaped cells)
- Tear-drop shaped cells (dacryocytes)
- Poikilocytosis (varying shapes)
- Sickle cells (collapsed, C-shaped cells)

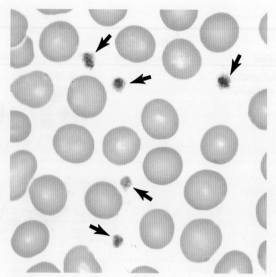

FIG. 5.16 Platelets *(arrows)* among the red blood cells. (From Carr JH, Rodak BF: *Clinical hematology atlas*, ed 4, St. Louis, 2013, Saunders.)

Abnormal colors:
- Hypochromic RBCs (faded color cells)
- Basophilic stippling
- Polychromatic RBCs (multicolored cells—bluish/red in color)

Platelet Description

Platelets (thrombocytes) are also assessed while scanning the slide (Figure 5.16). Their quantity is approximated by the hematologist while observing various fields under oil immersion.

Theory of Hemostasis

The cardiovascular system is equipped with a remarkable mechanism that swiftly stops blood from escaping out of a damaged blood vessel. First the blood vessel constricts, slowing the rate of blood flow. Then platelets concentrate around the damaged site and initiate a clot made of a sticky fibrin mesh (refer to Figures 5.8 and 5.9). The fibrin strands are the result of a complex chain reaction of 13 clotting factors, including the two plasma proteins—**fibrinogen (factor I)** and **prothrombin (factor II)**. It should also be noted that the critical vitamin used by the liver to produce clotting factors (prothrombin) is vitamin K. The formation of the sticky fibrin can be simplified into four steps, as illustrated in Figure 5.17.

After the clot is formed and has fulfilled its purpose, the body stops the reaction to prevent excessive clotting.

Coagulation and Testing

Most coagulation tests are performed at the hospital or reference laboratory to help determine why a patient is bleeding, bruising, or forming clots abnormally.

A patient who is prone to **thrombosis** (an abnormal condition of clotting) may need to take anticoagulant drugs such as warfarin (Coumadin is the brand name). Patients receiving anticoagulant therapy must be monitored on a predetermined schedule, sometimes weekly and then moving to monthly over time. They are tested to see the amount of time a sample of their

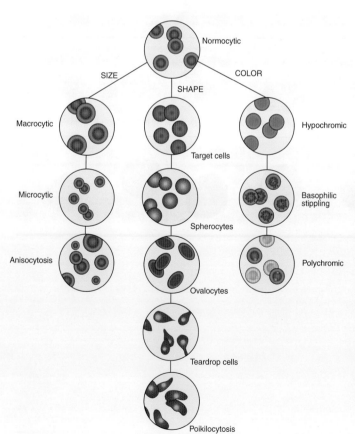

FIG. 5.15 Flow chart with the terms relating to variations in red blood cell size *(left)*, shape *(middle)*, and color *(right)*. (From Stepp CA, Woods M: *Laboratory procedures for medical office personnel*, Philadelphia, 1998, Saunders.)

1. **TISSUE FACTOR, CLOTTING FACTORS, and PLATELETS**

activate

2. **FACTOR X**

which, with calcium and other factors, stimulates the conversion of

3. **PROTHROMBIN** → to → **THROMBIN (an enzyme)**

which changes

FIBRINOGEN → to → **FIBRIN CLOT**

4.

FIG. 5.17 Four steps of the formation of fibrin. (From Chabner D: *The language of medicine,* ed 10, St. Louis, 2014, Saunders.)

blood takes to coagulate. If their blood coagulates too rapidly, they may have an underdosage of their anticoagulant, which may lead to a life-threatening blood clot. If, on the other hand, the blood coagulates too slowly, it may indicate an over dosage of their anticoagulant, which may cause a fatal hemorrhage.

The CLIA-waived testing method for monitoring these patients' coagulation times is called the prothrombin time, or protime test or **PT**. The result of the test is expressed as the number of seconds it takes for the prothrombin to form a fibrin clot in the laboratory. This result is then converted to an international normalized ratio (**INR**). The INR is a mathematical calculation that standardizes the PT result to account for differences between the manufacturer's thromboplastins used to obtain the PT result. The INR provides the physician a standardized test result to determine if the patient's anticoagulation therapy puts the patient in the appropriate range to prevent clot formation. A *normal* INR reading on *all* test methods will

usually have a value of 1. The goal for a patient receiving anticoagulant therapy, on the other hand, is to keep the INR at a standardized 2 to 2.5 and occasionally higher. A therapeutic PT at this level prolongs the clotting time enough to prevent unwanted clotting but not so long that the patient is in danger of abnormal bleeding.

Summary of Fundamental Concepts

This section presented the function, formation, and distinguishing characteristics of the cells and coagulation factors in blood. Procedure 5.1 describes the steps involved in staining a smeared blood specimen. After the specimen has been stained, the physician may identify the cells under the microscope using the WBC and RBC atlases as guides.

The next section, CLIA-Waived Hematology Tests, describes the most common hematology and coagulation tests performed in physician office laboratories (POLs).

PROCEDURE 5.1   Diff-Quick Staining Procedure

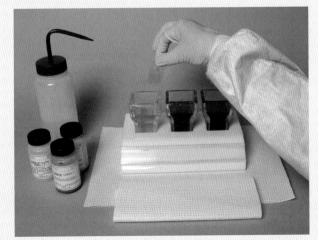

A, The side is dipped in fixative three times and *allowed to dry completely.*

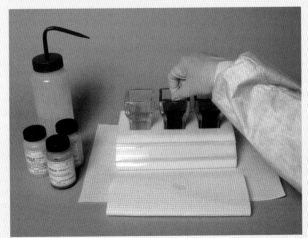

B, The side is dipped into the red eosin dye three to five times.

Continued

PROCEDURE 5.1 Diff-Quick Staining Procedure—cont'd

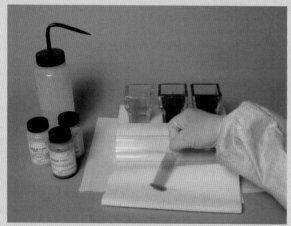

C, The excess dye is allowed to run off onto an absorbent paper.

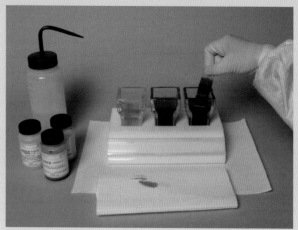

D, The slide is dipped into the blue baso dye three to five times.

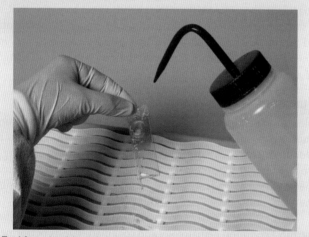

E, After the blue dye is blotted away, the slide is gently and thoroughly rinsed with water on both sides and dried and then brought to the microscope for viewing under the oil immersion lens.

Equipment and Supplies

Diff-Quick stain: fixative, red eosin dye, blue baso dye; staining rack; water source (bottled or running water); bibulous paper

Procedure

1. Dip the slide in fixative three times and allow it to dry completely (Figure A).
2. Dip the slide into the red eosin dye three to five times (Figure B).
3. Let the excess dye run off and blot the rest away with absorbent paper (Figure C).
4. Dip the slide into the blue baso dye three to five times (Figure D).
5. After the blue dye is blotted away, rinse the slide thoroughly with water on both sides and allow it to air-dry (Figure E). It can also be pressed between two bibulous papers to help remove the water.
6. Observe the slide under the oil immersion lens of the microscope. Refer to the microscope skill sheet in Chapter 2 for the proper steps to bring the slide into focus under the oil immersion lens. The cells and platelets will be enlarged 1000 times (100× oil objective times the 10× ocular lens). The slide will show predominantly red blood cells with some small platelet clumps throughout. The challenge is to find the white blood cells (WBCs). The two most commonly found WBCs are segmented neutrophils and small lymphocytes. See the WBC Atlas for assistance in identifying the WBCs.

❖ CLIA-WAIVED HEMATOLOGY TESTS

The most common procedure associated with hematology is the CBC. A CBC generally consists of the following seven laboratory tests: RBC, WBC, platelet counts, Hgb, hematocrit (Hct), differential, and RBC indices. The Hgb and Hct are CLIA-waived tests. The other five tests are moderately or highly complex and are discussed at the end of this chapter.

Four hematology tests have been approved as CLIA-waived hematology tests and can be performed in Certificate of Waiver (CoW) offices: Hgb test, Hct test, erythrocyte sedimentation rate (ESR), and PT test. (Competency skill sheets for each procedure are provided in the workbook.)

Hemoglobin

The Hgb within the RBCs is measured by hemolysis (hemolyzing, or destroying the RBCs) and allows the conversion of Hgb into cyanmethemoglobin. The new color reaction is then expressed as grams per deciliter (g/dL), which represents the weight of the Hgb (g) per the volume of blood (dL). The result is compared with the reference range. Expected Hgb values are as follows:

Men	14–18 g/dL
Women	12–16 g/dL
Children	10–15 g/dL (increases with age)
Newborns	17–21 g/dL

Notice that the Hgb level ranges in women are lower than those in men because women lose blood during menstruation each month during their reproductive years. Newborns are born with high Hgb levels that fall during early childhood and then build up to the adult levels. When any of the patient results drop below their reference range, it is referred to as *anemia*.

Hemoglobin Testing Methods

Common procedural steps in all Hgb tests include the following:

1. Collecting blood into an appropriate testing device
2. Hemolyzing the RBCs to release their Hgb
3. Analyzing the amount of released Hgb by sending a light source through the specimen. The instruments have highly sensitive optical readers that receive the light after it either passes through or reflects off the specimen; the resulting measurement of the light then allows the instrument to calculate the amount of Hgb within the specimen
4. Reading and reporting the digital readout, expressed in grams per deciliter
5. The instruments require daily optics checks and first-time operator verification of competency by using liquid controls. The workbook appendix has a generic quantitative competency check sheet that may be completed to meet the procedural requirements of these test methods. All the control results and patient results must be logged and evaluated by comparing them with their provided reference ranges.

Three common CLIA-waived Hgb test methods approved by the Food and Drug Administration (FDA) that are used in ambulatory care settings are the HemoCue method (HemoCue Inc., Lake Forest, CA), the Hgb meter method, and the i-STAT method (Abbott Laboratories, Abbott Park, IL).

HemoCue Method

The HemoCue method procedure check sheet is provided in the workbook and is demonstrated in Procedure 5.2, at the end of this section.

i-STAT Method

The i-STAT method uses a handheld point-of-care instrument that can be brought to the patient for a rapid assessment of Hgb level and other blood test results (Figure 5.18). NOTE: The i-STAT procedure is presented in Chapter 6, "Chemistry."

Hematocrit

Hematocrit measures the percentage of packed RBCs that develop after centrifuging a specimen and comparing the volume of the packed cells with the total volume of the measured specimen. The packed RBCs are expressed as a percentage of whole blood. Hct expected values are the following:

Men	42%–52%
Women	36%–45%
Children	36%–41% (increases with age)
Infants	30%–40%
Newborns	44%–64%

Notice that the RBCs occupy almost 50% of the total volume of blood in Figure 5.19. Also notice that the numerical values of Hgb are approximately one third the numerical values of the Hct. If a patient's results fall below the expected Hct range, this is considered anemic. A patient with an abnormally high Hct level is referred to as polycythemic. Any abnormal results will be further evaluated by the physician to determine the diagnosis and treatment of the patient.

General Spun Microhematocrit Procedures

Steps common to all microhematocrit procedures include the following:

- Collecting blood into two appropriate capillary tubes containing an anticoagulant to prevent clotting of the specimens (NOTE: Occupational Safety and Health Administration

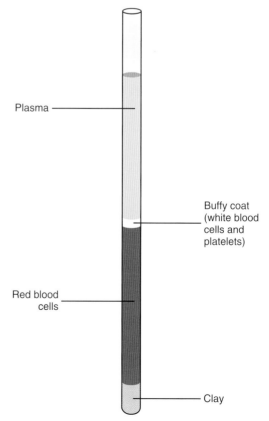

FIG. 5.19 Hematocrit tube layers: plasma, buffy coat, red blood cell layer, and clay sealant.

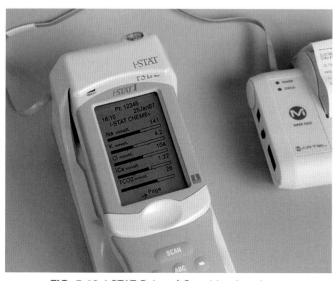

FIG. 5.18 i-STAT Point-of-Care blood analyzer.

safety precautions recommend using plastic capillary tubes, not glass, to prevent possible breakage and blood exposure incidents.)

- Sealing the capillary tubes with clay or a stopper at one end
- Centrifuging the specimens in an Hct centrifuge with the sealed end against the outer rubber gasket or down in the sleeved plastic holder for 5 minutes
- Observing the centrifuged layers: plasma, buffy coat, red cell layer, and sealant (see Figure 5.19)
- Determining the percent of RBC volume compared with the total blood volume by using a built-in scale or a variable volume scale

The results of the two capillary tubes should be within 2% of agreement, and the final result is recorded as the average of the two tubes. If the results of the two tubes are not within 2%, the test should be repeated. Also take note if the appearance of the plasma is red, indicating hemolysis; white, indicating lipemia (fat in the blood); or dark yellow-brown, indicating jaundice. If the specimen shows hemolysis (seen as pinkish-red plasma after centrifugation), a new specimen should be collected to prevent falsely decreased Hct result.

Procedure 5.3, presented at the end of this section, describes the general Hct procedure, and its corresponding check sheet is provided in the workbook.

HemataSTAT Procedure

Procedure 5.4 describes an alternate method for measuring blood Hct in which plastic-covered tubes are rapidly spun in a centrifuge for only 1 minute. The centrifuge has a built-in reading tray that provides a digital readout. A proficiency check sheet is provided in the workbook.

Erythrocyte Sedimentation Rate

The erythrocyte sedimentation rate (ESR) is the rate at which RBCs settle out of an anticoagulated blood specimen after 60 minutes. The result is reported in millimeters per hour. ESR expected values are as follows:

Men <50 years	0–15 mm/hr
Men ≥50 years	0–20 mm/hr
Women <50 years	0–20 mm/hr
Women ≥50 years	0–30 mm/hr

The ESR is a nonspecific screening test to help confirm and monitor changes in inflammatory diseases, autoimmune diseases, carcinomas, and certain forms of leukemia. Patients with these diseases will show ESRs greater than the expected values in the preceding list depending on the amount of inflammation occurring when blood is drawn.

The principle of the ESR is based on the effect of plasma proteins (especially globulins and fibrinogen) produced during inflammatory conditions. These proteins cause the RBCs to become sticky and stack or aggregate together in a rouleaux formation (resembling stacked poker chips) (Figure 5.20). The stacked RBCs fall at an increased rate that is directly proportional to the increased amount of proteins that were produced during inflammation.

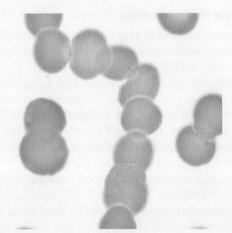

FIG. 5.20 Rouleaux formation causing a high erythrocyte sedimentation rate result. (From Carr JH, Rodak BF: *Clinical hematology atlas*, ed 4, St. Louis, 2013, Saunders.)

The shape and size of RBCs also affect the ESR results. For example, spherocytes fall, causing an increased rate; sickle cells fall at a slower rate, and macrocytes fall faster than microcytes.

Other technical factors, such as the following, can also interfere with obtaining accurate ESR results.

False Increased Rates

- Tilting the test tubes results in an erroneous increase in the ESR.
- Vibrations falsely increase the ESR.
- Extremely hot room temperatures falsely increase the ESR.
- Timing is critical; the results must be read at exactly 60 minutes because taking a reading after the specified time gives a result that is too high.

False Decreased Rates

- Extreme cold room temperatures falsely decrease the ESR.
- Taking a reading before the specified time gives a result that is too low.

Other Interferences

- Air bubbles in the tube interfere with sedimentation by breaking up the specimen and causing an erroneous lower value.
- The blood must be fresh, tested within 2 hours of collection or within 6 hours if the specimen has been refrigerated.

Sediplast ESR System

The Sediplast (Polymedco Inc., Cortlandt Manor, NY) ESR method uses a safe, disposable, calibrated plastic pipette that is inserted into a vial containing a mixture of transferred EDTA blood and a premeasured citrate solution. This closed-system test provides an ESR after allowing the pipette to stand in a vertical rack for 1 hour. The Sediplast procedure check sheet is provided in the workbook and is demonstrated in Procedure 5.5 at the end of this section.

Streck 30-Minute Manual ESR System

A new 30-minute test for ESR is now available. Blood may be collected directly into the black citrate tube or may be transferred from an EDTA tube to the citrate tube. The "Streck" tube is then suspended in the "Streck" rack for 30 minutes. The results are then manually read using the chart provided in the rack. See Procedure 5.6 in the workbook and demonstrated at the end of this section for this safe and timely way to test a patient's ESR.

Prothrombin Time

Prothrombin time is a commonly performed CLIA-waived test that measures the amount of time the blood takes to form a fibrin clot. The PT test uses thromboplastin as the active reagent to initiate the coagulation process by converting prothrombin to thrombin (refer to Figure 5.17 under Fundamental Concepts).

The PT test is used as a *screening* test for patients who lack clotting factors, have a liver disease, or are deficient in vitamin K (a critical element in the production of prothrombin). The PT of these patients will be prolonged, indicating they will be prone to bleeding. The PT test is also widely used to *monitor* patients who require anticoagulant therapy. These patients are taking anticoagulant drugs (warfarin, Coumadin) because they have had a tendency to produce internal clots, which could lead to strokes and heart attacks. The anticoagulant drugs suppress the liver from synthesizing prothrombin. The PT test measures both normal and therapeutic PTs in fresh whole blood.

Results are displayed in PT seconds and INR value. The PT reference range will vary depending on the manufacturer's method of testing and the amount of thromboplastin used in the test.

The normal PT reference range is usually approximately 10 to 13 seconds. The INR value is the patient's PT in seconds divided by the mean normal PT in seconds multiplied by the International Sensitivity Index (ISI). The PT rate for each test lot of thromboplastin is built into the test system. A normal INR should be close to 1.0

The INR is the coagulation value that more accurately compares to other PT test methods when a patient is monitoring his or her PT in a variety of settings. The therapeutic goal is to keep the patient's PT higher than normal at approximately 12 to 18 seconds (depending on the method used), or 2 to 2.5 INR (occasionally higher depending on therapeutic need).

Procedure 5.7, at the end of this section, presents the CoaguChek method, and a proficiency check sheet is provided in the workbook. The CoaguChek method uses a highly sensitive instrument that runs its optics check before each test.

Becoming Proficient at CLIA-Waived Hematology Tests

Now that you have learned about the significance of Hgb, Hct, ESR, and PT tests, take time to complete the following:

1. Answer the questions at the end of this chapter and the CLIA-waived portion in Chapter 5 of the workbook using your structured notes and text.
2. View the videos on-line to see Hgb and Hct testing performed.
3. Perform the Chapter 5 lessons on-line, which were designed to reinforce your knowledge of terminology and CLIA-waived test procedures.
4. Study Procedures 5.2 through 5.7 before your lab.

PROCEDURE 5.2 Hemoglobin HemoCue Method

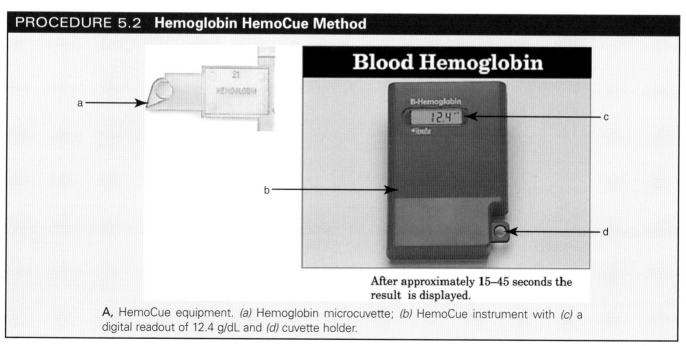

Blood Hemoglobin

B-Hemoglobin
12.4

After approximately 15–45 seconds the result is displayed.

A, HemoCue equipment. *(a)* Hemoglobin microcuvette; *(b)* HemoCue instrument with *(c)* a digital readout of 12.4 g/dL and *(d)* cuvette holder.

Continued

PROCEDURE 5.2 Hemoglobin HemoCue Method—cont'd

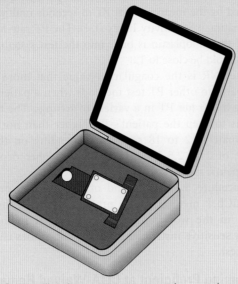

B, HemoCue calibration may use a red control cuvette. (NOTE: Newer models now have HemoCue internal controls.)

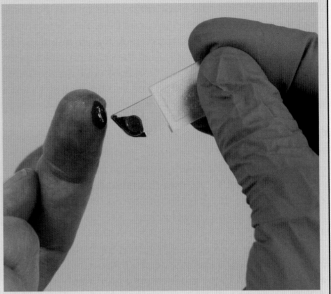

C, Fill the patient cuvette in one continuous process. It should never be topped up after the first filling. Wipe off the excess blood on the outside of the cuvette tip. Make sure that no blood is drawn out of the cuvette in this procedure.

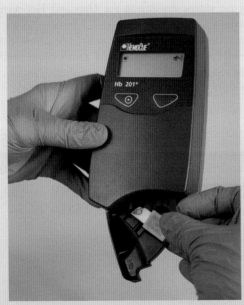

D, Place the filled cuvette into the cuvette holder immediately and push it into measuring position.

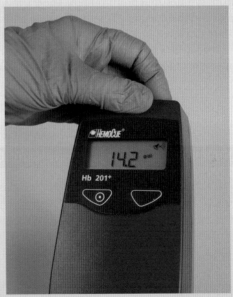

E, Hemoglobin result of 14.2 is digitally displayed.

Hemoglobin Procedure – Preparation -Pre-Analytical

1. Sanitize the hands and put on a fluid-impermeable gown and gloves.
2. Review test information. Figure A
3. Assemble all blood collecting and testing supplies.

Procedure – Analytical

4. Run and log the results of the control cuvette. Figure B
5. Collect patient specimen into the test cuvette. Figure C
6. Place test cuvette into the instrument. Figure D
7. Observe the test results displayed on the Hemocue instrument. Figure E

Follow-Up – Post-analytical

8. Record patient results on the lab log and chart results in the patient record.
9. Properly dispose of the lancets and cuvettes in biohazard waste container & disinfect the work area.
10. Remove personal protective equipment and sanitize hands.

PROCEDURE 5.3 Hematocrit General Procedure

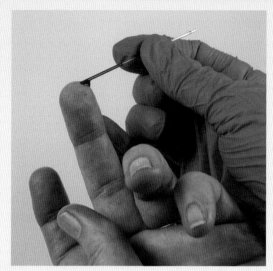

A, Hold the capillary tube in a horizontal position or slightly tipped downward to allow capillary action to pull blood into the tube.

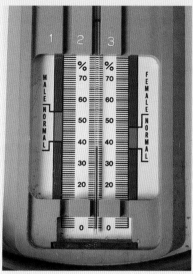

B, When using a built-in hematocrit scale as seen in the illustration, the capillary tube must be filled to the designated line on the capillary tube. (From Bonewit-West K: *Clinical procedures for medical assistants,* ed 10, St. Louis, 2018, Elsevier.)

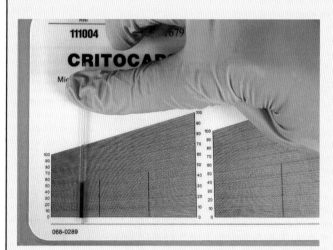

C, This spun blood sample is being read on a variable reader to determine the percentage of total blood occupied by the red blood cells.

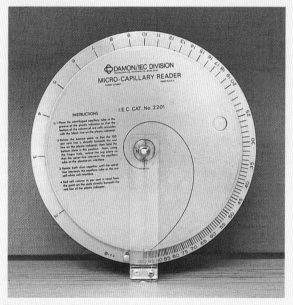

D, This Micro-Capillary Reader is also able to adjust and read various volumes of blood collected and spun during the hematocrit test. (From Rodak BF: *Hematology: clinical principles and applications,* ed 3, St. Louis, 2007, Saunders.)

Equipment and Supplies

- Hematocrit centrifuge with locking cover for safety when spinning the specimens
- Plastic capillary tubes and sealing clay (or self-sealing plastic protected capillary tubes)
- Two liquid controls to check accuracy of high and low hematocrit readings
- Blood specimens used in test—either venous blood collected in *lavender EDTA tube* or *capillary blood* from finger using a lancet, alcohol, and sterile gauze

Preparation—Preanalytical

1. Sanitize the hands and put on a fluid-impermeable gown and gloves.
2. Check the expiration date and storage requirements of all supplies and controls.

3. All first-time operators should run and log results of the controls to check that their technique produces accurate results. Controls should also be run whenever new supplies are used and on days when patients will be tested.

Continued

PROCEDURE 5.3   **Hematocrit General Procedure—cont'd**

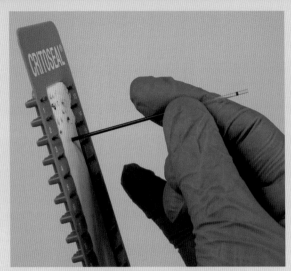

E, Seal the blood end of the tube with clay before centrifuging.

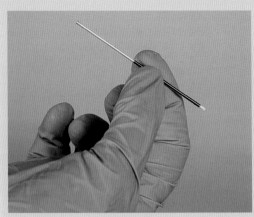

F, This is a safety tube that is coated with plastic and able to self-seal. The capillary collected blood is being tilted toward the sealing clay. When the blood reaches the clay, it automatically seals itself within 15 seconds of contact while holding it in a vertical position.

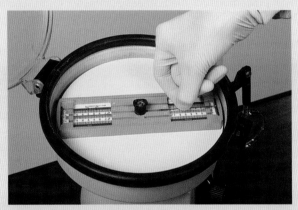

G, The filled tubes are placed opposite each other to balance the centrifuge while it spins the red cells to the bottom of the tube. (From Bonewit-West K: *Clinical procedures for medical assistants*, ed 10, St. Louis, 2018, Elsevier.)

- If a variable scale reader that can adapt to any volume of blood is being used (Figure C or Figure D), the tubes may be filled approximately ½ to ¾ full.
5. Seal the clean end of both tubes with clay, as seen in Figure E, or tip the blood toward the presealed end of the tubes as seen in Figure F, and then hold the capillary tube vertical for 15 seconds to ensure a good seal.
6. Place the tubes opposite each other with their clay ends toward the outside of the hematocrit centrifuge to create a balanced centrifuge (Figure G).
7. Lock the cover firmly against the capillary tubes to prevent breaking and centrifuge for 5 minutes.
8. Use the built-in scale or the variable scales to adjust your total volume (starting where the clay meets the cells and where the plasma meets the air at the top). Then determine the percentage of the total volume occupied by the red cells based on where they align with the plasma on the scale that is being used.
9. Check both readings to see if they are within 2% of each other and then record the average of the two tubes. (NOTE: See the two readings in Figure C: Do their results fall within 2% of each other?)

Procedure—Analytical
4. Collect two heparin-anticoagulated capillary tubes with blood from a finger or an EDTA tube of blood.
- Hold the capillary tube in a horizontal position or slightly tilted down to allow capillary action to pull the blood into the tube, as shown in Figure A.
- Avoid allowing bubbles into your specimen and fill exactly to the line if using a built-in centrifuge scale, as seen in Figure B.

Follow-Up—Postanalytical
10. Results of control and patient should be logged, and the patient results should be charted in the patient record.
11. Properly dispose of the lancets and capillary tubes in the biohazard sharps container and any other blood-contaminated supplies in the biohazard waste container. Disinfect the work area.
12. Remove personal protective equipment and sanitize the hands.

PROCEDURE 5.4 Hematocrit HemataSTAT Method

The HemataSTAT (Separation Technology, Inc., Altamonte Springs, FL) is a rapid portable microhematocrit system that uses replaceable plastic holders and plastic capillary tubes for increased operator safety. It has a built-in reading system that supplies a digital readout.

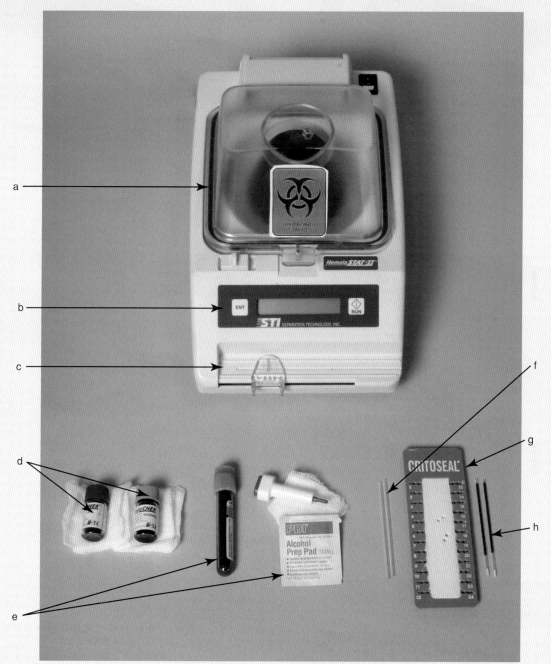

A, HemataSTAT instrument and supplies. *(a)* HemataSTAT centrifuge area; *(b)* HemataSTAT input controls; *(c)* capillary tube reading tray with plastic slider; *(d)* two liquid controls; *(e)* blood specimens used in test; *(f)* two plastic capillary tubes; *(g)* Critoseal plastic sealant; *(h)* two capillary tubes filled with blood and sealed before centrifuging.

Continued

PROCEDURE 5.4 Hematocrit HemataSTAT Method—cont'd

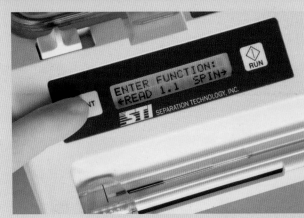

B, HemataSTAT tube reading procedure. With both the capillary tube sealed end and the movable slider all the way to the left, press ENT to "read" according to the display.

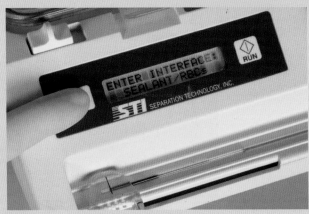

C, Follow the display command to move the slider so the line is directly above the sealant–red blood cell (RBC) interface and press ENT.

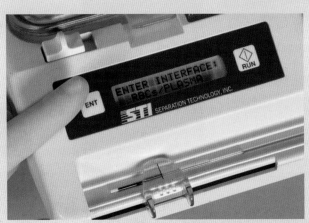

D, Follow the display command to move the slider so the line is directly above the RBC–plasma interface and press ENT.

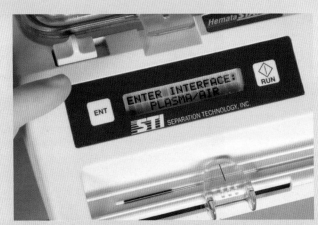

E, Follow the display command to move the slider so the line is directly above the plasma-air interface and press ENT.

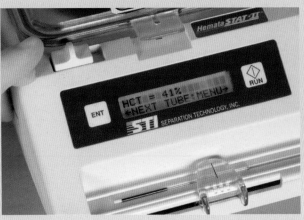

F, Read the final result on the display, record, and press ENT for the next tube.

Equipment and Supplies (see Figure A and Observe the Following)

- HemataSTAT centrifuge with locking cover for safety when spinning the specimens
- Input controls on each side of the digital screen
- Capillary tube reading tray with plastic slider
- Two liquid controls to check accuracy of high and low hematocrits
- Blood specimens used in test—either venous blood collected in lavender ethylenediaminetetraacetic acid (EDTA) tube or capillary blood
- Blood from finger using the lancet, alcohol, and sterile gauze
- Two plastic capillary tubes
- Critoseal plastic sealant for sealing one end of each capillary tube after collecting the blood specimen
- Two capillary tubes that have been filled with blood and sealed before centrifuging

Preparation—Preanalytical

1. Sanitize the hands and put on a fluid-impermeable gown and gloves.
2. Check the expiration date and storage requirements of all supplies and controls.

PROCEDURE 5.4   **Hematocrit HemataSTAT Method—cont'd**

3. All first-time operators should run and log results of the controls to check that their technique produces accurate results. Controls should then be run and logged periodically and whenever new supplies are used.

Procedure—Analytical

4. Collect two capillary tubes of anticoagulated blood; then seal and centrifuge them as directed.
5. Read the two tubes in the HemataSTAT instrument by following the digital screen instructions:
    - With the tube and slider all the way to the left, press ENT to "Read" (Figure B).
    - Move the slider so the line is directly above the sealant–RBC interface and press ENT (Figure C).
    - Move the slider so the line is directly above the RBC–plasma interface and press ENT (Figure D).
    - Move the slider so the line is directly above the plasma-air interface and press ENT (Figure E).
    - Observe the final digital result, record, and press ENT to set the instrument for the next tube (Figure F).
6. Repeat the preceding procedure with the second tube. Check both readings to see if they are within 2% of each other and then record the average of the two tubes.

Follow-Up—Postanalytical

7. Log and chart all results.
8. Properly dispose of biohazard waste materials and disinfect the work area.
9. Remove personal protective equipment and sanitize the hands.

PROCEDURE 5.5   **ESR Sediplast System Procedure**

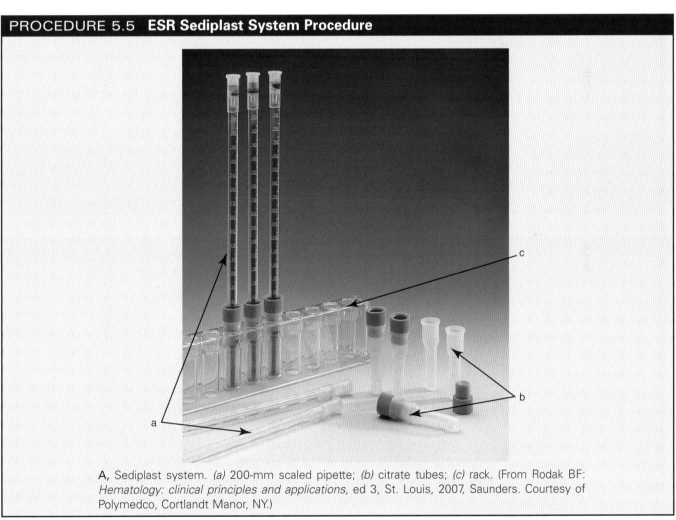

A, Sediplast system. *(a)* 200-mm scaled pipette; *(b)* citrate tubes; *(c)* rack. (From Rodak BF: *Hematology: clinical principles and applications,* ed 3, St. Louis, 2007, Saunders. Courtesy of Polymedco, Cortlandt Manor, NY.)

Continued

PROCEDURE 5.5 ESR Sediplast System Procedure—cont'd

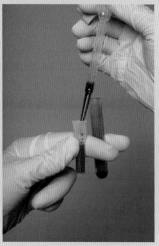 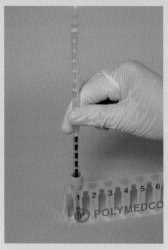

B, Transfer whole blood from the ethylenediaminetetraacetic acid (EDTA) Vacutainer tube to the indicated line on the citrate tube.

Equipment and Supplies (Figure A)
200-mm scaled Sediplast pipette; citrate tubes and rack; fresh venous blood specimen in EDTA (lavender top) Vacutainer tube

Procedure
1. Sanitize the hands and don personal protective equipment.
2. Transfer the whole blood from the EDTA tube to the indicated line on the citrate tube (Figure B).
3. After replacing the citrate tube's pink top and mixing the specimen, place the tube in the rack.
4. Slowly press the Sediplast pipette down fully into the citrate tube so that the blood rises up and over the top of the pipette (Figure C).

C, After replacing the citrate tube's pink top and mixing, place it in the rack. Press the pipette down fully into the citrate tube so that the blood rises up and over the top of the pipette. After 1 hour, measure the red blood cell sedimentation (note the three readings in Figure *A*).

5. After 1 hour, measure the number of millimeters the red blood cell (RBC) fell in the pipette. This number is the RBC ESR (note the three different readings in Figure A).

Follow-Up
6. After recording the results as millimeters per hour (mm/hr) in the patient chart, dispose of the biohazardous pipettes properly and disinfect the work area.
7. Remove personal protective equipment and sanitize hands.

PROCEDURE 5.6 ESR Streck 30-Minute Procedure

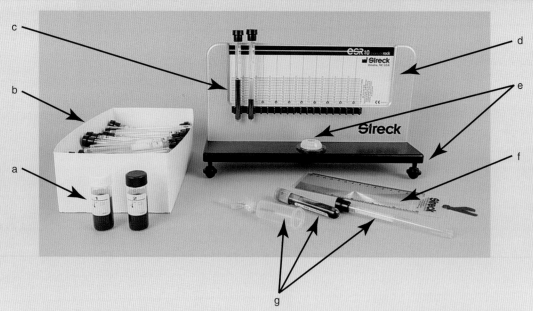

A, Streck 30-minute erythrocyte sedimentation rate (ESR) system: *(a)* liquid normal and high controls; *(b)* black Streck citrate tubes; *(c)* results of normal and high control tubes after 30 minutes; *(d)* Streck rack with mm scale for reading the ESR; *(e)* bubble level indicator and adjustable legs for assuring rack is perfectly upright; *(f)* magnifier for reading results; *(g)* Vacutainer system for drawing ethylenediaminetetraacetic acid (EDTA) tube and/or black citrate tube.

PROCEDURE 5.6 **ESR Streck 30-Minute Procedure—cont'd**

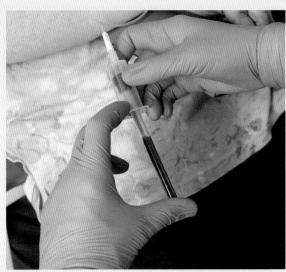

B, Collect the blood in a black-topped Streck citrate tube, making sure to push and hold the tube stopper firmly against the holder. Position the tube in an angle that allows the blood-stream to hit the wall before mixing with the citrate solution to minimize the formation of blood foam. The blood will stop flowing near the indicated line on the bottom of the Streck tube's label. Immediately remove the tube and tilt 8 to 10 times.

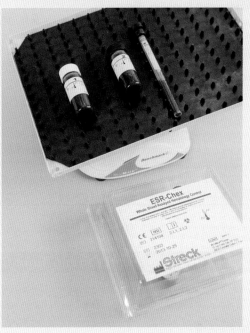

C, Allow the liquid controls and the labeled blood specimen to come to room temperature while mixing thoroughly on a rotating blood mixer for 15 minutes.

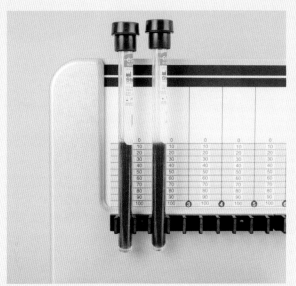

D, Place the ESR vacuum tube in any free position in the ESR-10 manual rack with the stopper in the upright position. Each tube position is marked with a red circle numbered 1 through 10. Align the tube so that the bottom of the liquid's curved meniscus is in line with the zero position on the measuring scale. (NOTE: Do not adjust the position of the tube by pulling on the stopper.)

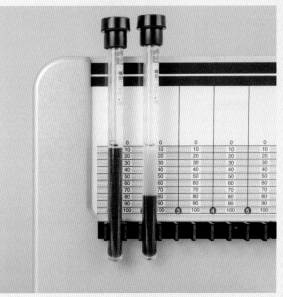

E, After 30 minutes, record the numerical value at the top of the column of sedimented erythrocytes. Report the result as mm/hr Modified Westergren method. The tube on the left shows the red blood cells (RBCs) settled to 4 mm/hr, and the tube on the right (the high control) shows an ESR of 84 mm/hr.

Continued

PROCEDURE 5.6   ESR Streck 30-Minute Procedure—cont'd

Equipment and Supplies (Figure A)

Streck equipment and supplies: black citrate tubes, normal and high liquid controls, balanced rack with built-in reading scale, magnifying reader, supplies for drawing the citrate tube or the EDTA tube to be transferred to the citrate tube

Procedure

1. Sanitize the hands and don personal protective equipment.
2. Collect whole blood into the black ESR citrate tube to the exact volume. (NOTE: If using a butterfly needle, a waste tube will be needed to clear the air from the tubing [Figure B].) Blood from an EDTA tube may also be used. It will need to be transferred into the black tube. In both cases, the blood must be mixed immediately after drawing.
3. The ESR citrate tubes and liquid controls must be mixed on a rotating mixer for 15 minutes to come to room temperature (Figure C).
4. Place the ESR tubes in the ESR-10 manual rack with the stopper in the upright position. Align the tube so that the bottom of the liquid meniscus is in line with the zero position of the measuring scale. NOTE: Do not adjust the position of the tube in the rack by pulling on the stopper (Figure D).
5. Allow the tube to settle in an undisturbed, vertical position for 30 minutes. Then record the numerical value at the top of the column of sedimented erythrocytes (Figure E). Report the result as millimeters per hour using the Modified Westergren method.

Follow-Up

6. After recording the results as millimeters per hour (mm/hr) in the patient chart, dispose of the biohazardous tubes of blood properly and disinfect the work area.
7. Remove personal protective equipment and sanitize hands.

PROCEDURE 5.7   Prothrombin Time CoaguChek XS PT Test Method

CoaguChek is a portable, battery-operated instrument. Its intended use is to determine quantitative prothrombin time (PT) testing in fresh capillary whole blood with the CoaguChek system. The CoaguChek system is intended for use by health care professionals or properly trained patients to monitor oral anticoagulation therapy.

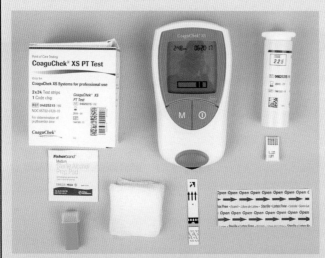

A, CoaguChek XS instrument and supplies (from *left* to *right* and *top* to *bottom*). *Top row,* CoaguChek box holding two containers of 24 test strips each and a Code chip; CoaguChek XS instrument displaying a symbol to insert strip container with code number "220" and 25 strips inside with its corresponding code chip "220" below it (the chip will be placed in the bottom left side slot of the instrument prior to testing). *Bottom row,* Alcohol, lancet, and gauze; test strip in position to be inserted into the CoaguChek XS; bandage.

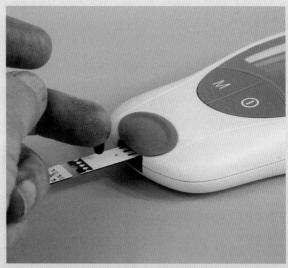

B, After inserting the test strip as far as you can into the meter, incise finger and apply 1 drop of blood to the strip in the meter.

PROCEDURE 5.7 Prothrombin Time CoaguChek XS PT Test Method—cont'd

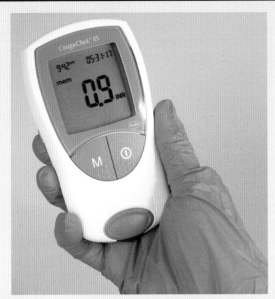

C, The result will appear in approximately 1 minute.

Equipment and Supplies

Figure A

  CoaguChek meter *(E)* with digital readout screen that guides the operator through the procedure

- CoaguChek test strips and code chip

  Alcohol, gauze, lancet, and bandage for capillary puncture site care *(C)*

- Biohazard sharps container *(F)*

Preparation—Preanalytical

1. Sanitize the hand, and don personal protective equipment.
2. Calibration check: If you are using test strips from a new, unopened container, you must change the Test Strip Code Chip. The three-number code on the test strip container must match the three-number code on the code strip.
3. Check the Controls and log.
4. Prepare puncture site by warming and gently massaging.

Procedure—Analytical

Below is a summary of the CoaguChek procedure. A more thorough explanation is found in the workbook skill sheet for Prothrombin Time—CoaguChek Method.

5. When you are ready to test, remove 1 test strip from the container and immediately close the container. Make sure it seals tightly. Do not open the container or touch the test strips with wet hands or wet gloves.
6. Insert test strip as far as you can into the meter. This powers the meter ON.
7. Press Patient Test on the meter display. The meter warms the test strip. Then the meter begins a count down. You have 180 seconds to apply a blood sample to the test strip.
8. Disinfect the finger with alcohol and wipe dry. Perform the finger stick.
9. Hold the incised finger very close to the target (clear area of the test strip) and apply 1 drop of blood to the top or side of the target area and wait until you hear the beep (Figure B). You must apply a hanging drop of blood to the test strip within 15 seconds of lancing the finger. Do not add more blood. Do not touch or remove the test strip while the test is in progress. The flashing blood drop symbol changes to an hourglass symbol when the meter detects sufficient sample.
10. The result appears in approximately 1 minute. The results may be displayed in two ways: the international normalized ratio (INR) or PT seconds (Figure C).

PROTHROMBIN TIME EXPECTED VALUES FOR NORMAL AND THERAPEUTIC WHOLE BLOOD

	INR	PT (in seconds)
Normal	0.8–1.2	6.5 to 11.9 sec for INRatio method*
Low anticoagulation therapy	1.5–2.0	Varies with method used
Moderate anticoagulation therapy	2.0–3.0	Varies with method used
High anticoagulation therapy	3.0–4.0	Varies with method used

*Laboratory reports and manufacturers must supply their own reference ranges along with each patient's results. This is because different methodologies may create different reference ranges as well as different units of measurement.

Follow-up—Postanalytical

1. Discard the strip and any biohazard materials appropriately. The meter will turn off automatically after 10 minutes. Identify any critical values and take appropriate steps to notify the physician.
2. Dispose of waste in the appropriate biohazard containers and disinfect the work area.
3. Remove personal protective equipment and sanitize the hands.

INR, International normalized ratio; *PT,* prothrombin time.

❖ ADVANCED CONCEPTS

Complete Blood Count

Many physicians order a CBC because they want a more complete picture of the internal status of the blood cells. The CBC specimen usually requires a lavender-topped Vacutainer tube with EDTA. EDTA acts as a preservative that maintains the integrity of the blood cells and works as an anticoagulant. Because the CBC consists of some moderately to highly complex tests, the blood specimen is usually sent to a reference laboratory to be tested with highly sophisticated instruments. See the laboratory requisition form in Chapter 1 (see Figure 1.7) and locate the place on the form denoting where to order the CBC and determine the tube that should be used. Then look at a subsequent laboratory report form in Chapter 1 with the results of a CBC seen in Figure 1.1. Notice the elevated WBC count and the elevated neutrophils. This advanced section helps explain what these results may mean.

A CBC generally consists of seven or more laboratory tests that reflect the total count, analysis, and microscopic descriptions of the various cellular elements (seen in the left column): RBCs, WBCs, and platelets (Table 5.1).

1. *RBCs* are counted and reported in millions per cubic millimeter or as a whole number times 10 to the ninth power per liter (International Units [SI]). Totals are then compared with reference ranges established for neonates (newborns), infants, children, men, and women. (Refer to table 5.1.)

TABLE 5.1   Reference Ranges for Complete Blood Count

Test	Neonates	Infants (6 mo)	Children	ADULTS Men	ADULTS Women
1. RBCs (million/mm³)	4.8–7.1	3.8–5.5	4.5–4.8	4.5–6.0	4.0–5.5
2. Hematocrit (%)	44–64	30–40	35–41	42–52	36–45
3. Hemoglobin (g/dL)	17–21	10–15	11–16	15–18	12–16
4. RBC indices					
MCV (μm)	96–108	—	—	82–98	
MCH (pg)	32–34	—	—	26–34	
MCHC (g/dL)	31–33	—	—	31–37	
5. White blood cells (/mm³)	9000–30,000	6000–16,000	5000–13,000	4000–11,000	
6. Differential WBC count					
Neutrophils	≥45% by 1 week of age	32%	60% of children 2 years and older	50%–65%	
Bands (%)	—	—	—	0–7	
Eosinophils (%)	—	—	0–	1–3	
Basophils (%)	—	—	1%–3%	0–1	
Monocytes (%)	—	—	4–9	3–9	
Lymphocytes	≥41% by 1 week of age	61%	59% for children 2 years or older	25.40%	
7. Platelets (/mm³)	140,000–300,000	200,000–473,000	150,000–450,000	150,000–400,000	

From Stepp CA, Woods M: *Laboratory procedures for medical office personnel*, Philadelphia, 1998, Saunders.
MCH, Mean cell hemoglobin; *MCHC*, mean (average) cell hemoglobin concentration; *MCV*, mean cell volume; *RBC*, red blood cell; *WBC*, white blood cell.

2. *Hct* measures the percentage of packed RBCs compared with the total blood volume.
3. *Hgb* within the RBCs is measured. The value is expressed as grams per deciliter and is compared with the reference range.
4. *RBC indices* are mathematic ratios of the three aforementioned tests (Hgb, Hct, RBC count). These RBC tests are valuable for identifying various forms of anemia (a condition in which the RBC or Hgb levels are below normal) and polycythemia (abnormal condition of increased RBCs).
   - The *mean (average) cell Hgb concentration* (**MCHC**) This ratio is commonly calculated in the ambulatory care setting because Hgb and Hct are both CLIA-waived tests. The reference ranges for MCHC in Table 5.1 show a 1:3 ratio of Hgb to Hct, which is approximately 33%. If the patient's values fall below the reference range, the RBCs contain less Hgb than normal. This is often the case in iron deficiency anemia, chronic blood loss anemia, macrocytic anemia, and hypochromic anemia. All these conditions can be confirmed during the microscopic examination of a stained blood smear.
   - The *mean cell volume* (**MCV**) and *mean cell Hgb* (**MCH**) indices compare the Hct volume and the Hgb value with the total RBC count, respectively. By comparing the patient's MCV with the reference range, the *general size of the RBCs* can be determined. If the MCV is less than 80 μm, for example, the RBCs are microcytic (small); if the MCV is greater than 100 μm, the RBCs are macrocytic (large). The MCH indicates the *concentration of Hgb* compared with the average size of the RBCs.
5. *WBCs* are counted and reported in thousands per cubic millimeter or as a whole number multiplied by 10 to the ninth power per liter in SI units. The total WBC count is compared with reference ranges, such as those in Table 5.1.
6. A *differential count* uses a stained blood smear (Figure 5.21). It is performed by identifying and counting each of the five types of leukocytes and then reporting the percentage of each cell after 100 cells have been identified. Locate the five listed rows of leukocytes in Table 5.1 under #6 Differential white blood cell count. The percentage of each WBC type is compared with the reference values shown in the columns for neonates, infants, children, men, and women. The appearance of the RBCs and platelets is also observed and described in the report. The WBC tests are valuable in identifying leukocytosis (an abnormal increase in the number of WBCs), forms of leukemia (various cancers of the WBCs), and leukopenia (an abnormal decrease in the number of WBCs).
7. *Platelets* are counted by approximation on the stained slide or by an automated instrument; platelet counts are expressed in hundreds of thousands per cubic millimeter or in SI units as a decimal fraction multiplied by 10 to the 12th power per liter. The patient's results are compared with a reference range, such as seen in the bottom row of Table 5.1. This information is useful in diagnosing various bleeding and clotting disorders.

Abnormal Complete Blood Count Findings

The CBC gives a complete picture of the RBCs, WBCs, and platelets. High-quality medical care requires that laboratory values always be correlated with the clinical state. For example, if a patient exhibits signs and symptoms of fatigue and hypoxemia (lack of oxygen in the blood), the physician may suspect that a

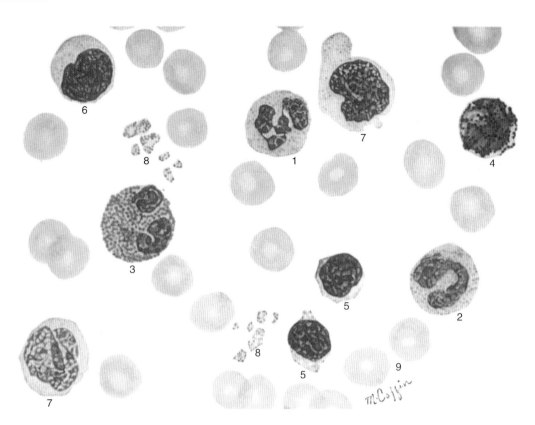

FIG. 5.21 Examples of the seven peripheral blood cells seen in a differential: *1,* segmented neutrophil; *2,* banded neutrophil; *3,* eosinophil with large red granules; *4,* basophil with dark blue granules; *5,* small, mature lymphocytes; *6,* atypical lymphocyte (seen in mononucleosis and acute viral infections); *7,* large monocytes with large convoluted nuclei; *8,* small fragmented platelets; *9,* red blood cells. (From Custer RP: An atlas of the blood and bone marrow, ed 2, Philadelphia, 1974, Saunders)

form of anemia is present. Remember, *anemia* is a condition in which the concentrations of RBCs or Hgb are less than normal. By ordering a CBC and observing all the RBC test results (RBC count, Hgb, Hct, and indices), the physician can then make a differential diagnosis.

Anemias

Below are six examples of causes of anemia in patients.

- *Iron deficiency anemia:* The hypochromic (less than normal color) and microcytic (small) RBCs result from the inability to build healthy Hgb. This is the most common type of anemia and is caused by blood loss or inadequate iron in the diet.
- *Hereditary spherocytosis:* Because of a genetic abnormality, the RBCs have a spherical shape rather than the normal disk shape.
- *Aplastic anemia:* All the blood cell elements show a decrease in aplastic anemia as a result of the inability to produce cells in the bone marrow.
- *Pernicious anemia:* The cells appear enlarged, fragile, and abnormally shaped because the diet is deficient in vitamin B_{12} or because intrinsic factor (a chemical that allows vitamin B_{12} to be absorbed into the blood from the digestive tract) is lacking.
- *Sickle cell disease:* The RBCs collapse into a sickle shape under certain circumstances. This condition is caused by an inherited Hgb-S molecule.
- *Thalassemia* and *hemolytic anemia* produce an increase of reticulocytes (immature RBCs) in the peripheral blood due to RBC destruction (hemolysis) caused by the inherited thalassemia or other hemolytic causes.

White Blood Cell Disorders

The WBC count and differential can also be correlated to the patient's clinical state. For example, if a patient has an infection, the total WBC count may rise as the body fights the infection (leukocytosis). The type of infection can be determined by observing the percentage of each type of WBC in the differential. For example, an increase in the number of neutrophils would indicate a bacterial infection as opposed to an increase in the number of lymphocytes, which would indicate a viral infection. Also, the viral infection referred to as *mononucleosis* is known for the presence of atypical lymphocytes that appear larger than normal. Malnutrition can also result in a decrease in certain types of WBCs, weakening the immune system.

An abnormally low WBC count (leukocytopenia) may be a sign of aplastic anemia, HIV/AIDS, or patients undergoing chemotherapy. An extremely high abnormal WBC count with a decrease in the RBC and platelet counts may indicate leukemia. Again, the stained blood smear will shed more light on the disease process that is occurring. As previously stated, all the blood cells come from one stem cell or hemocytoblast. There are four main classifications of leukemia based on cell type (myeloid or lymphocytic) and on presentation (acute or chronic). The classifications are as follows: acute myeloid leukemia (**AML**—myeloblasts)), chronic myeloid leukemia (**CML**), acute lymphocytic leukemia (**ALL**—lymphoblasts), and chronic lymphocytic leukemia (**CLL**)

CLIA-Nonwaived (Moderately Complex) Automated Hematology Systems

For offices that require more hematologic information than just the waived Hgb and Hct measurements, semiautomated hematology instruments that are CLIA approved as moderately complex may be appropriate. When performing this level of diagnostic testing, the laboratory professional will need to complete the registration, accreditation, and certification process via the Centers for Medicare and Medicaid Services (CMS) and comply with more rigorous quality control and assurance standards, including the documented training of operators and additional quality assurance standards, to include documentation of the following:

- Daily instrument calibrations and standards
- Two levels of controls run routinely
- Maintenance checks of the instrument, temperature, and supplies
- Proficiency testing

To pass the required proficiency testing, the office must run a sample from an outside proficiency laboratory twice a year and submit its results to see if they are within the acceptable range established by the accreditation agency. If the results are not in the acceptable range, the office must take the appropriate steps to correct the problem.

QBC STAR Centrifugal Hematology System

The QBC STAR centrifugal hematology system (Becton Dickinson) provides the ambulatory care setting with more than just Hgb and Hct values. It also provides information regarding the WBC count, platelet count, and distribution of granulocytes (neutrophils, basophils, and eosinophils) versus nongranulocytes (lymphocytes and monocytes). This additional WBC information is helpful when dealing with infections. Whereas neutrophils predominantly fight bacterial infections, lymphocytes fight viral infections. If the patient shows a high total WBC count (leukocytosis), the physician can determine which WBC demonstrates a higher percentage and act accordingly. This information is especially valuable to a pediatrician who needs to know whether a child should start taking antibiotics for a bacterial infection. Laboratory values must always be correlated with the clinical state.

The QBC system spins down a capillary sample of blood into its various layers (RBCs, buffy coat, and plasma). A fluorescent dye and a miniature float within the tube can stain and disperse the buffy coat of WBCs and platelets into three additional layers (granulocytes, nongranulocytes, and platelets). Figure 5.22

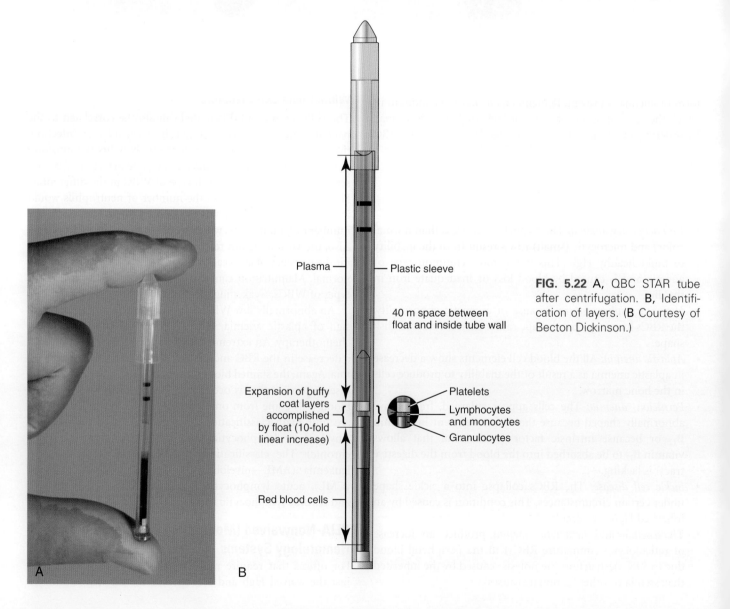

Plasma — Plastic sleeve

40 m space between float and inside tube wall

Expansion of buffy coat layers accomplished by float (10-fold linear increase) — Platelets — Lymphocytes and monocytes — Granulocytes

Red blood cells

A　B

FIG. 5.22 A, QBC STAR tube after centrifugation. **B,** Identification of layers. (**B** Courtesy of Becton Dickinson.)

shows the relative size of the centrifuged capillary specimen and the distribution of the centrifuged cell layers. A laser beam or a tungsten-halogen light beam is then directed at the separated layers of blood cells in the capillary tube to analyze each layer. The light beam strikes the cell layers at an angle, allowing sensors to detect the amount of light scattered and the amount absorbed by the cells. Each type of cell creates a different angle of scatter based on its volume, shape, and refractive index. After all the blood cell layers have been analyzed, the results are displayed and printed.

Quality Assurance

The QBC is a moderately complex instrument that requires regular monitoring with the high and low liquid controls. The control test results must be logged and plotted to detect any shifts, trends, or signs of inaccuracy. Proficiency testing with a specimen from an outside laboratory must also be done twice a year.

■ REVIEW QUESTIONS*

1. Which of the following is not a formed element in the blood?
   a. Platelets
   b. Prothrombin
   c. RBCs
   d. WBCs

2. Match the following terms with their descriptions:
   a. granulocytes
   b. anticoagulant
   c. erythrocytes
   d. megakaryocyte
   e. plasma
   f. platelet
   g. EDTA

   _____ complex liquid in which blood cells are suspended
   _____ most numerous blood cells (occupying almost 50% of the blood)
   _____ WBC group made up of neutrophils, eosinophils, and basophils
   _____ agent that prevents clotting of whole blood
   _____ cellular element important in hemostasis
   _____ most common anticoagulant used in routine hematology procedures
   _____ large bone marrow cell from which platelets are derived

3. Match the following terms with their definitions:
   _____ red cell
   _____ neutrophil
   _____ eosinophil
   _____ basophil
   _____ lymphocyte
   _____ monocyte
   _____ platelet
   _____ band cell

   a. immature neutrophil
   b. has coarse orange-red granules
   c. smallest WBC
   d. largest WBC
   e. has blue-black granules
   f. made of fragments of cytoplasm
   g. biconcave disk
   h. nucleus has two to five segments, and cytoplasm is pink or lavender with granules

4. Provide the missing terms found in the final steps of the common pathway of coagulation:

   _____ → Thrombin

   Fibrinogen → _____

5. Prothrombin (factor II) is a plasma protein dependent on vitamin _____.

6. Match each testing method with its appropriate test:
   ___ HemoCue
   ___ QBC
   ___ Westergren
   ___ HemataSTAT
   ___ Protime

   a. CBC
   b. ESR
   c. coagulation test
   d. Hgb
   e. Hct

7. Match each RBC index with its ratio elements:
   ___ MCV
   ___ MCHC
   ___ MCH

   a. Hgb/RBC
   b. Hct/RBC
   c. Hgb/Hct

8. Match each anemia with its cause:
   __ iron deficiency anemia
   __ hemolytic anemia
   __ aplastic anemia
   __ sickle cell anemia
   __ pernicious anemia

   a. destruction of circulating RBCs
   b. seen with blood loss (menses, ulcers, hemorrhaging)
   c. inherited abnormal Hgb-S molecule
   d. destruction of stem cells in bone marrow from toxins
   e. caused by decreased vitamin B_{12}

9. Match these leukocyte disorders with their descriptions:
   _____ leukocytopenia
   _____ ALL
   _____ mononucleosis
   _____ CML
   _____ leukocytosis

   a. presence of atypical "reactive" lymphocytes
   b. increase in WBCs (usually from infection)
   c. long-term cancer of granulocytes in bone marrow
   d. sudden cancer of a nongranulocyte
   e. abnormal decrease of WBCs

*Answers to these Review Questions are located in the Appendix on p. 278.

Chemistry

OBJECTIVES

After completing this chapter, you should be able to do the following:

1. Define and match key terms and abbreviations in this chapter.

Fundamental Concepts

2. Identify the plasma components in peripheral blood and describe their function and significance.
3. Describe the proper specimen collection and processing for various chemistry tests.
4. Explain the basic principles of glucose and fat metabolism.

CLIA-Waived Chemistry Tests

5. Describe the Beer-Lambert law and the principle supporting the way in which chemical analytes are measured by photometry.
6. Explain the importance of performing instrument calibrations, optics checks, quality controls, and Westgard's rules of quality control monitoring.
7. Perform the following Food and Drug Administration–approved, CLIA-waived tests according to the most current Occupational Safety and Health Administration safety guidelines and the test's objectives, conditions, and standards that are listed in the Procedure Sheets found in the student workbook:
   a. Glucose
   b. Hemoglobin A_{1c}
   c. Lipid panel
   d. i-STAT basic metabolic panel
   e. Fecal occult blood

Advanced Concepts

8. Discuss the use of the handheld i-STAT analyzer for point-of-care blood testing and list the eight critical chemistry tests performed during medical emergencies as seen on the i-STAT CHEM8+.
9. Match chemistry panels with the tests performed.
10. Identify when laboratory reports show chemistry values out of the expected range by comparing patient results with the laboratory's reference range and then use the chart of basic blood chemistry tests to identify a possible disease condition related to high or low patient test results.

KEY TERMS

absorbance photometry: indirect measurement of the amount of light that a solution absorbs

analytes: substances being tested, such as glucose or cholesterol in a blood specimen

anions: negatively charged ions

atherosclerosis: disease in which plaque accumulates along the inside walls of blood vessels resulting in hardening and narrowing of arteries

Beer-Lambert law or Beer's law: states that the concentration of a substance is directly proportional to the amount of light being absorbed at a particular wavelength

carbohydrates: organic compounds, including sugars, starches, and cellulose

catalysts: chemical substances that help speed up the rate of a chemical reaction without any permanent change in themselves

cations: positively charged ions

clinical diagnosis: diagnosis based on the patient's initial signs and symptoms

clot activator: chemical additive that accelerates the clotting of a blood specimen

definitive diagnosis: final, confirmed diagnosis based on clinical signs and symptoms and the results of diagnostic tests

dyslipidemia: abnormal amounts of lipids (fats) and/or lipoproteins in the blood

endogenous cholesterol: cholesterol manufactured in the liver

exogenous cholesterol: cholesterol derived from the diet

galvanometer: instrument capable of measuring small electric currents

glucagon: hormone produced by the pancreas to raise blood glucose levels by converting glycogen into glucose and noncarbohydrates into glucose

glycogen: stored form of glucose found especially in muscles and the liver

glycosylated hemoglobin: hemoglobin A molecule within red blood cells that becomes permanently bound to glucose

gout: form of arthritis caused by accumulation of uric acid crystals in the synovial fluid

hyperglycemia: elevated blood sugar levels

hyperinsulinemia: excessively high blood insulin levels

hyperlipidemia: excessive lipids in blood that may give the blood plasma a milky appearance

hypoglycemia: low blood sugar levels

insulin: hormone produced by the pancreas to move glucose from the blood into the body cells

insulin resistance: condition in which insulin is not effective at moving the glucose from the blood into the cells (seen in type 2 diabetes)

ions: electrolytes consisting of positively or negatively charged particles

ketoacidosis: acidosis caused by an accumulation of ketones in the body, a result of the excessive breakdown of fats; occurs primarily as a complication of type 1 diabetes mellitus

lipoproteins: protein-linked lipids

occult: hidden or not visible to the naked eye

panels: groups of tests that focus on blood cells, particular organs, or metabolic functions

reflectance photometry: indirect measurement of the light that reflects off a solution

synovial fluid: liquid found in joints

trans fats: synthetic hydrogenated fats

transmittance photometry: measurement of the amount of light passing through a solution

troponins I and T: heart-specific indicators of a recent myocardial infarction (heart attack)

ABBREVIATIONS

2-hr PP: 2-hour postprandial (after eating)

A1c: the abbreviated test name for hemoglobin A1c, glycosylated hemoglobin, or glycated hemoglobin

ALP or AP: alkaline phosphatase (also abbreviated as alk phos)

ALT (SGPT): alanine aminotransferase

AST (SGOT): aspartate aminotransferase

BUN: blood urea nitrogen

Ca^{2+}: calcium ion

Cl$^-$: chloride ion

CK or CPK: creatine kinase

DM: diabetes mellitus

FBG: fasting blood glucose

FPG: fasting plasma glucose

GGT: gamma-glutamyltransferase

GTT: glucose tolerance test

HCO$_3$$^-$: bicarbonate ion

HDL: high-density lipoprotein(s), or "healthy" cholesterol

IDDM: insulin-dependent diabetes mellitus (type 1)

iFOB: immunochemical fecal occult blood

Ig: immunoglobulins (antibodies)

IGT: impaired glucose tolerance

K$^+$: potassium ion

LDL: low-density lipoprotein(s), or "lousy" cholesterol

Na$^+$: sodium ion

NIDDM: non–insulin-dependent diabetes mellitus (type 2)

OGTT: oral glucose tolerance test (2-hour postprandial blood sugar)

SST: serum separator tube

T$_3$: triiodothyronine

T$_4$: thyroxine

TC/HDL ratio: total cholesterol compared with high-density lipoprotein

TCO$_2$: total carbon dioxide concentration

TSH: thyroid-stimulating hormone

VLDL: very-low-density lipoprotein(s) (e.g., protein and triglyceride)

❖ FUNDAMENTAL CONCEPTS

Clinical chemistry is the testing of the chemical analytes found in various body fluid specimens, such as urine, whole blood, serum, plasma, synovial fluid (from joints), pleural fluid (from the chest cavity), pericardial fluid (from the sac surrounding the heart), peritoneal fluid (from the abdominal cavity), and cerebrospinal fluid. The specimens most commonly tested in the ambulatory setting are urine and blood.

Chapter 5 details the various *cellular elements* found in blood (i.e., red blood cells [RBCs], white blood cells [WBCs], and platelets) and the blood coagulation process. This chapter deals with the *liquid* portion of blood: plasma.

Blood Plasma

Plasma is a pale yellow, sticky fluid occupying slightly more than 50% of the total blood volume. For a complete understanding of the numerous blood chemistry tests and their significance, the composition of plasma must be reviewed. Refer to the numbered flow chart (Figure 6.1) on the next page regarding each component.

Approximately 90% of plasma *(1)* is water *(2)*, with hundreds of dissolved substances and gases, including the following:

- *Salts (3)*—electrolytes consisting of positively and negatively charged particles (ions) that maintain water balance (e.g., sodium, chloride, potassium, calcium, magnesium, and bicarbonate)
- *Nutrients (4)*—derived from the gastrointestinal (GI) tract after it digests and absorbs carbohydrates (sugars and starches) into glucose, fats into fatty acids, and proteins into amino acids, along with essential vitamins and minerals
- *Waste products (5)*—from cellular and molecular metabolism; carried in the plasma and excreted by the urinary system (e.g., urea, creatinine, uric acid)
- *Hormones (6)*—from various endocrine glands (e.g., thyroid, pancreas)
- *Enzymes (7)*—catalysts produced by living cells that speed up chemical reactions without being chemically changed themselves
- *Proteins (8)*—a major portion of plasma that can be divided into three categories: albumin, globulin, and clotting proteins
- *Albumins (9)*—hold the water within the blood vessels, thus preventing water from leaking into tissues
- *Globulins (10)*—simple proteins further classified into *alpha (11), beta (12),* and *gamma (13);* gamma globulins are also called immunoglobulins (**Ig** or antibodies)
- *Fibrinogen (14)* and *prothrombin (15)*—clotting proteins produced by the liver (when these clotting factors have been

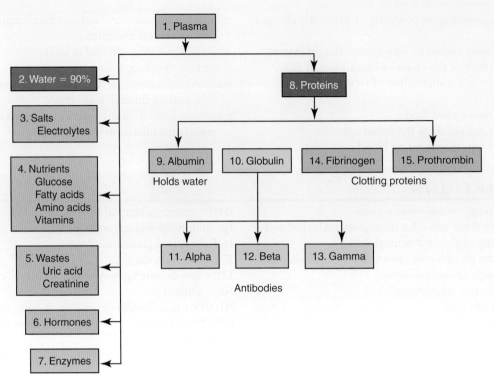

FIG. 6.1 Plasma flow chart.

removed from plasma during the clotting process, the remaining fluid is referred to as *serum*

Blood plasma is a dynamic, ever-changing fluid that reflects the inner workings of internal organs and tissues. In good health, the body is constantly producing or removing various chemical products within the plasma to maintain homeostasis. When disease strikes a particular organ or body system, homeostasis is interrupted, and a change is seen in the blood chemistry. The measured change in blood chemistry allows a physician to detect or confirm the clinical diagnosis (diagnosis made on the basis of the patient's initial signs and symptoms). Follow-up chemistry tests allow the physician and patient to monitor the progress of the disease.

Blood Chemistry Specimens
Reference Laboratory Specimens for Blood Chemistry Testing

Blood chemistry tests derived from a reference laboratory generally require a *serum specimen,* which is obtained from a coagulated (clotted) blood specimen. The vacuum tube of choice for serum specimens is usually the gold serum separator tube (**SST**) containing a gel and a clot activator (a chemical additive that accelerates the clotting of the blood specimen). To form a dense clot, the SST containing the blood specimen must sit for a minimum of 30 minutes after being drawn. The clotted specimen is then centrifuged for 20 minutes at a speed of 3000 revolutions per minute (rpm). Note: The specified time and rpm and the G-force (*g*) are dictated by your reference lab and your centrifuge. For example, Becton Dickinson's recommendations are the following: centrifuge at "full speed" (between 1100 *g* and 1300 *g*) for 10 minutes using swing-head centrifuges

or centrifuge for 15 minutes with fixed-angle centrifuges using balanced tubes in the centrifuge.

The centrifugation forces the clotted cells to the bottom of the tube. Also during centrifugation, the gel migrates up over the cells, separating the serum from the clot. Figure 6.2A and B, show the SST specimen (gold-topped tube) before and after centrifugation, and Figure 6.2C, shows the serum from a centrifuged red-topped "clot" tube.

Some chemical analytes may be affected by the clot activator or gel in the SST tube, so the laboratory may request to collect the serum specimen in a plain red-topped tube that allows the blood to clot with no additives (see Figure 6.2C). The serum would then be separated off the clot into a properly labeled tube.

Be sure to check the reference laboratory requisition (or the laboratory reference manual) to confirm the correct tube to draw for the ordered analyte(s). In the sample laboratory requisition illustrated in Figure 6.3, located on page 148 note the required tubes for individual chemistry tests based on their indicated color codes (seen in the bottom left of the requisition):

- G for gold or gel found in the SSTs—yields a serum specimen that is separated from the clot
- R for red-topped "clot" tubes—yields a serum specimen with no clot activators or gel
- P for purple ethylenediaminetetraacetic acid (EDTA) anticoagulant tubes—note the listed hematology tests that were performed in Chapter 5 that require an EDTA tube ("P")
- Light (Lt.) blue for sodium citrate anticoagulant—for coagulation testing (prothrombin time and activated partial thromboplastin time [APTT])

Also, notice the list of *panels* on the sample reference laboratory requisition on page 148. Panels are groups of tests that

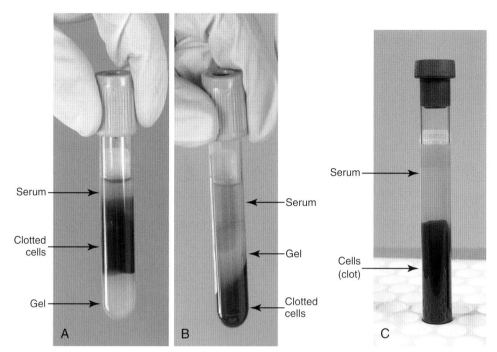

FIG. 6.2 A, Gold serum separator tube (SST) before centrifugation. Note the position of the gel on the bottom. **B,** Gold SST after centrifugation. Note that the gel now separates the serum from the clotted cells. **C,** Centrifuged red-topped "clot" tube with no gel or clotting additive. (Modified from Bonewit-West K: *Clinical procedures for medical assistants,* ed 10, St. Louis, 2018, Elsevier.)

give results on either blood cells (e.g., complete blood count [CBC] panels), particular organs (e.g., Hepatic Panel), or metabolic functions (e.g., Met. Panel, Basic, and Complete Met. Panel [CMP]). A panel of tests can usually be run on one analyzer with one serum specimen at a much lower cost than a series of individual tests. (The various panels of tests run in reference laboratories are discussed later in this chapter.) The listings of the panels, urine tests, and individual blood tests are each organized in alphabetical order on the requisition.

The required blood specimens for chemistry testing differ depending on which analyte is being tested and what testing method is used at the reference laboratory or ambulatory setting. See Figure 6.4 on page 149 showing the proper specimen collection and handling requirements for a comprehensive metabolic profile as presented in a laboratory directory or an electronic medical record. It is critical that *all* the steps are followed to obtain accurate and reliable results. Also note the causes for rejection of a specimen.

Physician's Office Laboratory Specimens for CLIA-Waived Chemistry Tests

The most common specimen in the physician's office laboratory (POL) for waived chemistry tests is a capillary puncture *whole blood* specimen. The blood is usually collected in a capillary tube containing an anticoagulant or directly into a testing device within a specified time frame. Testing devices may test the whole blood specimen directly, or they may separate the plasma from the whole blood before testing. The manufacturer's instructions must be read and followed for each procedure

to determine the exact type of specimen that should be used for each waived test.

Some waived tests may also use a venous anticoagulated whole blood specimen in place of the capillary blood specimen. Once again, only tubes designated by the manufacturer should be used. The following are examples of CLIA-waived specimens:

- *Glucose testing* may be run with the whole blood from a capillary puncture or venous blood specimen collected in a *gray-topped tube* or *lavender (purple) topped tube.* The gray tube contains an antiglycosylating additive that prevents the glucose from being metabolized by RBCs. NOTE: Some point of care glucose monitors do not work with the gray-topped blood specimens but do work with the lavender-topped tubes. Therefore, always refer to the manufacturer's directions regarding the appropriate colored tube to use.
- Glycosylated hemoglobin (hemoglobin A_{1c} molecule within RBCs that becomes permanently bound to glucose) can be performed with a capillary puncture specimen or a venous blood specimen collected in a *lavender-topped hematology tube.*
- *Cholestech* (Cholestech Corp., Hayward, CA) lipid tests must be run with whole blood from either a capillary puncture specimen or a venous blood specimen collected in a *green-topped tube* containing the anticoagulant *lithium heparin.* (NOTE: Green-topped *sodium* heparin tubes should *not* be used because they will interfere with the Cholestech testing method.)
- The *i-STAT instrument* provides basic metabolic chemistry tests from whole blood drawn into a *green lithium heparin tube* that is then transferred to a syringe for loading the blood into the test cassette.

Patient Name:_____ DOB:_____ SS#:_____

Ordering Physician Signature:_____ Date:_____

Routine:_____ Standing Order:_____ Fasting:_____ Nonfasting:_____

Diagnosis Code: 1._____ 3._____
                2._____ 4._____

Copy to:

_____

Panels		**Prostate Testing**	
_____ CBC w/Diff	P	_____ PSA Diag	G
_____ CBC without Diff	P	_____ PSA M-Screening	G
_____ Electrolyte Panel	G		
_____ Hepatic Panel	G	**Thyroid Specific Testing**	
_____ Hgb and Hct	P	_____ TSH	G
_____ Lipid Panel	G	_____ T4 (Thyroxine)	G
_____ Met. Panel, Basic	G	_____ T3 Uptake	G
_____ Met. Panel, CMP	G	_____ Thyroid Panel w/TSH	G
_____ Renal Function Panel	G		

Urine Testing		**Testing by Alpha**	
_____ U/A w/Micro		_____ 2 hr GTT	G
_____ Urinalysis-dip only		_____ 3 hr GTT	G
Individual Chemistry		_____ 5 hr GTT	G
_____ Alk Phos (ALP)	G	_____ Albumin	G
_____ BUN	G	_____ Amylase	G
_____ Calcium, Serum	G	_____ APTT	Lt. Blue
_____ Cholesterol	G	_____ Bilirubin-Dorest	G
_____ CK, Creat. Kinase Tot.	G	_____ Bilirubin-Total	G
_____ FSH	G	_____ Chloride	G
_____ Glucose	G	_____ CO_2	G
_____ Hemoglobin, A1c	P	_____ Digoxin	R
_____ H. Pylori	G	_____ HDL Cholesterol	G
_____ Iron	G	_____ LD Lactate Dehyd.	G
_____ Iron Panel, incl. binding	G	_____ Mono Test	R
_____ K (potassium)	G	_____ Phenytoin	R
_____ Magnesium	G	_____ Platelet Count	P
_____ Na (sodium)	G	_____ Preg. Test	G
_____ Phosphorus	G	_____ RPR	G
_____ Prothrombin Time	Lt. Blue	_____ Protein, Total	G
_____ Rheumatoid Factor	G	_____ Tegretol	G
_____ RA Titer	G	_____ TIBC	G
_____ Sed Rate	P	_____ Triglycerides	G
_____ SGOT (ALT)	G	_____ Valproic Acid	R
_____ SGPT (AST)	G		
_____ Uric Acid	G		

G = Gold gel (SST tube)
R = Red (clot tube)
P = Purple (EDTA tube)
Lt. Blue = (sodium citrate)

FIG. 6.3 Sample lab requisition showing the required patient information at the top; two columns of tests divided into panels, individual tests, and alpha tests; and the codes for the colored tubes at the bottom left.

Comprehensive Metabolic Profile

CPT Code:	80053

Tests included: albumin, albumin/globulin ratio (calculated), alkaline phosphatase, ALT, AST, BUN/creatinine ratio (calculated), calcium, carbon dioxide, chloride, creatinine, globulin, glucose, potassium, sodium, total bilirubin, total protein.

Type of specimen:	Serum
Amount:	4 ml
Collection supplies:	SST (send entire tube)
Collection techniques:	Let SST stand for 30 minutes. Centrifuge SST within 45 minutes of collection to separate serum from cells with gel barrier.
Patient preparation:	Patient should fast for 12 to 14 hours prior to collection.
Handling and storage:	Refrigerate or store at room temperature. Stable at room temperature for 24 hours and stable in the refrigerator for 72 hours.
***Causes for rejection:**	Nonfasting specimen, hemolysis, improper labeling of tube
Reference range:	Values given with report.

Use:
The CMP is used as a screening test to assess the overall health of an individual. It is used to detect any changes in the body's biologic processes that may be present, although the patient may not have had any symptoms to indicate these changes have occurred. Also see uses of individual tests.

Limitations:	See individual tests for limitations.
Methodology:	See individual tests for methodologies.

FIG. 6.4 Note all the criteria for collecting an acceptable blood specimen for a comprehensive metabolic profile (CMP) dictated by the laboratory's directory. Also note the causes for rejecting a specimen. *ALT,* Alanine aminotransferase; *AST,* aspartate aminotransferase; *BUN,* blood urea nitrogen; *SST,* serum separator tube. (From Bonewit-West K: *Clinical procedures for medical assistants,* ed 10, St. Louis, 2018, Elsevier.)

Glucose and Lipid Metabolism

In the ambulatory care setting, the most common CLIA-waived chemistry tests are designed to screen and monitor glucose and lipid metabolism. These in-office tests allow the physician to receive results immediately and counsel patients while they are still in the office. The physician may then order additional diagnostic tests from the reference laboratory to reach a definitive diagnosis (the final, confirmed diagnosis based on the initial clinical signs and symptoms of the patient compared with the results of the tests from the reference laboratory).

Glucose Metabolism

Glucose is a simple six-carbon sugar that all cells and tissues require for life-giving energy. Glucose enters the blood after the digestion of carbohydrates. When glucose is in the blood, it is distributed, metabolized, and processed in the following cells, tissues, and organs:

- Body cells—all absorb blood glucose for energy
- Muscles—use glucose for energy and store excess glucose as glycogen (a stored form of glucose found especially in the muscles and liver) for future needs
- Adipose tissues (fat)—absorbs triglycerides, which are the storage form of excess energy.
- Liver—converts excess glucose into glycogen or combines excess glucose with fatty acids to produce triglycerides

Glucose levels in the blood must be maintained within a homeostatic range of 70 to 100 mg/dL. The monitoring and control of glucose levels within this range are regulated by two

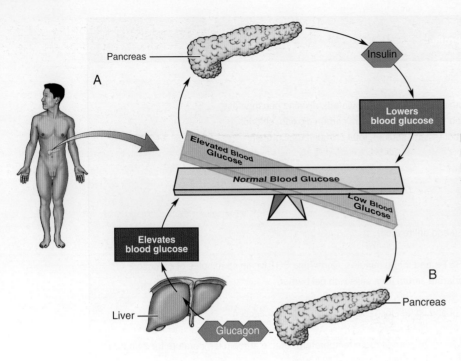

FIG. 6.5 Homeostatic balancing of glucose levels. **A,** When the glucose level is too high, insulin lowers it to normal. **B,** When the glucose level is too low, glucagon raises it to normal. (From Herlihy M: *The human body in health and illness,* ed 5, St. Louis, 2014, Saunders.)

hormones: insulin and its antagonist, glucagon (Figure 6.5). Both hormones are produced by the islets of Langerhans within the pancreas to prevent hyperglycemia (abnormally high blood sugar levels) and hypoglycemia (abnormally low sugar levels).

When glucose levels rise, as seen after eating, the hormone insulin is secreted from the beta cells within the islets of Langerhans to lower the glucose levels and prevent hyperglycemia. *Insulin reduces the level of plasma glucose* by (1) promoting movement of glucose from the blood into body cells, (2) stimulating the conversion of glucose to glycogen in the liver and muscles, and (3) stimulating the conversion of glucose and fatty acids into triglycerides within the liver and adipose tissues.

When blood glucose levels decrease, as during fasting, the hormone glucagon is secreted from alpha cells within the islets of Langerhans to raise blood glucose levels and prevent hypoglycemia. *Glucagon increases plasma glucose* levels by stimulating the conversion of the stored glycogen in the liver and muscles back into glucose and then releasing the glucose into the blood.

Diabetes Mellitus

Diabetes mellitus (**DM**) is a disorder of carbohydrate metabolism characterized by hyperglycemia (elevated blood sugar levels) and glycosuria (sugar in the urine) resulting from the inadequate production or use of insulin. DM occurs when the pancreas is unable to produce enough insulin to move the glucose from the blood into the body cells.

There are several types of diabetes.

Insulin-dependent diabetes mellitus (type 1). Insulin-dependent diabetes mellitus (**IDDM**) occurs in 5% to 10% of the diabetic population. It is the result of an autoimmune destruction of the pancreatic beta cells, which are then unable to produce insulin. Without insulin, the body cannot move glucose out of the blood and into the tissues. Consequently, patients

with IDDM must constantly monitor their blood sugar levels and inject the appropriate amount of insulin to prevent the harmful effects of hyperglycemia. If glucose levels remain high for long periods, the following severe complications may occur:

- *Microvascular problems* can lead to kidney disease and renal failure; retinopathy and blindness; and poor circulation in the extremities (e.g., the feet), resulting in recurring infections that may result in gangrene and amputation
- *Cardiovascular problems* make the heart vessels more prone to formation of fatty plaque along the inside walls of the arteries may lead to atherosclerotic heart disease, hypertension, and stroke.
- Ketoacidosis, a dangerous blood condition, may lead to diabetic coma. Ketoacidosis occurs in IDDM when insulin is not present and the cells do not receive their glucose. It is the result of the body's effort to obtain its energy from fat rather than glucose. The byproducts of the fat breakdown are ketones, which eventually make the blood dangerously acidic. When blood acidity and glucose levels are excessive, the patient may become comatose.

By frequently monitoring glucose levels, the patients with IDDM are able to administer insulin to keep blood glucose levels in a normal range, thus preventing the harmful effects of hyperglycemia and ketoacidosis. These patients can also keep glucose levels in control by following a low-carbohydrate diet and exercising.

Non–insulin-dependent diabetes mellitus (type 2). Non–insulin-dependent, or type 2, diabetes mellitus (**NIDDM**) accounts for 90% to 95% of the diabetic population. It has become epidemic in the United States because of the increasing numbers of obese, sedentary individuals. These individuals generally produce insulin, but it cannot effectively move the glucose from the blood into the cells, a condition known as insulin resistance. This ineffectiveness of insulin's response to

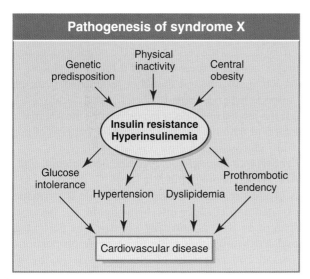

FIG. 6.6 Pathogenesis of syndrome X, also known as *metabolic syndrome.* (Courtesy of Dr. P E Belchetz and Dr. Peter J Hammond. From Belchetz P, Hammond P: *Mosby's color atlas and text of diabetes and endocrinology,* St. Louis, 2003, Mosby.)

TABLE 6.1 Comparison of Type 1 and Type 2 Diabetes Mellitus		
	Type 1	**Type 2**
Features	Usually occurs before age 30 Abrupt, rapid onset Little or no insulin production Thin or normal body weight at onset Ketoacidosis often occurs	Usually occurs after age 30 years Gradual onset; asymptomatic Insulin usually present 85% are obese Ketoacidosis seldom occurs
Symptoms	Polyuria (glycosuria promotes loss of water) Polydipsia (dehydration causes thirst) Polyphagia (tissue breakdown causes hunger)	Polyuria sometimes seen Polydipsia sometimes seen Polyphagia sometimes seen
Treatment	Insulin	Diet; oral hypoglycemic or insulin

From Chabner D: *The language of medicine,* ed 10, St. Louis, 2014, Saunders.

glucose is referred to as *impaired glucose tolerance* (**IGT**). Over time, IGT may then lead to hyperinsulinemia (excessive blood insulin levels). Hyperinsulinemia causes abnormal amounts of fat levels in the blood (dyslipidemia) that lead to atherosclerosis (the formation of plaque along the inside walls of blood vessels) and hypertension. The cascade effect of NIDDM that begins with insulin resistance and hyperinsulinemia, which then leads to high blood pressure and heart disease, has been described as *metabolic syndrome* (Figure 6.6).

If individuals with NIDDM do not maintain control of their high glucose levels, they incur the same microvascular and cardiovascular complications as patients with uncontrolled IDDM. Research has shown that if individuals with NIDDM are diagnosed early, they can begin diet management, exercise, and the use of oral hypoglycemic medication to bring their sugar levels down. They may then avoid developing any of the negative complications caused by abnormally high blood sugar levels.

Table 6.1 summarizes the differences between type 1 and type 2 diabetes.

Prediabetes. Prediabetes is the state that occurs when blood glucose levels are higher than normal but not high enough for a diagnosis of diabetes. Studies have shown that type 2 diabetes develops in most people with prediabetes within 10 years. Studies have also shown that people with prediabetes can prevent or delay the development of type 2 diabetes by up to 58% through changes in lifestyle that include modest weight loss with diets containing fewer refined carbohydrates (i.e., sugars and processed flour) and regular exercise.

Gestational diabetes. Gestational diabetes occurs during pregnancy. The mother's IGT usually subsides after delivery of the baby. Signs and symptoms of gestational diabetes include glucosuria, hyperglycemia, excessive weight gain in the mother, and a baby weighing 9 lb or more. Women who have gestational diabetes are also prone to developing type 2 diabetes later in life.

Transient diabetes. Individuals may have diabetes during acute illness or when being administered steroid therapy. This form of diabetes usually lasts as long as the condition or treatment continues and then subsides.

Blood Glucose Screening and Monitoring Tests

The American Diabetes Association recommends three tests to identify type II diabetes and prediabetes in the early stages: the fasting plasma glucose (**FPG**) test, the oral glucose tolerance test (**OGTT**), and the A1c. The blood glucose levels measured from these tests determine whether an individual has prediabetes or diabetes. The POL may perform CLIA-waived whole blood glucose tests that act as a screening test for potential patients with diabetes. If the results of the screening tests are high, they must be confirmed by the plasma test or serum test methods that are usually performed by moderately complex reference laboratories.

Fasting blood glucose. For a fasting blood glucose (**FBG**) test, a patient's fasting sample is usually taken in the morning after a fast of 10 to 14 hours. Patients cannot have any food from 10 PM on the night before until the test the next morning. Usually, they may drink only water, but check your institutional protocol for fasting preparations regarding proper timing, dietary restrictions, and medications. The patient's FBG level should be less than 100 mg/dL. If the FBG level is between 100 and 126 mg/dL on 2 different days, the patient is considered prediabetic. If the FBG level is greater than 126 mg/dL, the patient is considered diabetic (based on American Diabetes Association criteria). CLIA-waived glucose tests are for screening only and should be followed up with the more complex plasma tests for blood glucose measurements. A definitive diagnosis is usually made with a venous specimen that has been collected in a gray-topped tube.

Oral glucose tolerance test or 2-hour postprandial blood sugar. Another method of screening for diabetes mellitus is the

OGTT, also called a 2-hour postprandial blood sugar (**2-hr PP**). The OGTT begins with the measurement of FBG level. If the results are within an acceptable range after the initial test, the patient is given a glucose-rich drink (75 g of glucose), or a high carbohydrate meal and retested after 2 hours. Normal blood glucose levels should be lowered to less than 140 mg/dL 2 hours after the drink or a meal. If the glucose level does not fall below 140 mg/dL but is not greater than 200 mg/dL, the patient is considered prediabetic. If the glucose level is greater than 200 mg/dL after 2 hours, the patient is considered diabetic.

Random glucose test. A blood specimen can also be collected at any time to see if the glucose level is within the normal range of less than 140 mg/dL. A glucose level of 140 to 200 mg/dl is considered prediabetic. A random blood specimen with a glucose level greater than 200 mg/dL is indicative of diabetes.

Glucose tolerance test. A more thorough test for measuring an individual's glucose metabolism is the full glucose tolerance test (**GTT**), in which blood glucose levels are measured at fasting and then at 1-hour intervals for 2 to 6 hours. The test generally takes place at a reference laboratory or hospital outpatient laboratory.

The GTT can be used to screen for type 2 diabetes. It begins the same way the OGTT does, in that the patient is fasting and is initially tested for blood glucose level. If the results of the fasting test show a high glucose level (greater than 126 mg/dL), no further testing is done. If the results are within an acceptable range, the patient is given a 75- or 100-g dose of glucose to drink. Blood specimens are collected and tested for glucose levels after the first half hour and then every hour for a specified period of time. In some laboratories, urine may also be tested to see if and when the blood glucose levels exceed the renal threshold level for glucose

of 160 to 180 mg/dL. When the renal threshold level is exceeded, glucose is present in the urine.

During this test, the patient should be monitored for signs of fainting or nausea. If these occur, or if the blood glucose levels exceed 300 mg/dL, the test should be terminated. If the physician suspects hyperglycemia (diabetes), it is typically a 3-hour GTT. If the physician suspects hypoglycemia, the test may continue for 5 or 6 hours. Figure 6.7 shows the patterns of normal and faulty glucose metabolism during a GTT.

Glycosylated hemoglobin, glycated hemoglobin, Hgb A$_{1c}$, or "A1c". When hemoglobin A in the RBCs is exposed to high levels of glucose, the hemoglobin molecule is permanently glycosylated and changes into hemoglobin A$_{1c}$. Because the life span of an RBC is normally 120 days, the percentage of glycosylated hemoglobin molecules will be proportional to the overall concentration of glucose levels in the blood over the average life span of the RBCs (approximately 3 months). The percentage range of glycosylated hemoglobin in a whole blood specimen from adults without diabetes is below 5.7%. A prediabetic adult would be in the range of 5.7% to 6.4%, and a diabetic adult would have an A1c result of 6.5% or higher.

The A1c test result is especially valuable to the person who is diagnosed with diabetes or prediabetes because it provides an accurate long-term index of the patient's average blood glucose level. Also, A1c test results are not subject to the daily fluctuations that occur in plasma glucose monitoring. Therefore, the American Diabetes Association recommends the A1c as the best test to determine whether a patient's blood sugar level has been under control during the previous 2 to 3 months. For example, if an A1c test result of a diabetic person rises above the recommended 6% to 8%, the patient is at risk of developing the

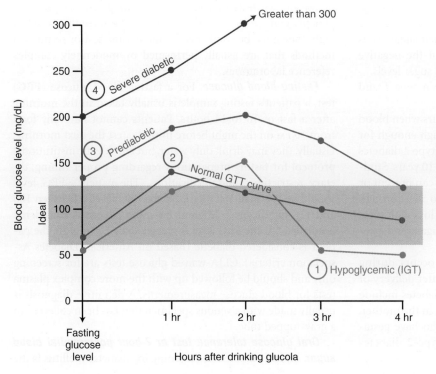

FIG. 6.7 Comparative patterns of glucose tolerance test (GTT) results. Compare the blood glucose levels for each condition during the initial fasting test and then the subsequent levels for each hourly test after consumption of the glucose drink. *IGT,* Impaired glucose tolerance.

microvascular and cardiovascular complications previously discussed. This information can be used to encourage the patient to better understand and follow the treatment plan to prevent these complications.

Patients should be aware that the higher their A1c percentage rises, the less control they have in maintaining proper glucose levels. This information can be used to encourage the patient to better understand and follow the treatment plan to prevent those complications.

Approved A1c tests for screening and diagnosis of diabetes have been referenced to the National Glycohemoglobin Standardization Program and certified. NOTE: The CLIA-waived A1c devices used in physician office laboratories are not accurate enough to diagnose diabetes but can be used to monitor treatment per Food and Drug Administration (FDA) regulations.

Lipid Metabolism and Testing

Lipids, or fats, are essential to the body. They are an alternate source of energy when blood glucose levels are low, and they are critical to cellular health. Research has shown that poor lipid metabolism and cardiovascular disease are directly linked. In an effort to help correct the growing problems of obesity and heart disease in the United States, annual lipid screening and monitoring tests are recommended. Lipid screening is approved as a CLIA-waived test.

Lipid Metabolism

Lipid metabolism begins with the ingestion of fats. Dietary fats and oils are digested into glycerol and fatty acids, which are transported to the tissues where they are further broken down and can be used for energy. Some of the essential functions and uses of lipids are the following:
- Production of steroidal hormones
- Absorption and transportation of fat-soluble vitamins (vitamins A, D, E, and K)
- Insulation against extreme temperatures
- Maintenance of healthy skin
- Protection of vital organs and nerves
- Potential source of energy when glucose is not available
- Reduction of feeling hungry

The two plasma lipids most routinely tested are cholesterol and triglycerides. These two lipids can be further categorized

and tested according to the three ways they are transported in the blood in the form of lipoproteins (protein-linked lipids): high-density lipoproteins (**HDL**), low-density lipoproteins (**LDL**), and very-low-density lipoproteins (**VLDL**). Cholesterol, triglyceride, and lipoprotein levels are frequently ordered together in a lipid panel.

Cholesterol. Cholesterol is found in all cells of the body and is a major constituent of cell membranes and the myelin sheath on nerves. Cholesterol is also required in the production of vitamin D. Most of the cholesterol found in the blood is manufactured in the liver and is called endogenous cholesterol. In fact, the liver is able to produce all the cholesterol the body needs.

Another source of cholesterol, exogenous cholesterol, comes from what we eat. Foods high in saturated fats and trans fats tend to raise the blood level of cholesterol. Trans fats are synthetic hydrogenated fats found in partially hydrogenated margarines and oils used in cooking and baking. Saturated fats are found in meat, egg yolks, milk, and other dairy products that are usually hard or semisolid at room temperature. Both trans fats and saturated fats are known to elevate cholesterol levels, causing atherosclerosis (Figure 6.8).

Not all dietary fats have the adverse effects of saturated fats and trans fats. Research has found that mono*unsaturated* fats and poly*unsaturate*d fats, which are naturally liquid at room temperature, actually lower the blood level of cholesterol. These may help reduce plaque buildup on blood vessel walls. Examples of "good" monounsaturated fats are canola oil, olive oil, and omega-3 oil from fish. Examples of good polyunsaturated fats are soybean, safflower, corn, and cottonseed oils.

Lipoproteins. Cholesterol and triglycerides are lipids that do not mix with the water in plasma. Consequently, the liver attaches a protein to these lipids, which then become lipoproteins. The following three types of lipoproteins are manufactured in the liver and are classified on the basis of their density:
- HDL is referred to as the "healthy" cholesterol because it has the lowest fat content and appears to protect against the accumulation of fatty deposits in blood vessels. In fact, HDL is capable of removing excess cholesterol from the interior walls of the blood vessels and carry it back to the liver to be excreted.
- LDL is referred to as the "lousy" cholesterol because when LDL levels are high, it can contribute to the formation of plaque on

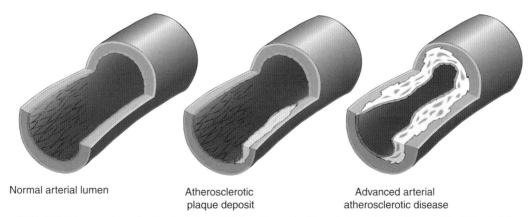

Normal arterial lumen   Atherosclerotic   Advanced arterial
                               plaque deposit   atherosclerotic disease

FIG. 6.8 Atherosclerosis, the buildup of fatty plaque in the arteries. (From Stepp CA, Woods M: *Laboratory procedures for medical office personnel,* Philadelphia, 1998, Saunders.)

the interior walls of the blood vessels (atherosclerosis). LDL becomes elevated in the blood after saturated fats and trans fats are ingested. Some individuals are also genetically predisposed to producing LDL endogenously within the liver.

- VLDL is made predominantly of proteins linked to triglycerides. VLDL is also directly linked to the formation of plaque and atherosclerosis.

Total cholesterol/high-density lipoprotein ratio. The total blood cholesterol level (TC) is compared with the HDL level in the form of a ratio. This ratio provides an important index for determining the cardiac risk a patient faces because of atherosclerosis. The TC/HDL ratio takes into account whether a high level of TC is made up of the HDL "healthy" cholesterol or the undesirable LDL cholesterol. A ratio of 3.5:1 is considered optimal. A ratio greater than 4.5:1 indicates that the person either is not producing enough good HDL or is producing too much bad LDL. The Association (AHA) suggests that physicians use LDL with patients instead of the cholesterol ratio to monitor heart risk. In either case, the individual with a high TC/HDL ratio will need to do the following to lower cardiovascular risk:

- Exercise routinely, which will cause the HDL level to rise and the triglyceride level to decrease.
- Change eating habits in favor of foods that are low in refined carbohydrates and high in fiber (e.g., whole grains, vegetables, fruits), which will lower glucose and triglyceride levels.
- Lower the dietary intake of trans fats and saturated fats found in baked goods, dairy products, and fatty meats. This will lower the LDL levels.
- Change to a diet containing natural monounsaturated fats and polyunsaturated fats found in olive, canola, soybean, safflower, and other oils. This will raise HDL levels.
- Take cholesterol-lowering medications (e.g., statins) as prescribed by the physician.

Triglycerides. Triglycerides are a direct result of diets rich in carbohydrates. Triglycerides account for 95% of the fat stored in adipose tissue. High levels of triglycerides are also associated with atherosclerotic risk. Like cholesterol, triglycerides are transported in the plasma bound to proteins as either LDL (15%) or VLDL (85%). When elevated, triglycerides produce a milky-white appearance in the plasma, a condition called hyperlipidemia. Triglyceride levels rise significantly in the blood after sweets or alcohol are ingested and blood insulin levels are high (hyperinsulinemia). Therefore, when testing for triglyceride levels in the blood, laboratories require the patient to fast 12 to 14 hours before testing and to refrain from alcohol 2 days before testing. Triglyceride levels can be lowered by exercising and decreasing dietary intake of sweets and alcohol.

The Lipid Panel

The lipid panel of tests consists of TC, HDL, LDL, VLDL, triglycerides, and the TC/HDL ratio. Medical research has established a direct link between blood lipid levels and coronary artery disease that may lead to subsequent myocardial infarcts (heart attacks). Myocardial infarction is the leading cause of death in the United States. An individual's cardiovascular risk can be determined by comparing the results of the tests in the lipid panel with the individual's age, weight, height, blood pressure, and smoking habits. Early detection of an at-risk individual

can reduce the risk of cardiovascular disease and heart attack if the individual begins an appropriate preventive treatment plan consisting of exercise, diet, and medication therapy.

Also, a high triglyceride result in the panel may indicate metabolic syndrome in patients with central obesity. It is important to remember that the patient must not have alcohol for 48 hours before being tested for triglycerides because alcohol raises the triglyceride levels.

❖ CLIA-WAIVED CHEMISTRY TESTS

Most of the CLIA-waived blood chemistry tests that are performed or observed in ambulatory settings are *quantitative* analyses. The numerical blood levels of glucose, lipids, glycosylated hemoglobin, electrolytes, blood urea nitrogen (BUN), and creatinine are all quantified by electronic photometers. The CLIA-waived fecal occult blood (hidden or not visible to the naked eye) test is a *qualitative* analysis that simply detects the presence or absence of blood in a fecal specimen.

Principle of Photometers and Spectrophotometers

Each blood chemistry testing method in this section involves collecting a capillary puncture whole blood specimen into a testing device containing premeasured reagents that react with the analyte being tested. The reagents change color as they react to the analyte in question (similarly to the color changes occurring in urine dipsticks). The testing devices are inserted into an electronic analyzer that sends a spectrum of light through the specimen. A photometer located within the analyzer measures the amount of light that passed through the specimen or is reflected off the specimen. The concentration of a substance is directly proportional to the amount of light being absorbed or reflected at a particular wavelength. This equation is known as the Beer-Lambert law or Beer's law.

The chemical analyzers used in blood chemistry testing are highly sensitive photometers and spectrophotometers that directly measure the amount of light passing through the solution (transmittance photometry), indirectly measure the amount of light that the solution absorbs (absorbance photometry), or indirectly measure the amount of light the solution reflects (reflectance photometry). When the light passes through the solution (or reflects off the specimen), it activates a photodetector that activates a galvanometer (an instrument capable of measuring small electric currents). The galvanometer sends the information to an electronic program that converts the measurement of electric current into a quantitative dial or digital readout (Figure 6.9).

Quality Assurance When Using Optical Instruments

Optical tests depend on all the elements in the light path functioning correctly to receive accurate and reliable results. To accomplish this, each analyzer provides an "optics check" or calibration device or setting that ensures the instrument's optics are working correctly.

Be sure to observe and document all the quality assurance and quality control steps in the instruction manuals for the chemical analyzer being used to. The skill check sheets and corresponding logs for the tests covered in this text are located in

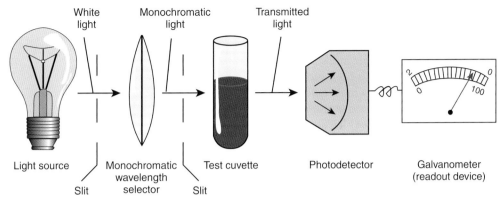

FIG. 6.9 Principles of photometry: A spectrum of light passes through the specimen and strikes a photodetector. The intensity of light received by the photodetector is then sent to a readout device that is able to convert the light intensity to a quantitative concentration of the analyte being tested. The concentration of the substance is directly proportional to the amount of light being absorbed at a particular wavelength (based on the Beer-Lambert law). (From Stepp CA, Woods M: *Laboratory procedures for medical office personnel*, Philadelphia, 1998, Saunders.)

the workbook and online in Evolve. They all have the following preanalytical requirements:

- Instruments must be calibrated *daily*, and the calibration results must be documented in the calibration log. Newer analyzers may self-calibrate with each specimen and will not require documentation.
- Run liquid controls for each test method according to the manufacturer's recommendations to check the technique and accuracy of the various testing devices, such as the glucose strip, the Hgb A_{1c} cartridge, and the Cholestech cassette. Document the results of the controls on their control logs. If they do not fall within the manufacturer's acceptable range, check the following:
  1. Was the control specimen processed poorly, or was the testing technique poor?
  2. Were the reagents or liquid controls stored at the wrong temperature? Had they expired?
  3. Was the instrument dirty or faulty?
- Always check the expiration date of the testing device and do not use it to run the test if the expiration date has passed.
- Because the testing device kits for each test must be stored and tested within a specific temperature range, record and monitor the daily room temperature and refrigerator temperature on a log sheet, as found in the workbook appendix. Also pay strict attention to the length of time it is necessary to wait for a testing device that has been stored in the refrigerator to come to room temperature.
- Always retain the most current package inserts that come with the liquid controls and the testing kits and attach them to the procedure sheets for each test method.

Westgard's Rules for Monitoring Quality Control Results

In Chapter 2, the weekly documentations of the liquid control results were placed onto a Levey-Jennings graph and analyzed for excessive scatter, trends, and shifts (see Figures 2.3 through 2.6). The control's mean (average) value and its reference range (± 2 standard deviations [SDs]) were compared with a target that would show if the daily results were consistently accurate and precise (see Figure 2.7). In this chapter, each of the chemical

analyzers requires the periodic running of one to three liquid controls to determine whether the testing procedure is able to consistently detect both the normal values and the abnormal values of the analytes being measured.

By plotting the daily, weekly, or monthly control results onto a Levey-Jennings graph, one can see if any of the following rules have been broken, which indicates a faulty testing system. If the testing system is faulty, do not run patient tests; contact the manufacturer if any of the following patterns appear on the Levey-Jennings chart:

1. Both levels of control results are outside the manufacturer's reference range.
2. 1 control exceeds ± 3 SD
3. The same control level falls outside of the ± 2 SD in two successive runs.
4. One of the controls falls outside of the ± 1 SD in four successive runs.
5. The range between 2 points exceeds 4 SDs.
6. One of the controls consistently falls above the mean value or consistently falls below the mean value for 10 consecutive runs.

A monthly Levey-Jennings graph and exercise are provided in Chapter 6 of the workbook. Also, when running the tests in the lab class, plot the results of the controls for all the students and analyze their accuracy and precision to see if the plotted results pass the criteria for reliability.

CLIA-Waived Glucose Tests

Present blood glucose levels can be readily screened and monitored with simple handheld glucometers. Blood glucose levels over time can also be monitored by testing the percentage of glycosylated hemoglobin (A1c) in a whole blood specimen.

Glucose Monitoring Devices

Numerous brands of glucose meters have been approved for home use and for point-of-care monitoring and screening. Technology continues to make it easier to collect blood specimens and obtain the glucose results in seconds. For example, multiple-site lancets can now be used to collect a very small amount of blood from sites other than the finger, such as the forearm. NOTE: Although forearm testing can give sensitive fingertips a break from testing, forearm testing is not recommended whenever the blood sugar levels may be running low, such as before meals, after exercising, and after administering insulin. It has been proved that fingerstick blood samples show hypoglycemia more quickly than forearm testing, thus alerting the patient to possible insulin shock.

Noninvasive infrared absorption technology has also made it possible to measure the blood glucose levels with no stick at all.

Glucose meters are also becoming more and more sophisticated, with computerized readouts that graph the patient's glucose readings throughout each day of the week. The computerized visual data help the patient and physician see exactly when glucose levels become unmanageable during the week. The patient may then take the appropriate steps to prevent those problems. The Contour (Bayer, Pittsburgh, PA) procedure check sheet is provided in the workbook and is demonstrated in Procedure 6.1, located at the end of this section. This monitor is similar to the OneTouch Ultra (LifeScan, Milpitas, CA). Both devices can be viewed on the Internet (along with many other glucose monitoring methods) by accessing the various manufacturers' websites. (NOTE: Never run the supplies or controls from one manufacturer on a different manufacturer's analyzer.)

Glycosylated Hemoglobin (A1c)

The CLIA waived A1c test is only used for monitoring patients with diagnosed diabetes or prediabetes at 3- and 6-month intervals to ensure they are keeping their long-term glucose levels under control. Several brands of analyzers measure A1c levels, and manufacturer inserts should clearly state that the A1c analyzer is not to be used for screening or diagnosing diabetes. The Bayer A1CNOW+ procedure check sheet is provided in the workbook and is demonstrated in Procedure 6.2 located at the end of this section. It uses a dedicated testing meter that is packaged with 20 test cartridges and 20 sampling packets that all share the same code as the meter. When the 20 tests are completed, the meter is deactivated. Another kit with a new dedicated meter and its 20 coded cartridges and sampling packets is then purchased for the next set of 20 A1c tests.

Cholesterol and Lipid Profiles with the Cholestech LDX

Total blood cholesterol testing and lipid profiles have become standard screening tests in POLs. The Cholestech LDX is a popular analyzer capable of measuring either single blood cholesterol levels or the full panel of lipids plus glucose. Its procedure check sheet is provided in the workbook and demonstrated in Procedure 6.3 located at the end of this section.

Liver Enzyme Testing with the Cholestech LDX

The Cholestech is also approved for CLIA-waived testing for two liver enzymes: alanine aminotransferase (**ALT [SGPT]**) and aspartate aminotransferase (**AST [SGOT]**). Levels of these enzymes may become elevated if a person is taking statin drugs (i.e., cholesterol-lowering drugs such as Zocor or Lipitor) and is consequently experiencing liver damage. If enzyme results are elevated, the physician may consider a different therapeutic drug. NOTE: Because levels of these enzymes are also elevated during muscle damage, the physician must interpret the significance of the

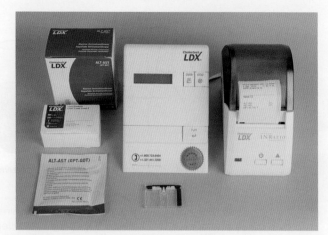

FIG. 6.10 Cholestech system with supplies and results showing elevated liver enzymes: alanine aminotransferase (ALT or SGPT) = 59 units/L; aspartate aminotransferase (AST or SGOT) = 43 units/L.

results on the basis of an entire clinical evaluation of the patient. See Figure 6.10 showing the supplies and equipment for measuring the two liver enzymes, ALT and AST.

i-STAT CHEM8+

The i-STAT system consists of a handheld analyzer and single-use disposable cartridges (Figure 6.11). The analyzer automatically controls all functions of the testing cycle, including fluid movement within the cartridge, calibration, and continuous quality monitoring. Its procedure check sheet is provided in the workbook and is demonstrated in Procedure 6.4 located at the end of this section.

The CLIA-waived i-STAT CHEM8+ cartridge can be used to test all the following blood chemistries and provide the results in minutes:

- Sodium (Na^+)
- Potassium (K^+)
- Chloride (Cl^-)
- Ionized calcium (Ca^{2+})
- **TCO_2**
- Glucose (Glu)
- BUN
- Creatinine (Crea)
- Hematocrit (Hct)
- Hemoglobin (Hgb)
- AnGap (anion gap)

See Figure 6.11 showing five of the i-STAT results.

Fecal Occult Blood Testing—Three Methods

Fecal occult blood testing is a simple, inexpensive test to detect blood that may be hidden or not visible to the naked eye (occult) on or in a stool specimen. It is a useful aid in the diagnosis of a number of GI disorders and is typically part of a routine physical examination or a mass screening clinic of the population for colorectal cancer.

The presence of blood in fecal matter may be the result of bleeding from hemorrhoids, polyps, diverticulitis, dysentery, parasites, fissures, colitis, stomach ulcers, or colorectal cancer. If a positive result is obtained, additional follow-up diagnostic tests are performed,

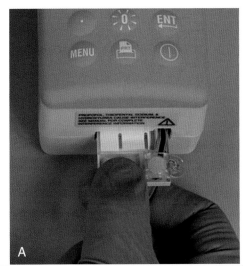

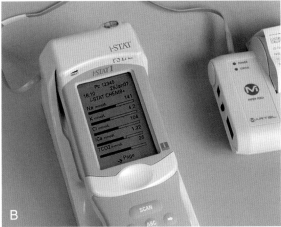

FIG. 6.11 A, i-STAT Cartridge with patient specimen inserted into i-STAT meter. **B,** Digital readout showing five chemistry results.

such as proctosigmoidoscopy, colonoscopy, barium enema x-ray studies, or endoscopy, to determine the cause of the bleeding.

Cancer of the colon is one of the leading causes of death in the United States. The early stages of colon cancer are usually painless and asymptomatic. By the time an individual becomes aware of the condition, the cancer is typically at the metastasizing phase. Therefore, early detection is especially critical while it is still localized and curable. The American Cancer Society recommends that a fecal occult blood test be a routine part of the physical examination of adults. Some patients are embarrassed about the collection of a fecal specimen and must be encouraged to collect such a specimen and submit it for testing.

Occult Blood Testing with the Guaiac Slide Method

The principle of the test is to apply samples from various fecal specimens to paper slides coated with guaiac (a wood resin that reacts with blood). The paper slides are contained within cardboard testing devices that are then mailed or returned to the testing site. If blood is present, the hemoglobin will react with the guaiac and turn blue when a developing solution (hydrogen peroxide) is applied. False-positive test results can occur if the patient's diet is high in red meat, turnips, horseradish, or bananas. Certain therapeutic drugs, such as nonsteroidal anti-inflammatory drugs, aspirin, iron preparations, and anticoagulants, may also cause positive findings because of their effects on the GI tract. The procedure for fecal occult blood check sheet is provided in the workbook and is demonstrated in Procedure 6.5 located at the end of this section.

ColoCARE Method Using Test Pads

An alternative patient-friendly method of testing for occult blood consists of simply floating a test pad in the toilet after a bowel movement. The test pad is checked for a change in color that is produced when blood is in the toilet water. When blood is present, the test pad will show areas of blue or green. See Procedure 6.6 for this ColoCARE method of testing for fecal occult blood.

NOTE: Results are dependent on the patient's interpretation. This method may be less sensitive than the guaiac slide method but may be more acceptable to patients who tend to be noncompliant in submitting a fecal specimen.

iFOB (Immunochemical Fecal Occult Blood) Method (or "FIT" Fecal Immunochemical Test)

The QuickVue **iFOB** test is a rapid immunochemical diagnostic tool intended to detect the presence of blood in stool specimens. iFOB is the acronym for immunochemical fecal occult blood (Figure 6.12). This highly sensitive qualitative

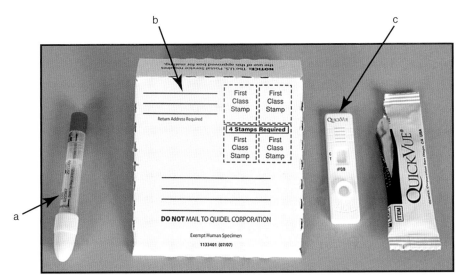

FIG. 6.12 The QuickVue immunochemical fecal occult blood (iFOB) test is a rapid immunochemical diagnostic tool intended to detect the presence of blood in stool specimens. *(a)* Fecal specimen collection tube; *(b)* mailer to send specimen to office; *(c)* in office test kit.

test uses an antibody–antigen reaction (rather than the guaiac methods described earlier) and uses a test kit similar to the lateral flow tests covered in Chapter 7: Immunology. This new method of testing occult blood is demonstrated in Procedure 6.7 at the end of this section, and a check sheet is available in the workbook.

Summary of CLIA-Waived Tests

All the CLIA-waived tests covered in the preceding sections are *screening* tests to detect possible risks to a patient's health. The glucose test detects possible diabetes, the lipid profile detects possible cardiovascular disease, the i-STAT detects possible chemical imbalances related to the body's homeostatic state, and the occult blood test detects possible colon cancer.

Diabetes and cardiovascular diseases have become so prevalent in the United States that in 2005 the Centers for Medicare and Medicaid Services approved coverage of glucose screening and preventive cardiovascular screening for all Medicare beneficiaries. The new coverage went into effect as part of the larger Medicare Prescription Drug, Improvement, and Modernization

Act of 2003. The approved cardiovascular screening includes three tests to detect early risk for cardiovascular disease: TC, HDL, and triglycerides. The TC/HDL ratio can also be determined by these tests, which can be ordered individually or as part of a lipid panel.

Becoming Proficient at CLIA-Waived Chemistry Testing

Now that you have learned about the significance of glucose, hemoglobin A$_{1c}$, lipid panels, basic chemical homeostasis, and occult blood tests, take time to complete the following:

1. Answer the CLIA-waived portion in Chapter 6 of the workbook using your Student Handout and text.
2. View the procedural videos online to see glucose test and cholesterol test.
3. Perform the Chapter 6 online lessons, which are designed to reinforce your terminology and CLIA-waived test knowledge.
4. Study Procedures 6.1 through 6.7 at the end of this section before performing your lab procedures.

PROCEDURE 6.1 Glucometer Procedure

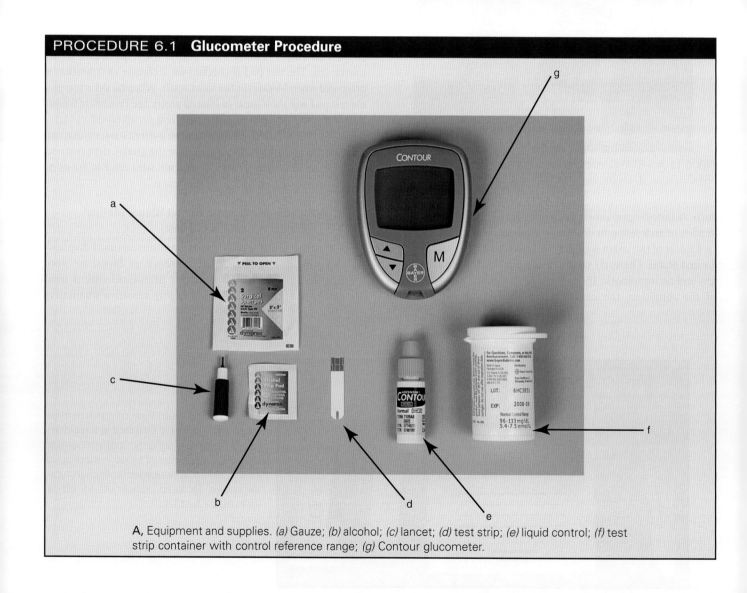

A, Equipment and supplies. *(a)* Gauze; *(b)* alcohol; *(c)* lancet; *(d)* test strip; *(e)* liquid control; *(f)* test strip container with control reference range; *(g)* Contour glucometer.

PROCEDURE 6.1 Glucometer Procedure—cont'd

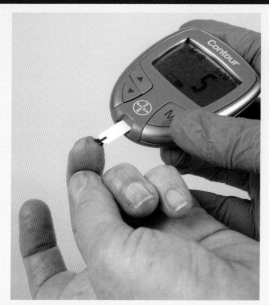

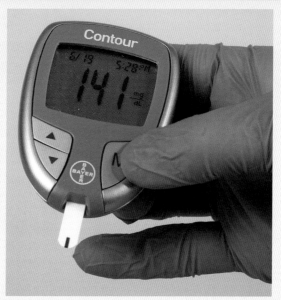

B, Glucometer procedure showing the specimen being pulled into the tip of the strip as it is held in the drop of blood. When a beep sounds, remove the finger from the strip.

C, The glucometer will display the glucose result after 5 to 30 seconds depending on the model (e.g., the newer Bayer *Contour* displays the result in 5 seconds, but older models display results in 30 seconds).

Equipment and Supplies (Figure A)
- Gauze and personal protective equipment (gloves and gown)
- Alcohol
- Lancet
- Test strips
- Liquid control
- Strip container with liquid control reference range
- Contour glucose monitor

Patient Specimen
NOTE if the patient's capillary specimen is random, fasting, or 2-hour postprandial. Each of these specimens will have a different reference range.

NOTE: The Contour pictured in Figure A is an upgraded version of the glucometer Elite seen in these pictures; the procedure steps remain the same.

Procedure
1. Sanitize the hands and put on gloves.
2. Turn on the meter by inserting the end of the strip that contains the metallic contact bars.
3. Perform a capillary puncture and wipe away the first drop. Then touch and hold the exposed end of the strip into the base of the second drop of blood. This allows the strip to "sip," or draw the blood in without interruption (Figure B). Do not smear or place blood on the top or bottom of the strip. When a beep sounds, quickly remove the strip from the blood to keep it from overfilling
4. After 5 seconds, the result on the Contour meter is displayed on the screen (Figure C).
5. Discard all the test materials in the appropriate biohazard containers.
6. Remove and discard gloves into the biohazard container. Sanitize hands.

The expected results for this test are as follows:

	Fasting	2-hr Postprandial (After Drinking Glucose-Rich Beverage)
Normal	<100 mg/dL	<140 mg/dL
Prediabetes	100–125 mg/dL	140–199 mg/dL
Diabetes	≥126 mg/dL	≥200 mg/dL

Quality Control Procedures
The "coding" or calibration of the Contour glucose monitors is set when each strip is inserted into the glucometer. Liquid controls are provided by the glucose meter manufacturer and should be run the same way patient specimens are run to ensure that your technique and the system are providing reliable results.

The glucose liquid controls must be run with each new shipment of glucose strips, with each new operator, and on the days when glucose testing is performed. Patient samples cannot be run if the control results are not acceptable. If the controls are run again and they are still not acceptable, there are three areas to investigate: (1) the *technique* used to process the specimen and run the test, (2) the liquid control and/or the *reagent* expiration dates and their temperature and time requirements, and (3) the *monitor's* optics and maintenance requirements. If all these areas are acceptable and a new set of controls still does not work, call the manufacturer.

A control log has also been provided in the workbook to track the results of multiple glucose control readings. The results can then be plotted on a Levey-Jenning's graph as seen in Chapter 2 to observe trends, shifts, randomized errors, and excessive scatter. An extra control log and a control graph are provided in the workbook appendix and on the Evolve website to plot the results of multiple control readings. Check the plotted control graph for signs that show when the multiple results are out of the control limits based on Westgard's rules.

Photo A by Zack Bent.

PROCEDURE 6.2 A1CNOW+ Glycosylated Hemoglobin Procedure

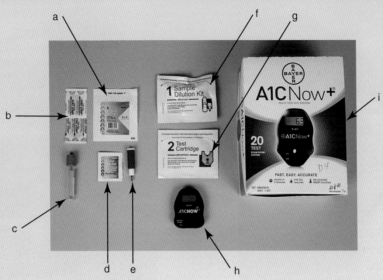

A, Supplies and equipment for the Test Kit Method for A1c. *(a)* Gauze; *(b)* bandage; *(c)* heparin tube for venous blood sample; *(d)* alcohol swab; *(e)* lancet for capillary blood sample; *(f)* sample dilution kit containing capillary tube collector and sampler body; *(g)* test cartridge; *(h)* A1c monitor programmed to work only with the 20 cartridges in the kit; *(i)* box containing 1 monitor and 20 sample dilution kits and 20 cartridges.

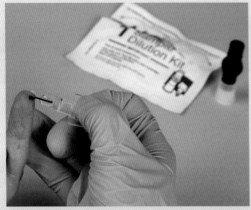

B, After lancing the finger and wiping away the first drop, gently touch the blood drop and fill the capillary blood collector from the #1 packet, as seen above.

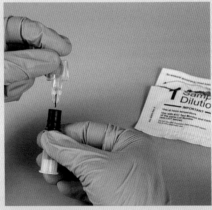

C, After wiping any blood from the outside of the capillary tube, firmly insert the blood collector into the top of the dilution sampler body, as seen above.

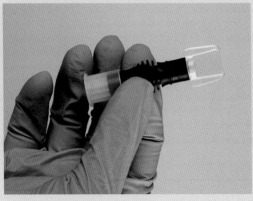

D, The fully inserted sample is then mixed with the dilution by tilting 6 to 8 times. Then stand the sampler on the table.

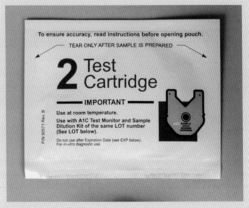

E, Open packet #2 and use within 2 minutes. Click the cartridge into the monitor from the same kit.

PROCEDURE 6.2 A1CNOW+ Glycosylated Hemoglobin Procedure—cont'd

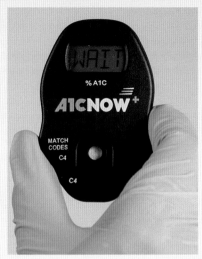

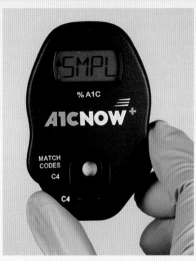

F, The inserted cartridge will start the monitor, which indicates a "WAIT" message.

G, Wait for the "SMPL" to appear before proceeding with the next step.

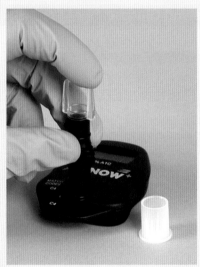

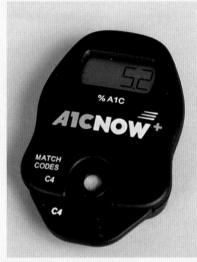

H, Remove the sampler from its base and push it down onto the white well of the cartridge. The monitor must be on a level surface and cannot be moved until the test is complete.

I, Next, the A1c result will appear along with an intermittent "QCOK," indicating that the test controls were within their normal limits and then a number indicating how many more tests are available in the kit.

Equipment and Supplies
See Figure A.

Patient Specimen
Use only *fresh capillary blood* or venous whole blood collected in a *green heparin tube*. Venous blood may be used only if the tube is less than 1 week old and has been under refrigeration during that time. The blood being tested should fill the small glass capillary tube located on the capillary holder provided in the kit (Figure B). Do not allow blood to touch the holder. If using the venous tube of blood, dispense the well-mixed blood onto a slide and obtain the blood by dipping the capillary tube into the drop at a 45-degree angle. After the glass capillary tube has been filled with the specimen, the analysis must begin within 5 minutes.

Procedure
1. Sanitize the hands and put on personal protective equipment (gown and gloves).

2. Remove the blood collector from the foil #1 sampler dilution kit. Touch the tip of the capillary tube that is attached to the holder into the small drop of blood from the fingerstick or the venous blood drop on the slide until the capillary is filled (Figure B).
3. Wipe the outer sides of the capillary tube with tissue, being careful not to draw out any of the blood sample within the tube.
4. Insert the capillary holder into the sampler body that also came from the #1 sampler dilution kit (Figure C). Push together and twist until the holder and sampler body snap into place.
5. The fully inserted sample is then mixed with the dilution by tilting six to eight times (Figure D). Then stand the sampler on the table.
6. Open the #2 test cartridge (Figure E) foil package and perform the following within 2 minutes: click the cartridge into the monitor that came in the same kit box and check code numbers, which must match.
7. While the monitor indicates "WAIT" (Figure F), prepare the sample by removing the base.

Continued

PROCEDURE 6.2   A1CNOW+ Glycosylated Hemoglobin Procedure—cont'd

8. Do not add the sample until the monitor indicates "SMPL" (Figure G).

9. Push sampler down onto the white well of the cartridge (Figure H). The monitor must be on a level surface and cannot be moved until the test is complete.

10. After several minutes, the monitor will indicate "QCOK" followed by the test result (Figure I), which in this case shows a result of 5.2 followed by the number of tests left in the kit..

11. Record the results from the display and report to the physician.

12. Properly dispose of all biohazard supplies, disinfect the area, remove gloves, and sanitize hands.

The expected results of an **A1c** test are the following:

Nondiabetics	3%–6%
Controlled diabetics	6.8%
Poorly controlled diabetics	As much as 20% or higher

NOTE: Because **A1c** is also affected by hemoglobin concentration, the patient's hemoglobin level should be tested to ensure that it is in the normal range.

Quality Control Procedures

The liquid controls must be run with each new shipment of test cartridges (foil package #2) and their accompanying monitor and the sample dilution kits (foil package #1). Use the capillary holder from one of the sampler dilution kits to collect the control specimens. Insert the filled capillary holder into the sampler body as for a patient specimen. Patient samples cannot be run if the control results are not acceptable. If the controls are run again and they are still not acceptable, there are three areas to investigate: (1) the *technique* used to process the specimen and run the test, (2) the liquid control and *reagent* expiration dates and their temperature and time requirements, and (3) the *analyzer's* optics and maintenance requirements. If all these areas are acceptable and a new set of controls still does not work, call the manufacturer.

Photos A through I by Zack Bent.

PROCEDURE 6.3   Cholestech Method of Measuring Lipids and Glucose

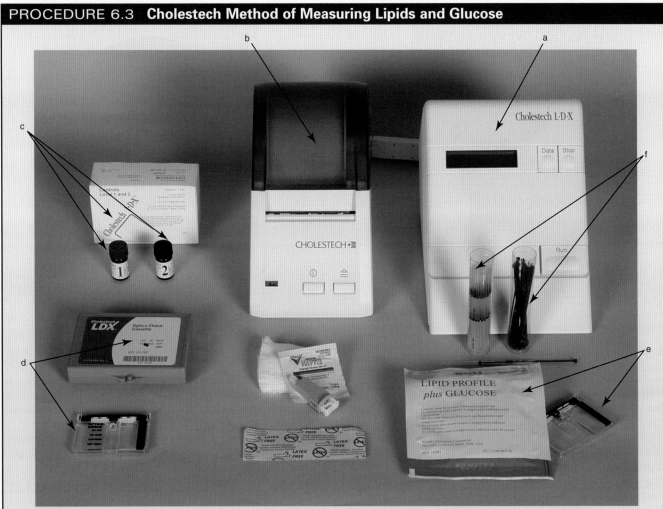

A, Cholestech analyzer and supplies. *(a)* Cholestech LDX analyzer; *(b)* printer with self-adhesive individual reports; *(c)* liquid control box with insert reference sheet of values for level 1 and level 2 controls; *(d)* optics check container and cassette for daily optics checks; *(e)* foil wrap and testing cassette; *(f)* capillary tubes and plungers for collecting and dispensing capillary blood samples.

PROCEDURE 6.3   Cholestech Method of Measuring Lipids and Glucose—cont'd

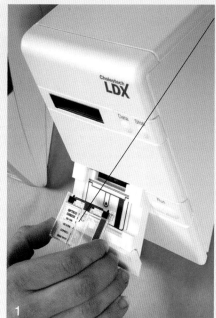

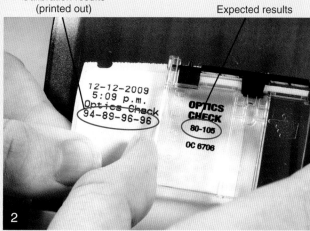

B, Calibration check. (1) Place the "Optics Check" calibration cassette in the drawer of the Cholestech. (2) The results of the optical reading in all four testing areas will be displayed and printed.

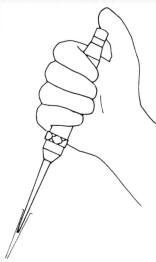

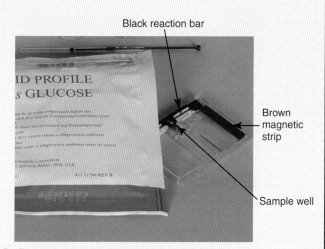

C, Micropipetter for obtaining and dispensing liquid controls and venous blood collected in a green lithium heparin tube. (1) First, press thumb down on plunger to dispense out the air before entering sample. (2) Release thumb while in sample, causing the pipette to fill. (3) Clean outside of pipette with gauze. (4) Press thumb down again to deliver the sample into the cassette and then remove the pipette from the device before releasing thumb to avoid pulling the specimen back into the pipette. (From Proctor D, Adams A: *The medical assistant: an applied learning approach,* ed 12, St. Louis, 2014, Saunders.)

D, Remove a new cassette from the foil without touching the brown magnetic strip or black reaction bar.

Continued

PROCEDURE 6.3   Cholestech Method of Measuring Lipids and Glucose—cont'd

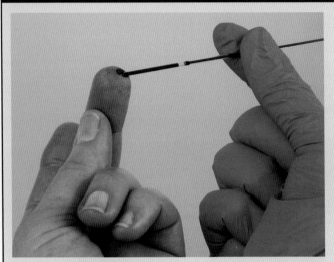

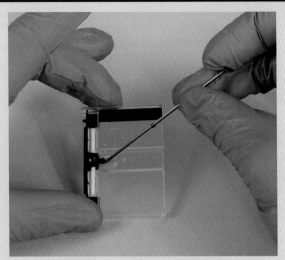

E, Collect blood into the capillary tube with the black plunger inserted into the red end of the capillary tube. Collection should be completed within 10 seconds.

F, Transfer the blood into the cassette test well using the plunger as seen above within the next 5 minutes (this avoids clotting of the specimen). Also, observe the positioning of the cassette with the testing bars to the left of the well and the hand on the cassette pointing down toward the well.

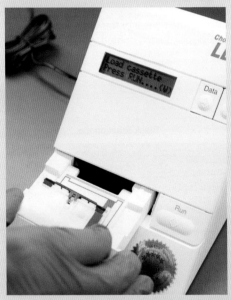

G, Immediately place the cassette with the specimen in the opened drawer and press RUN. Results will be printed after 5 minutes.

The test can be run with whole blood from a fingerstick that is collected in the appropriate capillary tube with its black plunger inserted. Whole blood from a green-topped lithium heparin tube can also be used. (NOTE: Green-topped *sodium* heparin tubes are not acceptable.) Cholestech provides an automatic micropipetter that consists of a disposable plastic-tipped pipette placed on the end of a plunger (Figure C). The plunger is pushed in before entering the tube of blood. When in the blood, the plunger is released, causing the correct amount of blood to flow into the plastic tip. The blood can then be transferred to the Cholestech testing device by pushing down on the plunger.

Equipment and Supplies (Figure A)

- Cholestech LDX analyzer
- Printer that provides individual self-adhesive patient readouts
- Control box with level 1 and level 2 liquid controls (stored in refrigerator)
- Optics check container and optics check cassette (Figure B) (stored at room temperature)
- Individual foil wrap and test cassette for running a test on a patient or a liquid control (stored in refrigerator)
- Cholestech capillary tubes and black plungers for collecting and transferring capillary blood samples (stored at room temperature)

Patient Sample

If a lipid panel including triglycerides is ordered, the patient should not drink alcohol for 48 hours before testing and should have fasted for 10 to 12 hours.

Procedure

1. Allow the refrigerated cassette to come to room temperature (at least 10 minutes before opening).
2. Make sure the analyzer is plugged in and warmed up.
3. Remove the cassette from its foil pouch and place it on a flat surface. Do not touch the black bar or the brown magnetic strip (Figure D). Hold the cassette by the short sides only.
4. Press RUN. The analyzer will perform a self-test, and the screen will display "Self-Test Running" and then "Self-Test OK."
5. The cassette drawer will open, and the screen will display "Load Cassette and Press Run." The drawer will remain open for 4 minutes, after which it will close with the message "System timeout. Run to continue." If the RUN button is not pushed within 15 seconds of the message, the drawer will close, and the screen will go blank. If this happens, simply press RUN and allow the analyzer to go through the self-test again; then proceed.
6. Collect a blood sample from a fingerstick into the Cholestech LDX capillary tube with its plunger in place (Figure E). (Or use the Mini-Pet pipette provided by Cholestech to collect the Vacutainer blood and the control samples.)
7. The blood or control sample must then be plunged into the cassette well within 5 minutes after collection, or the blood may clot (Figure F).
8. Immediately place the filled cassette into the drawer of the analyzer (Figure G).
   a. Keep the cassette level after the sample is applied.
   b. The black reaction bar faces toward the analyzer.
   c. The brown magnetic strip is on the right.
9. Press RUN. The drawer will close, and the screen will display "(Test names) Running."

PROCEDURE 6.3   Cholestech Method of Measuring Lipids and Glucose—cont'd

10. When the test is complete, the analyzer will beep, and the screen will display results. At the same time, the printer will provide the results. (NOTE: Pressing the DATA button will display the calculated results of all tests on the screen if you are running a panel of tests. The DATA button will also display questions that must be answered to determine the cardiac risk factor.)

The interpretation of the lipid panel as it relates to cardiovascular risk is as follows (based on American Heart Association recommendations):

Total Cholesterol Levels	What It Means
<200 mg/dL	Desirable
200–239 mg/dL	Borderline high risk for heart disease
≥240 mg/dL	High risk for heart disease

LDL Cholesterol Levels	What It Means
<100 mg/dL	Optimal
100–129 mg/dL	Near optimal
130–159 mg/dL	Borderline high
160–189 mg/dL	High
≥190 mg/dL	Very high

HDL Cholesterol Levels	What It Means
<40 mg/dL	High risk for heart disease
40–59 mg/dL	Less risk for heart disease
≥60 mg/dL	Desirable

TC/HDL ratio ≤4.5 is desirable.

Triglycerides	What It Means
<150 mg/dL	Desirable
150–199 mg/dL	Borderline high
200–499 mg/dL	High
≥500 mg/dL	Very high

Cholestech results when testing ALT (SGPT) and AST (SGOT) enzymes: ALT and AST are enzymes that are measured to help assess liver damage. ALT and AST levels are monitored in patients who are taking certain medications to lower cholesterol level, control diabetes, or treat other diseases. A normal ALT range is 10 to 40 units/L. A normal AST range is 7 to 56 units/L.

Quality Control Procedures

The calibration "optics check" cassette should be run daily. It does not require any specimen in its well. Simply place the cassette in the drawer of the Cholestech. The results of the optical reading in all four testing areas will be displayed and printed (see Figure B). Document the results on the calibration log and compare the numbers with the required range designated on the cassette. If any number falls out of range, patient tests cannot be run until the cause is determined and corrected.

The two levels of liquid controls should be run at least monthly, with a new user, or whenever a new set of cassettes is opened. Use the Mini-Pet pipette to transfer the control solution into the cassette well and run the control as you would a patient sample. Document the results on the control log and compare them with the control's package insert. If the results do not fall in the required range, patient samples cannot be run until the cause is determined and corrected.

PROCEDURE 6.4   i-STAT Chemistry Analyzer Procedure

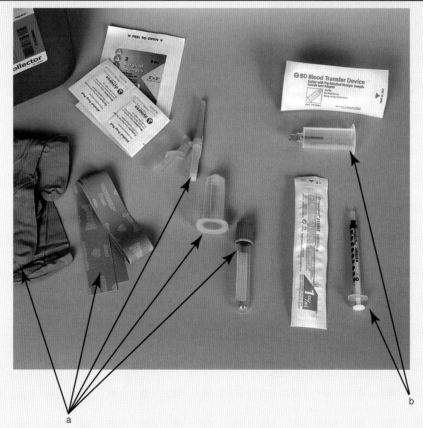

Preanalytical supplies: *(a)* Venipuncture items using a 4-mL lithium heparin tube and *(b)* the safety transfer device that will be used to transfer the blood from the Vacutainer tube to the 1-mL syringe.

Continued

PROCEDURE 6.4 i-STAT Chemistry Analyzer Procedure—cont'd

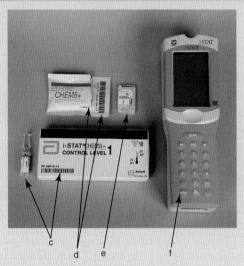

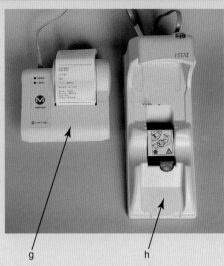

Analytical supplies and analyzer: *(c)* Liquid control ampule and package, *(d)* foil cartridge CHEM8+ package with bar code, *(e)* cartridge, and *(f)* the handheld analyzer.

Postanalytical supplies: *(g)* Printer and *(h)* recharging dock for analyzer.

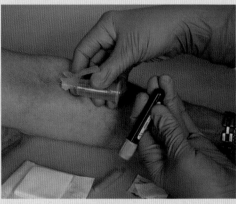

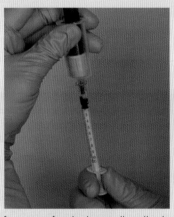

A, Collect blood, making sure the 4-mL heparin tube fills completely and that the blood is mixed by tilting 10 times. The specimen should be tested within 10 minutes. NOTE: During this time, enter in the operator and patient information followed by scanning the cartridge's bar code.

B, Using the safety transfer device, pull well-mixed blood from the tube into about half of a 1-mL syringe. If air enters the syringe, do not push it back into the blood tube.

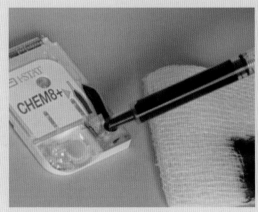

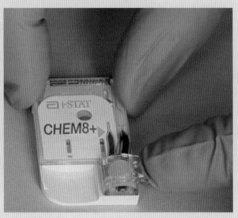

C, Remove any air at the tip of the syringe along with 3 drops of blood onto a gauze pad. Then carefully push the blood into the cartridge well until the blood reaches the arrow and there is still blood remaining in the well but not overflowing.

D, Swing the cover tab over the well from left to right using one finger. Do not press on the beige circle area directly over the well. Push down on the tab until it snaps into place.

PROCEDURE 6.4   i-STAT Chemistry Analyzer Procedure—cont'd

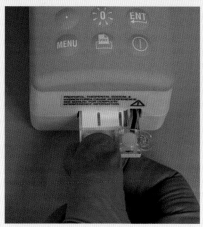

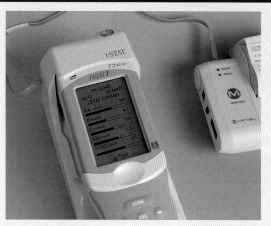

E, Use the grooved area to the left of the well or the sides of the cartridge to slowly insert it into the analyzer.

Equipment and Supplies

Specimen Collection—Preanalytical
- 4-mL lithium heparin tube
- Safety transfer device and 1-mL syringe

Testing Supplies and Analyzer—Analytical
- Liquid controls
- Foil cartridge package with bar code
- CHEM8+ cartridge
- Handheld analyzer

Print Equipment—Postanalytical
- Printer
- Recharging dock for analyzer

Patient Sample
The FDA-approved CLIA-waived i-STAT test requires a whole blood sample from a completely filled green-topped *lithium* heparin tube. (NOTE: Green-topped *sodium* heparin tubes are not acceptable.) The well-mixed blood is then transferred to a 1-mL syringe using the safety transfer device, and then it must be inserted into the test cassette within 10 minutes.

Procedure
1. Allow the cassette to come to room temperature (at least 10 minutes before opening).
2. Key in operator and patient information into the handheld analyzer followed by scanning the cartridge bar code until a beep is heard.
3. *Within 10 minutes* of drawing a 4-mL specimen of blood into a vacuum tube, perform the following (Figure A):
   - Mix the specimen by tilting 10 times.
   - Connect a safety tip or safety transfer device to a 1-mL syringe.
   - Invert the green top tube with the specimen and pierce the green stopper with the syringe safety tip or the transfer device.

F, After 2 to 3 minutes, the results will appear on the screen. Note the "→ Page" command on the bottom of the screen indicating more results will appear on a second screen. Press the print button to send the results to the printer via wireless transmission or via the docking device USB connection.

- *Slowly* pull back on the syringe plunger until it is about one-half full; note any air bubbles that enter syringe while transferring and do not push them back into specimen (Figure B).
- Disconnect syringe from vacuum tube and continue to hold it with tip pointed upward; then hold a gauze pad at the tip of the syringe to absorb blood while syringe plunger is slowly pushing out the air and approximately three drops of blood.
- Tear open the foiled cartridge pouch and remove the cartridge by holding the sides and placing it on a flat surface.
- Hold the syringe tip directly over and into the sample well and carefully push the blood into the cartridge until the blood reaches the blue arrow indicator and there is still blood remaining in the well but not overflowing (Figure C).

4. Move the tab over the well from left to right using one finger; do not press on the beige circle area directly over the well; push down on the tab until it snaps into place (Figure D).
5. Use the grooved area to the left of the well or hold the sides of the cartridge to slowly insert it into the analyzer (Figure E).
   - The handheld analyzer first displays "Identifying Cartridge" and then a "time-to-result" bar appears.
   - *Do not remove cartridge until the* "Cartridge Locked" message on the handheld analyzer is removed and results are displayed on screen.
6. Review results
   - After 2 to 3 minutes, the results will appear on the screen (Figure F). The "→ Page" command on the bottom of the screen indicates more results will appear on a second screen. Press the print button to send the results to the printer by wireless transmission or by the docking device USB connection.
   - The handheld device shows the numerical values and units with the results. It also shows bar graphs with tic marks for reference ranges.

Continued

PROCEDURE 6.4 i-STAT Chemistry Analyzer Procedure—cont'd

Test	Test Symbol	Units	Reportable Range	Reference Range	Results	Critical Low or High
Sodium	Na^+	mmol/L	100–180	138–146		
Potassium	K^+	mmol/L	2.0–9.0	3.5–4.9		
Chloride	Cl^-	mmol/L	65–140	98–109		
Total carbon dioxide	TCO_2	mmol/L	5–50	24–29		
Ionized calcium	iCa^{2+}	mmol/L	0.25–2.50	1.12–1.32		
Glucose	Glu	mg/dL	20–700	70–105		
Urea nitrogen	BUN	mg/dL	3–140	8–26		
Creatinine	Crea	mg/dL	0.2–20.0	0.6.1.3		
Hematocrit	Hct	% PCV	10–75	38–51		
Hemoglobin*	Hgb	g/dL	3.4–25.5	12–17		
Anion gap*	AnGap	mmol/L	10–99	10–20		

*These results are figured mathematically from the other results (not directly).

Quality Control Procedures

The calibration "optics check" is performed using the simulator provided by i-STAT. Simply place the simulator into the same port as the patient cassette. The results of the optical reading will be displayed and printed. If the result falls out of range, patient tests cannot be run until the cause is determined and corrected.

The two levels of liquid controls should be run at least monthly or whenever a new set of cassettes is opened. Use the syringe to transfer the well-mixed control solution into the cassette well and run the control as you would a patient sample. Document control results and compare them with the control package insert. If the results do not fall in the required range, patient samples cannot be run until the cause is determined and corrected.

Photos by Zack Bent.

PROCEDURE 6.5 Occult Blood ColoScreen III Method

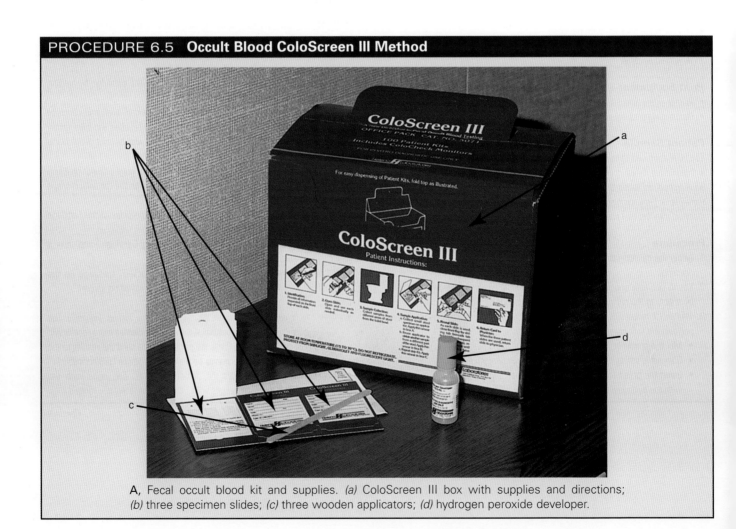

A, Fecal occult blood kit and supplies. *(a)* ColoScreen III box with supplies and directions; *(b)* three specimen slides; *(c)* three wooden applicators; *(d)* hydrogen peroxide developer.

PROCEDURE 6.5 Occult Blood ColoScreen III Method—cont'd

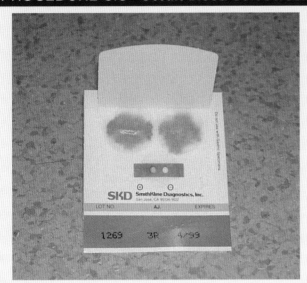

B, Observe the blue positive occult blood test results in the upper patient areas of the slide and confirm the control results at the bottom: positive blue *(left)* and negative white *(right)*. (From Stepp CA, Woods M: *Laboratory procedures for medical office personnel,* Philadelphia, 1998, Saunders.)

Equipment and Supplies for ColoScreen III Method (Figure A)
- ColoScreen III
- Three specimen slides
- Three wooden applicators
- Hydrogen peroxide developer

Check for proper storage (e.g., temperature, light). Check the expiration date. Locate the package insert and patient instructions.

Patient Preparation and Pretest Instruction

Two days before the test and during the specimen-collecting day, the patient should eat a high-fiber diet, including well-cooked poultry or fish; cooked fruits and vegetables; bran cereals; raw lettuce, carrots, and celery; and moderate amounts of peanuts and popcorn. The patient should refrain from ingesting the following items, which may interfere with the test results: red and partially cooked meats, turnips, cauliflower, broccoli, parsnips, melons (especially cantaloupe), alcohol, aspirin, and vitamin C.

When collecting specimens, the patient should use the slides, applicators, and the take-home instructions as follows:

1. After a bowel movement, use the wooden applicator to collect a small sample by scraping the surface of the feces and spread a thin layer in box A of the slide. Using the same applicator, collect a second sample from a different part of the feces and spread it in box B.
2. Discard the wooden applicator, reseal the cover of the slide, and complete the information requested on the outside of the cover.
3. Repeat the preceding steps with the next two consecutive bowel movements and the two remaining slides.

Test Procedure

4. Apply gloves and observe Universal Precautions. Confirm that all necessary information was written on slide covers.
5. Open the back sides of all three slides and place 2 drops of developer on each specimen. Any blue reaction in the specimen area indicates a positive result. A positive result may be read in as early as 30 seconds to 2 minutes but do not record a negative (no blue) until at least 2 minutes have passed.
6. Perform the monitor test (internal control) by placing one or 2 drops between the monitor boxes and waiting 30 seconds to 2 minutes to read the results and confirm that the positive turned blue and the negative did not.
7. Observe if there are positive blue specimen reactions and validate the results of the control monitors showing blue on the positive dot and no blue color on the negative dot (Figure B).

The example in Figure B is positive for occult blood and both controls had correct reactions.

PROCEDURE 6.6 Occult Blood ColoCARE Method

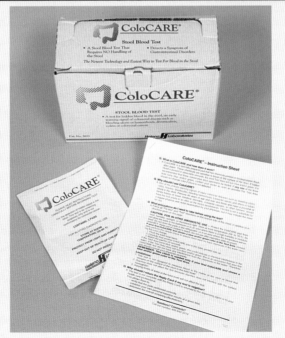

A, ColoCARE method for fecal occult blood. The patient receives a foil packet with three test pads, a reply card, and an instruction sheet.

Continued

PROCEDURE 6.6   Occult Blood ColoCARE Method—cont'd

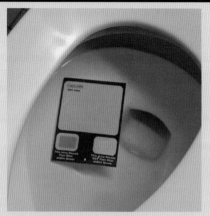

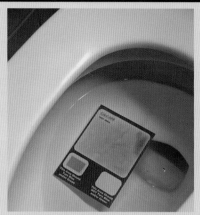

B, Negative occult blood test result with no color in the large test box. The controls show blue in the positive left lower corner and no color in the negative control box in the lower right corner.

C, Positive occult blood test showing blue color in the large test box. The controls again show blue in the positive left lower corner and no color in the negative control box in the lower right corner.

First Bowel Movement	Second Bowel Movement	Third Bowel Movement
Date _____	Date _____	Date _____

ColoCARE
Test area

ColoCARE
Test area

ColoCARE
Test area

This area should turn blue and/or green	This area should NOT turn blue and/or green	This area should turn blue and/or green	This area should NOT turn blue and/or green	This area should turn blue and/or green	This area should NOT turn blue and/or green

D, Patient marks the diagram on the reply card labeled "first bowel movement" with an "x" in each area of the pad that turned a blue or green color. The areas include the large test area and the two smaller areas at the bottom (the positive and negative control areas). The same directions apply to the second and third bowel movements.

Equipment and Supplies for ColoCARE Method

The patient receives foil packet containing three test pads and a reply card along with an instruction sheet (Figure A).

Patient Preparation and Pretest Instruction

Two days before the test and during the specimen-collecting day, the patient should eat a high-fiber diet, including well-cooked poultry or fish, cooked fruits and vegetables, bran cereals, raw lettuce, carrots, celery, and moderate amounts of peanuts and popcorn. The patient should refrain from ingesting the following items, which may interfere with the test results: red and partially cooked meats, turnips, cauliflower, broccoli, parsnips, melons (especially cantaloupe), alcohol, aspirin, and vitamin C.

At-Home Test Procedure

1. After a bowel movement, do not flush or put toilet paper in the toilet. **Perform the following steps within 5 minutes after bowel movement.**
2. Open foil pouch by tearing along the dotted line at the bottom of the pouch, being careful not to tear the pad inside and remove one ColoCARE pad from the pouch. Tape the pouch closed to protect the remaining pads from light and moisture.
3. Hold the ColoCARE pad with the printed side up. Carefully release the pad, allowing it to float on the water in the center of the toilet bowl.
4. Observe the ColoCARE pad for 30 seconds and note any blue or green appearance on the pad (see Figures B and C for possible negative and positive results).
5. After testing the first bowel movement, mark the diagram on the reply card (Figure D) labeled "First Bowel Movement" with an "x" in each area of the pad that turned a blue or green color. The areas include the large TEST AREA and the two smaller areas at the bottom of the pad (the positive and negative control areas). After recording the results on the reply card, flush the floating test pad down the toilet.
6. Repeat step 5 for the next two consecutive bowel movements and mark the second and third diagrams on the reply card according to the same instructions.
7. Fill out all the patient information required on the reply card and either mail it to the office or bring the card back to the office for interpretation.

Photos A, B, and C by Zack Bent.

PROCEDURE 6.7 Occult Blood iFOB Method

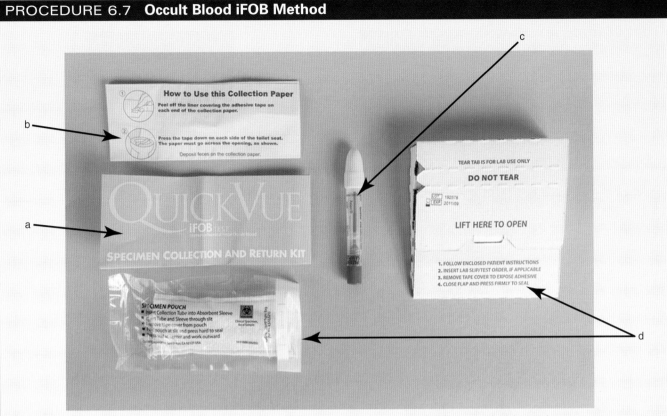

A, Patient supplies for collecting fecal specimen at home for iFOB method: *(a)* step-by-step illustrated instruction sheet; *(b)* specimen collection paper to place across toilet seat; *(C),* specimen collection tube with internal sampling probe to pierce the specimen; *(d)* plastic biohazard bag and mailer to send specimen to the lab or office.

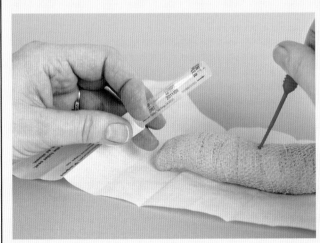

B, Demonstrating how to pierce the specimen using the collection tube's blue probe. The patient is then instructed to recap the blue sampler into the collection tube (on the left), firmly tighten, and shake well. The specimen is then inserted into the provided absorbent sleeve and then into the biohazard plastic bag. The bagged specimen is then placed into the cardboard mailer and returned to the office or laboratory within 24 hours.

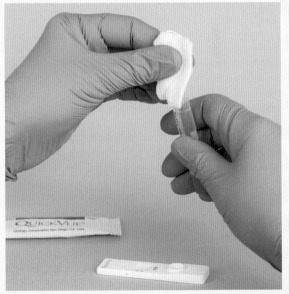

C, After receiving the patient's specimen, the medical assistant or lab tech shakes the specimen thoroughly, and then unscrews the pale blue–capped end of the collection tube. Using the absorbent sleeve or a gauze pad, quickly snap away the plastic tip of the collection tube as seen above.

Continued

PROCEDURE 6.7   Occult Blood iFOB Method—cont'd

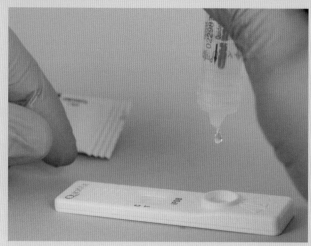

D, Next, holding the sampler collection tube vertically, squeeze 6 drops into the sampling well. Allow the sample to remain undisturbed for 5 to 10 minutes. (This allows the sample to flow laterally across the test area ["T"] and the control area ["C"].)

Patient Supplies for iFOB Method (Figure A)
- Instruction sheet
- Specimen collection paper to place across toilet seat
- Specimen collection tube with internal sampling probe to pierce the stool specimen
- Absorbent pouch, plastic biohazard bag, and mailer to send specimen to the lab or office

Patient Preparation and Pretest Instruction

The QuickVue iFOB test is specific to human hemoglobin. Therefore, the patient does not need to follow the food restrictions in the previous fecal occult tests. Patients with the following conditions, however, should not be considered for testing, because these conditions may interfere with test results:
- Menstrual bleeding
- Bleeding hemorrhoids
- Constipation bleeding
- Urinary bleeding

The patients with the aforementioned conditions may be considered for testing after such bleeding ceases.

Alcohol and certain medications such as aspirin, indomethacin, reserpine, phenylbutazone, corticosteroids, and nonsteroidal antiinflammatory drugs may also cause gastrointestinal irritation and subsequent bleeding in some patients.

Enter the Patient Identification Information on the Collection Tube Label

1. When collecting specimens, the patient should use the take-home instructions as follows:
   - Do not collect specimen if bleeding is present from hemorrhoids, constipation, urination, or menstruation.
   - Urinate before positioning collection paper (or a paper plate).
   - Do not urinate on fecal specimen or collection paper.
   - Position paper on rear half of toilet seat and press the tape down on each side.
   - Deposit fecal specimen on the collection paper.

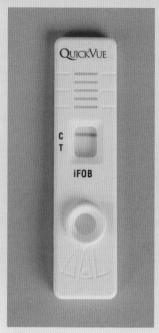

E, After 5 to 10 minutes, inspect the "T" area for a line indicating a positive result for fecal occult blood, or no line indicating a negative result for fecal blood. In both cases, the "C" (control) must show a line indicating the test kit results are "valid." This patient's results show a valid negative result for fecal occult blood.

2. Unscrew the dark blue sampler probe from the collection tube that contains a liquid buffer solution:
   - Using the probe, pierce the specimen in at least five different sites (Figure B).
   - Insert the sampler back into the collection tube, firmly tighten the tube, and then shake the tube well.
   - Flush remaining specimen and collection paper.
3. Make sure the patient's identification line has the patient's name on the label. Then, in the following order, insert the collection tube that has the well-mixed specimen and solution into the:
   - Absorbent sleeve
   - Plastic specimen pouch
   - Cardboard mailer
   - Mail or bring to the medical office or laboratory

Test Procedure After Receiving Specimen

4. Apply gloves and observe Universal Precautions. Confirm that all necessary information was written on the collection tube.
5. Shake tube well and unscrew pale blue cap.
6. Cover the tip with the absorbent sleeve or gauze and snap the tip away (Figure C).
7. Squeeze 6 drops into the test well (Figure D).
8. Read results as positive, negative, or invalid after 5 to 10 minutes (Figure E) based on the following criteria:
   - Positive result: A pink line appears next to the letter T and next to the letter C.
   - Negative result: Only one pink line forms next to the letter C.
   - Invalid test: If there is no pink line next to the letter C, the test results are invalid and should not be reported.

❖ADVANCED CONCEPTS

i-STAT

Additional CLIA-waived point-of-care chemistry analyzers, such as the i-STAT, have been approved for POLs. Originally, this handheld i-STAT device was designed for critical care situations in which blood chemistry test results were needed immediately *(stat)*. The technology was designed to ensure that a non–laboratory-trained health professional could run the chemistry tests at the patient's bedside and obtain reliable results. Table 6.2 shows the critical test values that are typically monitored during a patient's "crisis" situation. The reasons that these values are needed are discussed in the following paragraphs.

Almost all metabolic processes in the body are dependent on or affected by *pH, blood gas,* and *electrolyte levels.* The pH is critical for maintaining proper physiologic molecular structure and chemical reactions. The *electrolytes* (Na^+, K^+, Cl^-, and ionized Ca^{2+}) are involved with water distribution, proper muscle and nerve function, oxidation-reduction reactions, and enzymatic reactions. Proper concentrations of blood gases (oxygen and carbon dioxide) are also critical for maintaining correct tissue oxygenation and pH balance.

Glucose level determinations help in evaluating disorders of carbohydrate metabolism (i.e., hypoglycemia, hyperglycemia, and in establishing a diagnosis of diabetes).

Blood urea nitrogen and *creatinine* measurements are commonly used to evaluate, diagnose, and monitor renal disease. An abnormally high level of urea nitrogen in the blood is an indication of kidney impairment or kidney failure because of the kidney's inability to remove urea from the blood. Other causes of increased values for urea nitrogen include GI bleeding and a high-protein diet. Low BUN levels are not common and usually not significant. Causes of decreased urea values include pregnancy, severe liver insufficiency, overhydration, and malnutrition.

The whole-blood *hematocrit* and *hemoglobin* measurements are useful for determining if RBC quantity is sufficient to maintain a proper oxygen level. It is a key indicator of the body's state of hydration, anemia, or severe blood loss, as well as the blood's ability to transport oxygen.

Piccolo Xpress

Demands for improved patient care and greater cost control are driving profound changes in the structure of health care delivery. Within and outside of traditional hospital environments, evolving technology is permitting some types of diagnostic testing and patient monitoring to move from the clinical laboratory to the near-patient environment. Many health care professionals whose roles have traditionally involved hands-on patient care are now being asked to take a role in clinical chemistry testing as well.

Laboratorians, with their training and experience, know that rigorous quality control (QC) is an absolute necessity for accurate test results on which treatment decisions can confidently be based. The Piccolo Xpress point-of-care chemistry analyzer incorporates a process called iQC ("intelligent Quality Control") that meets established QC standards independently of the operator's skill level. iQC is a series of sophisticated automatic checks that verify the chemistry, optics, and electronic functions of the analyzer during each run and ensure that operators in a wide range of environments report only accurate and reliable results.

The Piccolo Xpress point-of-care chemistry analyzer is a lightweight portable instrument that processes whole blood, serum, or plasma samples in self-contained, single-use reagent disks. Transparent to the operator, iQC checks the analyzer, the reagent disk, and the sample during each run to verify correct electronic and chemistry performance. If it detects uncharacteristic performance, iQC automatically suppresses a single chemistry test result or the entire panel of results and immediately alerts the operator to any problems. From the self-test at power up to the recording and printing of patient results, the Piccolo Xpress conducts multiple QC checks automatically with each run; iQC ensures that the operator reports only accurate and reliable results.

Metabolic Panels: Basic and Comprehensive

Not all offices can afford the previously described chemistry analyzers. When physicians need to know blood chemistry values to arrive at a definitive diagnosis, they will have either the medical assistant or the phlebotomist draw a blood sample (usually a gold SST) and send it to a reference laboratory for

TABLE 6.2   Normal and Critical Blood Chemistry Results (on i-STAT Analyzer)

		Arterial	Venous	Critical Ranges
Reference Ranges	pH	7.35–7.45	7.32–7.42	<7.200 or >7.55
	Pco₂	35–45 mm Hg	41–51 mm Hg	<20 or >65 mm Hg
	Po₂	80–100 mm Hg		<50 mm Hg
	Sodium	136–146 mmol/L		<120 or >160 mmol/L
	Potassium	3.5–5.0 mmol/L		<2.5 or >6.0 mmol/L
	Chloride	101–114 mmol/L		<80 or >130 mmol/L
	Glucose	Fasting: 73–115 mg/dL		Adult: <40 or >500 mg/dL Newborn (birth to 3 months): <40 or >200 mg/dL
	Blood urea nitrogen	Adults (>12 years): 8–20 mg/dL		
	Hematocrit	Male subjects: 42%–52% Female subjects: 37%–47%		<15%
	Hemoglobin	12–17 g/dL		<7 g/dL

testing, or they will send the patient to the reference laboratory. Depending on what the physician needs to know, a metabolic panel, which typically consists of 6 to 12 or more chemistry tests, will be ordered. The panels are usually ordered as part of an annual physical examination, when a patient is being prepared for surgery, or when a patient is exhibiting specific symptoms. Metabolic panels provide the physician with a comprehensive picture of the patient's carbohydrate and lipid metabolism. They also provide information regarding the liver, kidney, heart, and thyroid functions. Typical tests in a metabolic panel include electrolytes, lipids, glucose, BUN, bilirubin, enzymes, and hormones. The report in Figure 6.13 shows each analyte's result along with the lab's reference range. Note that when an analyte is out of range, it is noted in a column next to the reported value. Laboratories are now required to indicate when analytes are outside of their particular reference range because ranges may vary between different methods of testing. The physician must interpret these chemistry results along with the rest of the patient's examination to make a definitive diagnosis.

Kidney or Renal Panel

The renal, or kidney, panel consists of tests that portray how the kidney is functioning. The kidney is responsible for excreting the following chemical wastes: urea, creatinine, and uric acid. By observing increases in **BUN**, blood creatinine, the physician can determine when the kidney has become impaired as well as the degree of impairment. This panel of tests is helpful in monitoring patients with diabetes who are at risk for kidney failure. Elevated uric acid levels within the kidney panel of tests may be associated with **gout** (a form of arthritis caused by the accumulation of uric acid crystals in the synovial fluid of joints).

Electrolyte Panel

The electrolyte panels give a picture of the patient's water-salt balance and the ability to maintain proper pH. The most common electrolytes measured in the serum are the following:
- K^+ and Na^+, two positively charged ions, or **cations**
- Cl^- and HCO_3^-, two negatively charged ions, or **anions**

DATE & TIME RECEIVED	ACCESSION NUMBER
10/20/2010 20:45	
LOCATION	DATE REPORTED
	10/21/2010

PHYSICIAN	PATIENT'S INFORMATION

TEST		RESULTS	REFERENCE RANGE	UNITS
CHEMISTRY 23 - PANEL B				
CALCIUM, TOTAL, SERUM	LO	7.4	8.5-10.5	mg/dL
PHOSPHORUS	LO	2.8	3.0-4.6	mg/dL
URIC ACID	LO	3.2	3.5-7.2	mg/dL
CHOLESTEROL	LO	123	151-240	mg/dL
TRIGLYCERIDE		121	58-258	mg/dL
LDH		217	118-242	IU/L
SGOT (AST)	HI	41	10-37	IU/L
SGPT (ALT)	HI	45	10-40	IU/L
GGTP	LO	8	11-51	IU/L
ALKALINE PHOSPHATASE		63	39-117	IU/L
BILIRUBIN, TOTAL		0.3	0.1-1.5	mg/dL
ALBUMIN	LO	2.4	3.7-5.2	g/dL
TOTAL PROTEIN	LO	3.6	6.0-8.5	g/dL
ALBUMIN/GLOBULIN RATIO		2.0	1.0-2.2	RATIO

FIG. 6.13 Example of an abnormal metabolic panel report. Notice the second column indicating if an analyte is "HI" or "LO" compared with its reference range. See text for abbreviations. (From Zakus SM: *Mosby's clinical skills for medical assistants,* ed 4, St. Louis, 2001, Mosby.)

Liver or Hepatic Panel

The hepatic panel is a series of tests to determine liver function and damage or disease. The liver is involved in the following metabolic functions:

- It metabolizes glucose from the GI tract into stored glycogen.
- It metabolizes amino acids from the GI tract into plasma proteins—albumin, some globulins, and the clotting proteins (fibrinogen and prothrombin).
- It metabolizes fatty acids from the GI tract into the various blood lipids.
- It processes bilirubin, a waste product from the breakdown of hemoglobin, and excretes it in the bile.
- When the liver is extremely impaired, the blood chemistry may reflect *increases* in bilirubin levels, and *decreased* levels of albumins and clotting proteins, owing to the impairment of protein production.

Enzymes are usually located within the cells of organs and tissues. Enzymes are catalysts that assist in the specific metabolic changes required of cells. An enzyme's name always ends with the suffix *-ase.* The word root preceding the *-ase* explains the chemical reaction in which the enzyme is involved. When a tissue or organ is damaged, it releases its specific enzymes into the blood. Because the liver is involved in so many intracellular metabolic reactions, levels of all the following enzymes may become elevated in the blood when it is damaged:

- Alkaline phosphatase (alk phos, **ALP**, or **AP**)
- Gamma-glutamyltransferase (**GGT**)
- Aspartate aminotransferase (AST)
- Alanine aminotransferase (ALT)
- Lactic acid dehydrogenase (LDH)

Patients who are taking medications (e.g., statin drugs that lower blood cholesterol) may have their ALT or AST levels tested to see if the liver is being damaged by the medication.

Other damaged organs may release some of these enzymes as well. Again, the physician must interpret the chemical results along with the complete clinical picture of the patient before making a definitive diagnosis.

Cardiac Panel

When the heart is injured, as in a myocardial infarction (heart attack), it releases the following into the blood:

- Troponins I and T— heart muscle proteins that, when elevated, are excellent heart-specific indicators of a recent myocardial infarction.
- Creatine kinase (**CK or CPK**)—an enzyme found in muscle and brain tissue becomes elevated soon after the heart is damaged. The use of this test to diagnose a heart attack has been replaced by the troponin test. Two other heart enzymes that were used in the past, LDH and AST (SGOT), may also become elevated. These have also been superseded by the troponin markers.

Thyroid Panel

The thyroid gland plays a critical role in body metabolism by producing two hormones, thyroxine (T_4) and triiodothyronine (T_3). Their production is regulated by the pituitary gland, which releases thyroid-stimulating hormone (**TSH**).

Individual Analytes and Their Disease Associations

The laboratory requisition, as previously seen in Figure 6.3 at the beginning of the chapter, listed many individual tests that can be ordered, as well as the panels of tests. Individual tests are preferred over panels after the diagnosis is made and the condition requires frequent monitoring. Table 6.3 lists the most common chemistry tests categorically, their expected ranges, and the possible disease associations if the test results are high or low.

TABLE 6.3 Common Chemistry Panels and Tests, and Their Possible Disease Associations

Tests and Panels	Expected Range*	POSSIBLE DISEASE ASSOCIATIONS	
		High Levels	Low Levels
Renal Panel—Kidney			
BUN (blood urea nitrogen)	8–26 mg/dL	Impaired kidney function Acute renal failure Cardiovascular failure Obstruction of urine flow	No clinical significance
BUN/creatinine ratio	10–20	Prerenal impairment Dehydration Congestive heart failure Gastrointestinal bleed	Renal tubular necrosis Liver disease
Creatinine	0.7–1.4 mg/dL	Impaired kidney function Acute glomerulonephritis Obstruction of urine flow	No clinical significance
Uric acid	3.6–8 mg/dL (male subjects) 2.5–6.78 mg/dL (female subjects)	Gout Decreased renal function Emotional stress Total fasting	Use of some drugs

Continued

TABLE 6.3 **Common Chemistry Panels and Tests, and Their Possible Disease Associations—cont'd**

Tests and Panels	Expected Range*	POSSIBLE DISEASE ASSOCIATIONS	
		High Levels	Low Levels
Electrolyte Panel			
Chloride	98–108 mmol/L	Congestive heart failure	Nephritis
		Dehydration	Diuretic administration
		Cushing disease	Starvation
		Diabetes insipidus	Severe vomiting
		Severe hyperaldosteronism	Severe hypoaldosteronism
Potassium	3.5–5.3 mmol/L	Urinary obstruction	Diarrhea
		Renal failure	Diuretic administration
		Ketoacidosis	Starvation
		Hypoaldosteronism	Hyperaldosteronism
			Renal tubular defects
Sodium	135–146 mmol/L	Severe dehydration	Metabolic acidosis
		Brain injuries	Diarrhea
		Diabetic coma	Renal tubular disease
		Cushing disease	Polyuria
		Hyperaldosteronism	Addison disease
		Lack of ADH	Overhydration
		Renal failure	Hypoaldosteronism
			Renal SIADH
Hepatic—Liver Panel			
Bilirubin	0.1–1.2 mg/dL	Massive hemolysis	No clinical significance
		Obstructive jaundice	
		Cirrhosis	
		Carcinoma	
		Renal calculi	
A/G ratio (albumin/globulin ratio)	1.1–2.5	No clinical significance	Viral hepatitis
			Ulcerative colitis
			Burns
			Multiple myeloma
			Sarcoidosis
			Metastatic carcinoma
			Nephrotic syndrome
			Diabetic ketosis
			Congestive heart failure
Albumin	3.5–5.0 g/dL	Dehydration	Impaired synthesis (cirrhosis, hepatitis)
			Hemorrhage
			Acute nephritis
			Protein-losing gastroenteropathies
			Inadequate protein intake
			Excessive protein breakdown
			Burns
Globulin	1.7–3.5 g/dL	Chronic active hepatitis	Celiac disease
		Multiple myeloma	Neoplasms
		Hodgkin disease	Hypogammaglobulinemia
		Collagen disease	Renal disease
		Tuberculosis	
		Brucellosis	
		Sarcoidosis	
Protein	6–8.5 g/dL	Multiple myeloma	Impaired kidney function
		Dehydration	
		Vomiting	
		Diarrhea	

TABLE 6.3 Common Chemistry Panels and Tests, and Their Possible Disease Associations—cont'd

Tests and Panels	Expected Range*	POSSIBLE DISEASE ASSOCIATIONS	
		High Levels	Low Levels
Blood Enzyme Panel			
ALP (alkaline phosphatase)	117–390 units/L (children) 39–117 units/L (adults)	Obstructive jaundice Paget disease Rickets Osteomalacia Hepatocellular disease Biliary obstruction Cirrhosis	Malnutrition Scurvy Hypothyroidism Zinc and magnesium deficiency Anemia
AST (SGOT) aspartate transaminase	0–37 units/L (male) 0–31 units/L (female)	Myocardial dysfunction Acute hepatitis Cirrhosis Mononucleosis	No clinical significance
ALT (SGPT) alanine transaminase	0–40 units/L (male) 0–31 units/L (female)	Viral hepatitis Biliary obstruction	No clinical significance
CK (creatine kinase)	10–90 units/L (depending on method of testing)	MI Duchenne muscular dystrophy Crush injuries	No clinical significance; may be seen in early pregnancy
GGT (gamma-glutamyltransferase)	11–50 units/L (male) 7–32 units/L (female)	Cirrhosis Congestive heart failure Alcoholism Obstructive jaundice Hepatocellular disease	No clinical significance
LD or LDH (lactic acid dehydrogenase)	118–242 units/L (male) 122–220 units/L (female)	Hemolytic anemia Pernicious anemia Infections Acute kidney disease Liver disease LD isoenzymes needed to identify specific tissue disorders (i.e., MI, lung infarction)	No clinical significance
Minerals			
Calcium	8.5–10.5 mg/dL	Dehydration Myeloma Hyperparathyroiditis Sarcoidosis Bone metastases Leukemia Lymphoma Paget disease Acute renal failure Hypervitaminosis D Addison disease	Regional enteritis Ulcerative colitis Diarrhea Hypoparathyroidism Cushing disease Pancreatitis Malabsorption Malnutrition Rickets Tetany (neonates) Vitamin D deficiency Some renal and intestinal disorders
Phosphorus	2.5–4.5 mg/dL	Addison disease Hypervitaminosis D Acromegaly Hypoparathyroidism Chronic renal failure	Hyperparathyroidism Vitamin D deficiency Rickets Malabsorption IDDM
Iron	40–160 mcg/dL	Hemolytic anemia Hemochromatosis Increased release from body stores Decreased use of iron (e.g., lead poisoning) Sideroblastic anemia	Iron deficiency anemia Pregnancy Insufficient dietary intake of iron

Continued

TABLE 6.3 Common Chemistry Panels and Tests, and Their Possible Disease Associations—cont'd

Tests and Panels	Expected Range*	POSSIBLE DISEASE ASSOCIATIONS	
		High Levels	Low Levels
Blood Gases			
Carbon dioxide	Dependent on method and if	Aldosteronism	Diarrhea
Oxygen	blood is arterial or venous	Respiratory acidosis	Metabolic acidosis
		Metabolic alkalosis	Respiratory alkalosis
Metabolism			
Cholesterol	140–200 mg/dL	Atherosclerotic disease	Malnutrition
	LDL <100 mg/dL	Alcoholism	
	HDL >50 mg/dL	Defects in lipoprotein metabolism	
		Hypothyroidism	
		Diabetes mellitus	
Glucose	65–100 mg/dL	Diabetes mellitus (hyperglycemia)	Hypoglycemia
		Cushing disease	Addison disease
Triglycerides	30–150 mg/dL	Atherosclerotic disease	Malnutrition
		Alcoholism	
		Hyperlipidemia	
		Hypothyroidism	
		Pancreatic disorders	
		Diabetes mellitus (poorly controlled)	

*The exact ranges vary because of testing method, population, location, and so on.
ADH, Antidiuretic hormone; *IDDM,* insulin-dependent diabetes mellitus; *MI,* myocardial infarction; *SIADH,* syndrome of inappropriate secretion of antidiuretic hormone.

Summary

Because blood chemistry is so crucial to diagnosis and patient care, technology will continue to provide POLs with new and improved, user-friendly chemical testing analyzers. Be sure to stay informed through local diagnostic test suppliers, vendor displays at professional association meetings, and the Internet for the latest in chemistry testing. The websites for each of the CLIA-waived testing methods presented in this chapter are also listed. Review the latest news at each site, as well as their educational departments and their demonstration videos.

■ REVIEW QUESTIONS*

1. What type of specimen is required for most blood chemistry tests in the POL? (Hint: Think of the waived tests.) When collecting blood for a reference laboratory?
2. When plasma glucose level is high, what hormone is secreted?
3. What percentage of diabetes mellitus cases in the United States are type 2, or non–insulin-dependent, cases?
4. The presence of sugar in the urine is called _____ _____.
5. A type of blood glucose test that requires no special fasting or other preparation is the
   a. GTT.
   b. fasting glucose.
   c. 2-hour postprandial glucose.
   d. random glucose test.
6. Explain the reason for testing Hgb A_{1c}.
7. List the two main sources of cholesterol in the blood.
8. Why is LDL cholesterol referred to as "lousy" cholesterol and HDL referred to as "healthy" cholesterol?
9. What is the purpose of calibrating a blood chemistry analyzer?
10. List three reasons that a control would not fall within its designated range.

11. List the ranges for each of the following total cholesterol categories:
    a. Desirable cholesterol level:
    b. Low-risk cholesterol level:
    c. High cholesterol level:
12. Match the following:

    _____ LDL
    _____ HDL
    _____ glycogen
    _____ hypoglycemia
    _____ hyperglycemia
    _____ lipoprotein

    a. an abnormal increase in the glucose level in the blood
    b. a complex molecule consisting of protein and a fat such as cholesterol
    c. the form in which carbohydrate is stored in the body
    d. a lipoprotein consisting of protein and cholesterol that removes excess cholesterol from blood vessel walls
    e. an abnormally low level of glucose in the blood
    f. a lipoprotein consisting of protein and cholesterol that adheres to blood vessel walls, forming plaque

13. What is the main reason for performing the fecal occult blood test? List the three methods for testing fecal occult blood.

14. Match the blood chemistry profiles for the various body organs or diseases with their corresponding chemistry tests:

    ___ renal panel   a. uric acid
    ___ liver panel   b. BUN, creatinine, electrolytes
    ___ cardiac panel   c. troponin I and T, CK
    ___ lipid panel   d. bilirubin, alkaline phosphatase, albumin, globulin, ALT (SGPT)
    ___ gout   e. cholesterol, LDL, HDL, triglycerides

*Answers to these Review Questions are located in the Appendix on p. 278.

WEBSITES

Bayer Contour information:
www.bayercontour.com/Blood-Glucose-Monitoring/Product-Portfolio

Demonstration video on how to use the LifeScan OneTouch
   Ultra glucose monitor from Johnson & Johnson:
www.lifescan.com

i-STAT information:
file:///C:/Users/Owner/Downloads/i-STAT_1_Quick_Reference_Guide_716942-00K.pdf
Information on iFOB testing:
www.quidel.com/assets/swf/iFOBTrainingvideoHQ.htm
Piccolo Xpress information:
www.abaxis.com/medical/

Immunology

OBJECTIVES

After completing this chapter, you should be able to do the following:

1. Define and match key terms in this chapter.

Fundamental Concepts

2. Explain the following concepts related to the immune process:
   - List the three lines of defense against harmful invaders.
   - Differentiate between cell-mediated immunity and humoral immunity.
   - Match the classes of immunoglobulins (antibodies) with their locations or functions.
   - List the four ways to acquire adaptive (acquired) immunity.
3. Discuss the principles of in vivo and in vitro immunology tests as they relate to allergy testing.

CLIA-Waived Immunology Tests

4. Give examples of direct and indirect immunology tests based on the detection of antigens or antibodies.
5. Describe mononucleosis, *Helicobacter pylori*, and HIV infections and explain how they are diagnosed.

6. Obtain specimens and perform the following CLIA-waived immunology tests according to the stated task, conditions, and standards listed in the Learning Outcome Procedure Sheets in the student workbook:
   - Pregnancy test
   - Infectious mononucleosis test
   - *H. pylori* test
   - HIV blood or oral test

Advanced Concepts

7. Discuss advanced immunologic techniques such as agglutination and enzyme-linked immunosorbent assay and a lateral flow immunochromatographic assay.
8. Explain the basic principles of ABO and Rh blood typing and discuss the relationship between hemolytic disease of the newborn and the Rh-negative status of the mother.
9. Explain how antibody titers are used by physicians in the diagnosis and prognosis of disease conditions.
10. Identify common immunology tests within three categories: bacterial infections, viral infections, and detection of other antigens such as hormones and cancer-related substances.

KEY TERMS

active immunity: long-term protection against future infections resulting from the production of antibodies that were formed naturally during a specific infection or artificially by vaccination

agglutination: clumping of blood cells or latex beads caused by antibodies adhering to their antigens

allergen: an antigen that causes an allergic reaction

antibodies: specific immunoglobulins produced to destroy foreign invaders (antigens)

antigens: substances that are perceived as foreign to the body and elicit an immune response; the production of antibodies

autoimmune diseases: destructive tissue diseases caused by antibodies produced against self-antigens

cell-mediated immunity: T-lymphocytic cell response to antigens

chromatographic assay: a visual color change that appears when enzyme-linked antibody–antigen reaction takes place during a testing procedure

complement proteins: proteins that stimulate phagocytosis and inflammation and are capable of destroying bacteria

erythroblastosis fetalis: a hemolytic anemia in newborns resulting from maternal–fetal blood group incompatibility

helper T cells (TH4 or CD4): antigen-activated lymphocytes that stimulate other T cells and invoke B cells to produce their antibodies

heterophile antibody: antibody that appears during an Epstein-Barr viral infection (mononucleosis) and has an unusual affinity to the antigens on the red cells from sheep, horses, or cows

histamine: chemical compound released by injured cells, and during allergic, and inflammatory reactions that causes the dilation of blood vessels

humoral immunity: B-lymphocytic cell response to antigens resulting in the production of specific antibodies to destroy a foreign invader; also called antibody-mediated immunity

***H. pylori*:** spiral-shaped bacteria believed to be the cause of most peptic ulcers

iFOB (immunoassay Fecal Occult Blood) and FiT (Fecal immunochemical Test): new immunology methods for testing fecal occult blood

immunosorbent: pertaining to the attachment of an antigen or antibody to a solid surface such as latex beads, wells in plastic dishes, or plastic cartridges

inflammation: overall reaction of the body to tissue injury or invasion by an infectious agent, characterized by redness, heat, swelling, and pain

interferons: proteins secreted by viral infected cells to prevent the further replication and spread of an infection into neighboring cells

in vitro: outside of the living body and in an artificial environment (i.e., the laboratory)

in vivo: within a host or living organism

killer T cells: antigen-activated lymphocytes that attack foreign antigens directly and destroy cells that bear the antigens; also called cytotoxic cells

memory B cells: antigen-activated B lymphocytes that produce antibodies upon the first encounter and then remember the antigen for future encounters

memory T cells: antigen-activated T lymphocytes that remember an antigen for future encounters

mucous membrane: thin sheets of tissue that line the internal cavities and canals of the body (i.e., gut and respiratory passages)

natural killer cells: special type of lymphocyte that attacks and destroys infected cells and cancer cells in a nonspecific way

normal flora: harmless microorganisms that normally inhabit the skin and mucous membranes

passive immunity: short-term acquired immunity created by antibodies received naturally through the placenta and the colostrum (first breast milk) to an infant or received artificially by injection

phagocytes: cells capable of engulfing, ingesting, and destroying microorganisms and cellular debris

phagocytosis: process of engulfing, digesting, and destroying microorganisms and cellular debris

plasma cells: B lymphocytes that produce the antibodies that travel through the blood specifically targeting and reacting with antigens

qualitative test: test that simply looks for the presence or absence of a substance

self-antigens: substances within the body that are capable of inducing the production of antibodies that attack an individual's own body tissues; also called autoantigens; they may result in an autoimmune disease

serology: branch of laboratory medicine that performs antibody–antigen testing with serum

suppressor T cells: also referred to as Regulatory T cells, antigen-activated lymphocytes that inhibit T and B cells after a sufficient number of cells have been activated

T cells: small lymphocytes associated with the thymus gland

titer: a quantitative test that measures the amount of antibody that reacts with a specific antigen

vaccination: process of injecting harmless or dead microorganisms into the body to induce immunity against a potential pathogen (also called immunization)

wheal: a reddish, raised induration (hardened tissue), such as a hive caused by an antibody–antigen reaction

❖ FUNDAMENTAL CONCEPTS

Overview of Immunology

The immune system is a remarkable defense system that protects the human body against invading pathogens, toxins, allergens, and cancer cells. When the body is under attack by any of these invaders, it has a full arsenal of defenses to destroy the invader, as well as protect itself from future attacks. A key ingredient in this defense mechanism is the body's production of antibodies (immunoglobulins produced specifically to destroy foreign invaders). These antibodies are produced after the body detects the presence of specific antigens (substances that are perceived as foreign to the body). After antibodies are produced, they attack the antigens, forming an antibody–antigen complex that destroys or renders the invader harmless.

Biotechnology research has made it possible to detect and measure specific antibodies and their specific antigens in blood and body fluids. Antibody–antigen testing is a rapidly expanding laboratory science called *immunology.* Because antibodies are usually found in serum, the laboratory department performing antibody–antigen testing may also be referred to as the serology *department.*

The science of immunology dates to the 1500s, when it was recorded that China had developed a technique of exposing individuals to a powder made from smallpox scabs to produce protection against the disease. The thought was that if children or young adults were exposed in a healthy state, the disease would not be as devastating; unfortunately, that did not always occur. In the late 1700s, Edward Jenner, an English country doctor, found that injecting individuals with material from cowpox provided effective protection against smallpox. This preventive process of injecting harmless or dead microorganisms into the body to induce immunity against a potential pathogen was known as vaccination or immunization.

The field of immunology has benefited from a tremendous amount of new research and subsequent knowledge over the past 100 years. In fact, the cells responsible for the body's immune response were not discovered until the 1960s. Another recent finding is that the body may respond to self-antigens (substances within the body that are capable of inducing the production of antibodies that attack an individual's own body tissues; also called *autoantigens*). Antibody or self-antigen reactions may cause a variety of destructive tissue diseases referred to as autoimmune diseases.

The Immune Process

The overall immune process that occurs as the body protects itself against foreign invaders can be viewed as three lines (or battlefields) of defensive mechanisms. Figure 7.1 is a simplified picture of these lines of defense. The potential foreign invaders are listed at the top of the flow chart. The next two rows are the body's first and second lines of defense and are considered

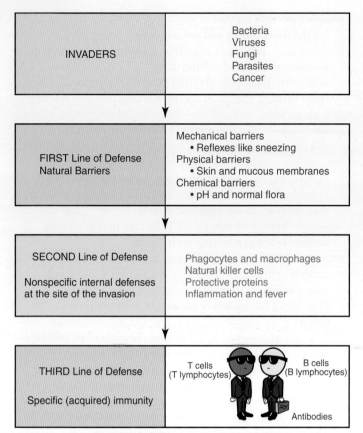

FIG. 7.1 Three lines of defense against harmful invaders. Non-specific immunity defenses are external barriers, and then internal responses to the invaders. Specific immunity (the third line of defense) involves "intelligent" T cells, B cells, and the production of antibodies. (Modified from Herlihy M: *The human body in health and illness,* ed 5, St. Louis, 2014, Saunders.)

"nonspecific immunity"—nonspecific because they fight all invaders in the same way. The third line of defense, at the bottom of the illustration, is referred to as "specific immunity" because it intelligently identifies each invader on the basis of its specific antigens. The intelligent T cells are able to give critical information to the B cells that are then able to produce a specific antibody capable of destroying the invader.

First line of defense: natural barriers. The first line of defense stops invaders from entering or growing on the body. The skin and **mucous membrane** (thin sheets of tissue lining the internal cavities and canals) serve as anatomical barriers that prevent the entry of pathogens into the body. They also secrete chemicals that discourage the growth of pathogenic bacteria. These secretions maintain a skin pH of 5.6, which allows the growth of **normal flora** (harmless microorganisms that normally inhabit the skin and mucous membranes) while inhibiting the growth of pathogens. In the respiratory tract, the mucous membranes contain mucus, which entraps foreign organisms. Coughing and sneezing help move foreign organisms out of the body.

Second line of defense: nonspecific internal response. The second line of defense is the internal nonspecific response to all invaders that have passed the natural barriers and entered the

body. When invaders break through the barriers, the body quickly responds by sending **phagocytes** (cells capable of engulfing, ingesting, and destroying pathogens and cellular debris) to the site of invasion. Two white blood cells—neutrophils and monocytes (which become macrophages in the tissue)—engulf, ingest, and destroy the invaders by the process of **phagocytosis**.

Natural killer cells are a special type of lymphocyte sent to the scene of invasion to attack and destroy the body's infected cells and cancer cells in a nonspecific way. Protective proteins such as interferons and complement proteins also play an important role at the site of invasion. **Interferons** are proteins secreted by infected cells to prevent the further replication and spread of the infection into neighboring cells. **Complement proteins** are proteins that further stimulate phagocytosis and **inflammation** (reaction of the body to tissue injury or invasion by an infectious agent) and are capable of destroying bacteria. Complement proteins swarm over a bacterium and punch holes in its membrane, causing it to fill with fluid and explode.

At the same time that these defenders are doing their jobs to destroy the invader, the injured tissues are initiating a nonspecific *inflammatory* response. The clinical signs of inflammation are heat, redness, swelling, and pain. Inflammation begins when **histamine** is released by the injured cells, causing the dilation of blood vessels. The increased blood flow to the affected areas results in redness and heat. Fluids in the plasma leak into the tissue because of the increased permeability of the vessels, causing the swelling and pain.

The second line of defense is generally seen within the first 12 hours of an infection. For example, the first signs and symptoms of influenza start with sore throat, dry cough, chills, aching muscles, and fever. These symptoms are the result of an active nonspecific battle against the invaders consisting of the phagocytes, natural killer cells, and protective proteins and the subsequent inflammatory response.

Third line of defense: acquired (adaptive) immunity. The third line of defense is activated when the first two lines have failed to bring the invasion under control. It is the "intelligent" identification of the invader based on its antigenic properties. The T cells and B cells work together to produce the specific antibodies that will destroy the invader or render it harmless. This adaptive process takes 6 to 10 days to accomplish. The T and B cells are also capable of developing immunologic memory so that a second encounter with the same organism will induce a heightened immune reaction.

Both these intelligent lymphocytes provide different immunologic functions, as described in the following sections.

Cell-mediated immunity. **T cells**, small lymphocytes associated with the thymus gland, are involved in **cell-mediated immunity**. They become involved at the site of the invasion, where they become activated after they receive an antigen presentation from the macrophages (Figure 7.2).

After they are activated, T cells rapidly duplicate themselves into clones that differentiate into the following four subgroups:
1. **Killer T cells**, or cytotoxic cells, are antigen-activated lymphocytes that attack foreign antigens directly and destroy cells that bear the antigens.

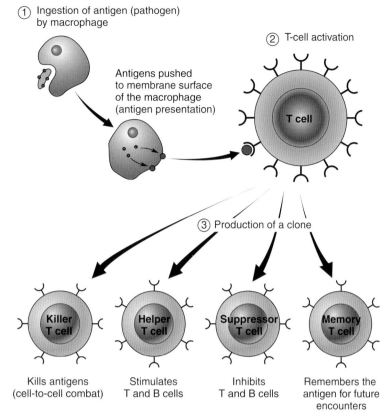

FIG. 7.2 Activation of T cells from the antigens provided by the macrophage resulting in cell-mediated immunity. The three-step process results in four subsets of T cells. (From Herlihy M: *The human body in health and illness,* ed 5, St. Louis, 2014, Saunders.)

2. **Helper T cells (TH4 or CD4)** stimulate other T cells and stimulate B cells to produce their antibodies. (NOTE: These are the cells that can become infected and destroyed by the human immunodeficiency virus [HIV].)

3. **Suppressor T cells** (Regulatory T cells) inhibit the T and B cells after a sufficient number of cells have been activated.

4. **Memory T cells** remember the antigen for future encounters. They are ready to respond to future exposures with increased speed and intensity.

Of the lymphocytes circulating in the blood, 70% to 80% are T cells.

Humoral immunity (antibody-mediated immunity). B cells are involved in **humoral immunity**. Humoral immunity begins with the interaction of a B cell with a specific antigen and the lymphokine (chemicals) from the T helper cell (Figure 7.3).

After it is activated, it rapidly duplicates into a clone and differentiates into the following two subgroups:

1. **Plasma cells** produce the antibodies (immunoglobulins) that travel through the blood specifically targeting and reacting with the antigens, resulting in the destruction of the invader.

2. **Memory B cells** remember the antigen for future encounters. They also are ready to respond to subsequent exposure to the specific antigens with increased speed and intensity.

Classes of antibodies (immunoglobulins). Biomedical researchers have found that antibodies are part of the globulin group of proteins that circulate in the blood. Because of their globulin properties, antibodies are referred to as *immunoglobulins*

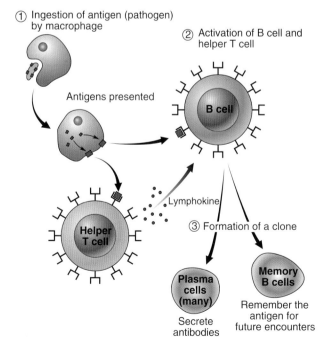

FIG. 7.3 Activation of B cells by antigens and T helper cells resulting in humoral (antibody) immunity. The three-step process results in the production of antibodies by the plasma cells. (From Herlihy M: *The human body in health and illness,* ed 5, St. Louis, 2014, Saunders.)

(Igs). The researchers have classified immunoglobulins into the following groups, based on their shapes, locations, and functions:

- IgE is the immunoglobulin involved in acute allergic reactions and parasitic infections.
- IgM is the primary responder in the first encounter with an invading antigen.
- IgG responds to the antigens in future invasions.
- IgA protects mucous membranes from bacterial and viral infections.
- IgD is involved in lymphocyte activation and suppression.

Ways to acquire specific immunity. When a specific antibody is present in the blood, the individual is said to be immune to its particular disease, pathogen, or antigen. There are four ways to acquire specific immunity: (1) active immunity acquired naturally, (2) active immunity acquired artificially, (3) passive immunity acquired naturally, and (4) passive immunity acquired artificially (Figure 7.4).

Active immunity is long-term protection against future infections that results from the production of antibodies that were formed naturally during an infection or artificially by vaccination. In both cases, the antibody is remembered in the memory B cells, making the individual immune to future encounters with the pathogen.

Passive immunity is short-term protection against infections created by antibodies received naturally through the placenta (or the colostrum to an infant) or artificially by the injection of antiserum or gamma globulins. Passive immunity is only temporary.

Two Types of Allergy Testing
In Vivo Testing

The body is capable of overreacting to antigens by producing too many antibodies resulting in allergic or autoimmune conditions such as asthma, hives, breathing difficulties, and gastrointestinal inflammation. Allergy tests have been performed to visualize the specific reaction between an allergen (an antigen that causes an allergic reaction) and its specific antibody. Tests are done in vivo (within a host or living organism) by injecting or pricking an antigen into the skin and seeing whether a wheal (a reddish, raised induration or hardened tissue, such as a hive) forms in response to the antibody–antigen reaction. Tuberculosis screening tests and allergy skin tests are examples of in vivo immunology tests.

In Vitro Testing

Laboratory immunology tests (also referred to as *serology tests*) are now being performed in vitro (outside of the living body). It is now possible to test the antigen–antibody reaction using only the serum from a tube of blood. Through this testing method, a multi-well plate is coated with various food proteins or inhalants (or both) that are possible allergens capable of

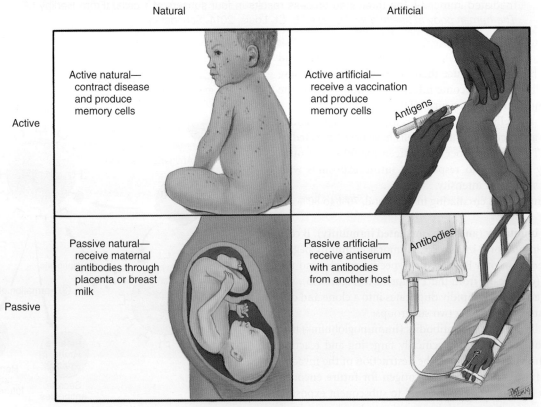

FIG. 7.4 Examples of the four combinations of active and passive immunity and natural and artificial immunity. NOTE: the "Active" row exposures generally produce permanent immunity, and the "Passive" row methods of immunity produce temporary immunity (because the individual does not "learn" to make their own antibodies). (From Applegate EJ: *The anatomy and physiology learning system,* ed 4, St. Louis, 2011, Saunders.)

causing allergic reactions. The patient's serum is then added to each well. If the patient's serum contains IgE or IgG antibodies to any of the specific food or inhalant proteins, a binding reaction occurs. The degree of antibody–antigen binding depends on the concentration of antibodies present in the patient's serum. The reaction is then detected through a color change and assessed spectrophotometrically. The wells showing a strong color reaction caused by high levels of IgG immunoglobulins will indicate an allergic response to the items in the wells. A typical serologic food panel test will indicate possible allergies in the following food groups: gluten; peanuts; dairy; meat or fowl; fruits; fish, crustacea, or mollusk; grains; vegetables; spices; and herbs.

❖ CLIA-WAIVED IMMUNOLOGY TESTS

CLIA-Waived Enzyme-Linked Immunoassays

Manufacturers produce a large variety of immunology testing devices. In most of these rapid screening tests, a liquid specimen is absorbed and travels across a testing area that enzymatically changes color if an antibody–antigen reaction takes place, referred to as a Chromatographic assay. The tests typically include an internal control that must also change color to prove the testing device is working. The control area is usually located just beyond the test area to make sure the solution has traveled all the way through the test area. This method is often referred to as a *lateral flow immunochromatographic assay.* Figure 7.5 shows the before and after reactions of a positive and a negative urine pregnancy test result.

The presence of specific antibodies or antigens associated with a specific disease can be detected in the blood or other body specimens by mixing them with their specific antigen or antibody and observing a reaction. The test kits usually provide a visual reaction when the antibody–antigen complex is formed. Biotechnology continues to develop numerous CLIA-waived test kits designed to rapidly detect the presence of an antigen (direct test) or an antibody (indirect test) associated with a particular disease or infection. These screening tests are usually displayed and interpreted via a visual color change that appears when the enzyme-linked antibody–antigen reaction takes place.

Table 7.1 lists the common CLIA-waived tests that use the lateral flow method to detect the presence of an antigen or antibody associated with a specific disease or condition. Some test kits provide the antibody and test for its antigen in the specimen (direct tests). Other test kits provide the antigen and test for its specific antibody in the specimen (indirect tests). In both cases, a color reaction occurs if both antibody and antigen are present, and the results are recorded as positive. If the color reaction does not occur in the test area, the result is recorded as negative. Also note that if a color does not develop in the internal control area, the patient's result is invalid, and the test must be repeated.

A variety of test kits are available for CLIA-waived screening tests for pregnancy, mononucleosis, *Helicobacter pylori* infections, HIV, and the new iFOB (immunoassay Fecal Occult Blood) and FiT (Fecal immunochemical Test) methods for testing fecal occult blood (as seen in Chapter 6). (NOTE: This text provides the directions that apply to the specific manufacturer's kits portrayed in the procedures. Never assume that the instructions from a new kit or a kit from another manufacturer are the same. The instructions packaged with each box of testing kits should be read thoroughly, followed, and saved as a reference for as long as there are kits to be tested with the box's lot number.)

Pregnancy Testing

Pregnancy testing is based on the detection of a hormone called *human chorionic gonadotropin (hCG)*, which is found in urine or blood. hCG levels in blood and urine may detect pregnancy

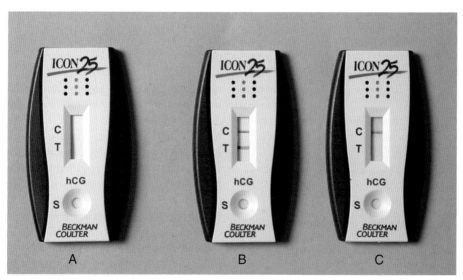

FIG. 7.5 In vitro pregnancy test showing the lateral flow immunochromatographic test method. **A,** Test device before adding specimen (*S,* specimen is placed in well; *T,* specimen travels through test area; *C,* control must turn color to prove device is functioning correctly). **B,** Positive result in test area and control area (two pink bands). **C,** Negative result in test area and positive reaction in control area.

TABLE 7.1 Common CLIA-Waived Tests That Use the Lateral Flow Method

	WHEN BOTH ANTIGEN AND ANTIBODY ARE PRESENT → POSITIVE RESULT	
Screening Tests	**Antigens (When Testing for Antigen in Specimen = Direct Test)**	**Antibodies (When Testing for Antibody in Specimen = Indirect Test)**
Pregnancy	hCG from mother's placenta in urine specimen (**direct**)	Anti-hCG antibodies in test kit
Bladder tumor–associated antigen (BTA)	BTA from bladder cancer in urine specimen (**direct**)	Monoclonal antibodies in test kit react with BTA
Mononucleosis	Heterophile antigens in test kit	IgM heterophile antibody produced against EBV found in blood specimen (**indirect**)
Helicobacter pylori	*H. pylori* antigens in test kit	IgG antibodies specific against *H. pylori* found in blood specimen (**indirect**)
HIV	HIV-1 antigens in test kit	Antibodies against HIV-1 found in blood or cheek cells (**indirect**)
Immunoassay for fecal occult blood (iFOB)*	Blood from fecal matter (**direct**)	Immunochemical color reaction occurs if positive
Influenza A and B†	Viral antigens from nasal swab specimen (**direct**)	Antiviral antibodies in test kit
Streptococcus A infection†	Streptococcal antigen extracted from throat swab (**direct**)	Antistreptococcal antibodies in test kit
Drug testing in urine‡	Drug will inhibit immune reaction	NOTE: Reaction does *not* appear in test area if positive

*iFOB is covered in Chapter 6.
†Antigenic direct testing for the presence of influenza A and B infection and streptococcus A infection is covered in Chapter 8.
‡Drug testing in urine is covered in Chapter 9.
EBV, Epstein-Barr virus; *hCG*, human chorionic gonadotropin; *HIV*, human immunodeficiency virus.

1 to 5 days after conception. hCG is produced by the chorionic villi of the developing placenta, with levels peaking between the 50th and 80th days of pregnancy. After this time, the levels decline and remain at a lower level and then disappear a few days after the birth.

The CLIA-waived immunoassay is a qualitative test that detects the presence or absence of hCG. The test takes approximately 5 minutes to perform and is easy to read. The following points are important to remember:

- The urine specimen container must be free of detergents; a clean, disposable urine container is best for collection.
- A first morning urine specimen is recommended because it will contain the highest concentration of hCG. Specific gravity testing should be performed to determine if the urine specific gravity is more than 1.010. An overly diluted specimen with a specific gravity less than 1.010 could cause a false-negative result.
- The urine should be refrigerated if testing cannot be performed within 1 hour. The urine must be brought back to room temperature before testing.
- Follow the manufacturer's recommendations for storage of the kit. If the kit is refrigerated, it also must be brought to room temperature before testing.
- Do not use expired kits.
- Do not use the supplies or reagents from one kit with another kit.
- Test results will show "negative" or "positive" but be sure to chart "negative for pregnancy" or "positive for pregnancy."
- Observe Health Insurance Portability and Accountability Act (HIPAA) guidelines regarding patient confidentiality.
- Observe Occupational Safety and Health Administration (OSHA) guidelines when dealing with specimens.

The **SureStep Pregnancy Test** procedure check sheet is provided in the workbook and is demonstrated in Procedure 7.1, located at the end of this section.

Automated urine pregnancy testing is also available on the Clinitek instrument presented in Chapter 3: Urinalysis. See Figure 7.6A, on the next page that shows the urine liquid controls containing the hCG hormone, and the testing supplies that are used to prepare the pregnancy cartridge for testing on the Clinitek instrument seen in Figure 7.6B.

Mononucleosis Testing

The causative agent of mononucleosis is the Epstein-Barr virus (EBV). The infection is often called the "kissing disease" because it is transmitted by direct oral contact through saliva. Mononucleosis is an acute infectious disease most frequently seen in children and young adults. *Clinical signs* and symptoms are mental and physical fatigue, severe weakness, headache, fever, sore throat, and swollen lymph nodes. *Hematologic findings* may show an increase in the number of reactive lymphocytes. *Immunologically,* the antibody that is produced during EBV infection is called a heterophile antibody. This heterophile antibody has an unusual affinity for antigens on animals cells (e.g., the red blood cells [RBCs] of sheep). The heterophile antibody is produced by patients infected with mononucleosis usually by the fifth to eighth day after infection. Within 3 weeks of infection, 80% of the patients have a detectable level of heterophile antibodies. In the 20% of patients who do not produce the antibody, the diagnosis depends solely on the clinical and hematologic findings. In the outpatient laboratory, rapid mononucleosis tests that detect heterophile antibodies are easy to perform and provide reliable results.

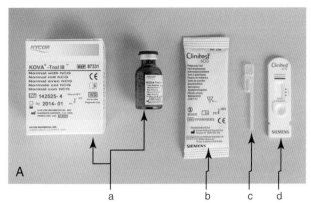

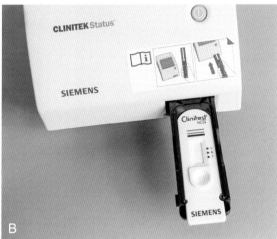

FIG. 7.6 Automated pregnancy test. **A,** *(a)* Urinalysis normal liquid control (containing human chorionic gonadotropin pregnancy hormone); *(b)* Clinitek pregnancy test packet containing *(c)* a urine pipette; and *(d)* a test cartridge. **B,** Pregnancy cartridge placed on Clinitek instrument that will electronically test and record the results.

The **QuickVue+ Mononucleosis Test** Procedure check sheet is provided in the workbook and is demonstrated in Procedure 7.2 at the end of this section.

Helicobacter pylori Testing

H. pylori are spiral-shaped bacteria believed to be the cause of most peptic ulcers (90% of duodenal and 80% of gastric ulcers). This organism weakens the mucous lining of the stomach and duodenum. Stomach acids and bacteria are able to penetrate the sensitive lining beneath the mucous layer and cause an ulcer. Symptoms of an ulcer include a gnawing pain in the abdominal area a few hours after eating and during the night. These symptoms are relieved by eating and taking antacids. Ulcers are now being treated with antibiotic drugs that kill the *H. pylori* bacteria along with drugs that reduce the amount of stomach acid.

The **QuickVue+ Helicobacter pylori gII** Test procedure check sheet is provided in the workbook and is demonstrated in Procedure 7.3, located at the end of this section.

Human Immunodeficiency Virus

HIV attacks and destroys the T helper (CD4) lymphocytes. As previously stated in this chapter, the T helper cells play a critical

role in protecting the body against infection by cell-mediated immunity. They also help the B cells produce their specific antibodies during humoral immunity. As more and more T helper cells are destroyed by the HIV infection, the body becomes less able to fight infections and becomes more susceptible to opportunistic infections. Acquired immunodeficiency syndrome (AIDS) is the condition that eventually occurs and is characterized by the presence of life-threatening infections and cancers (see Chapter 1 for more information on AIDS and this bloodborne pathogen).

At this time, there is no known cure once someone has an HIV infection. Therefore, in 2013 the Centers for Disease Control and Prevention and World Health Organization both advised prevention measures to control the disease. This requires early detection and early treatment of HIV-infected individuals. The sooner the virus is detected via immunologic testing, the sooner treatment with antiretroviral medications may begin. The current recommended treatment of just one tablet daily is able to keep the virus from duplicating and destroying the T cells, thereby halting the progression to AIDS and reducing the possibility of infecting others.

CLIA-waived HIV tests are now readily available to detect the presence of the HIV antibodies in blood and in oral specimens. The immunologic tests for HIV are able to detect HIV infection 3 months after a risk event. A risk event is defined by any of the following list of activities:

- Sex (vaginal or oral) with multiple sex partners
- Sex with someone who is HIV positive or whose HIV status is unknown
- Sex between a man and another man
- Use of illegal injected drugs or steroids
- Use of shared needles or syringes
- Participation in exchanged sex for money
- Diagnosis or treatment for hepatitis, tuberculosis, or a sexually transmitted disease such as syphilis

Patients who are "at risk" for HIV infection are now encouraged to take a 10- to 20-minute blood test in outpatient clinics or perform an oral self-test from a kit that is available at pharmacies.

Remember, HIV is a bloodborne pathogen. Therefore, it is critical that health care workers testing blood and body fluids adhere to the OSHA Bloodborne Pathogens Standard to avoid exposure during all testing processes. The CLIA-waived HIV blood and oral testing procedure check sheets are provided in the workbook and are demonstrated in Procedures 7.4 and 7.5 located at the end of this section.

In both testing methods, it is very important to provide the patient with information or counseling regarding HIV infection and its relationship to AIDS. They also need to understand the five possible test results (i.e., positive, negative, false positive, false negative, and invalid). Be aware that the patients being tested may be very fearful and that proper knowledge presented in a therapeutic way will help them dispel the fear and take positive action toward preventive behavior and treatment. Positive HIV test results need to be verified at the hospital or reference laboratory using the enzyme-linked immunosorbent assay (ELISA) test, with a confirmatory test called the Western immunoblot method.

PROCEDURE 7.1 SureStep Pregnancy Test Procedure

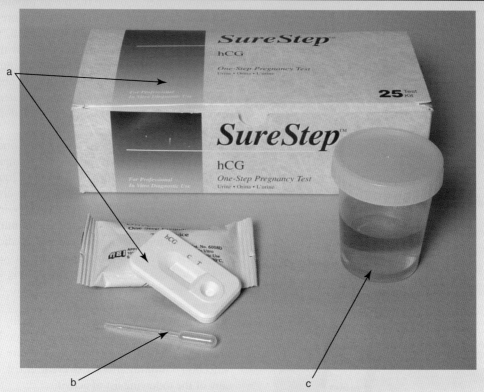

A, SureStep pregnancy test. *a*, Test device; *b*, pipette; *c*, urine specimen.

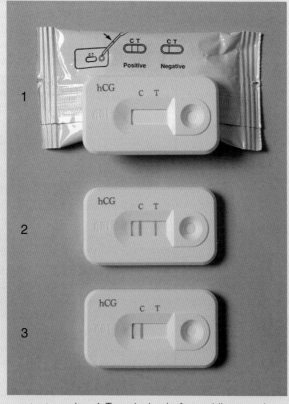

B, SureStep pregnancy test results. *1*, Test device before adding specimen (*C*, control; *T*, specimen travels through test area; well: holds specimen); *2*, positive reactions in test area and control area (two pink bands); *3*, negative reaction in test area and positive reaction in control area.

PROCEDURE 7.1   SureStep Pregnancy Test Procedure—cont'd

Equipment and Supplies (Figure A)—Preanalytical
- Test device from foil package stored in SureStep box
- Pipette from foil-wrapped package
- Urine specimen
- Gloves *(not pictured)*

Procedure—Analytical
1. Sanitize the hands and apply gloves.
2. Remove the test device from its protective pouch and label it with the patient's identification. Bring it to room temperature before opening to prevent condensation.
3. Draw the urine sample to the line marked on the pipette, approximately 0.2 mL. Use separate pipettes and test devices for each specimen and control.
4. Dispense the entire contents of the pipette into the sample well.
5. Wait for the pink bands to appear.
   - High concentrations of hCG can be observed as soon as 40 seconds.
   - Low concentrations may need 5 minutes of reaction time.
   - Do not interpret results after 10 minutes.
6. At 5 minutes, read and record the results (Figure B).
   - Positive test result: Two distinct pink bands appear, one in the patient test region *(T)* and one in the control region *(C)*.
   - Negative test result: Only one pink band appears in the control region *(C)*. No pink band is apparent in the patient test region *(T)*.
   - Invalid: Pink band is absent from the control region. Repeat the test with a new device. If the problem persists, call for technical assistance.

Follow-Up—Postanalytical
7. Properly dispose of biohazard waste material and disinfect the work area.
8. Remove personal protective equipment and sanitize the hands.
9. Document patient and control results on lab log.

Quality Control Procedure
In addition to the internal control region built into the test device, external positive and negative liquid controls should be performed when a new kit is used. Also, each operator of the test should perform a positive and negative control once with each testing method to confirm that his or her testing technique is correct. The results of the control tests should be documented on the hCG control log.

The positive liquid control procedure is performed in the same way as the patient procedure, with a new pipette and testing device. Observe and record the results in 5 minutes. Repeat the procedure with a drop of well-mixed negative control.

hCG, Human chorionic gonadotropin.

PROCEDURE 7.2   QuickVue+ Mononucleosis Test Procedure

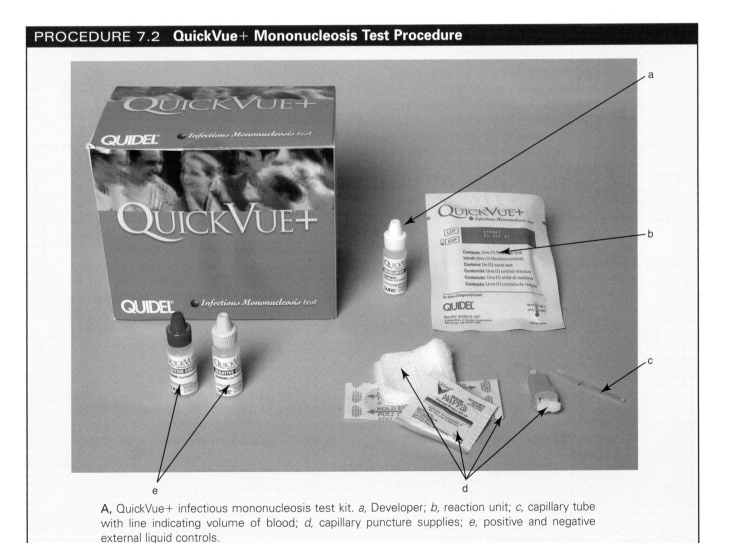

A, QuickVue+ infectious mononucleosis test kit. *a,* Developer; *b,* reaction unit; *c,* capillary tube with line indicating volume of blood; *d,* capillary puncture supplies; *e,* positive and negative external liquid controls.

Continued

PROCEDURE 7.2 QuickVue+ Mononucleosis Test Procedure—cont'd

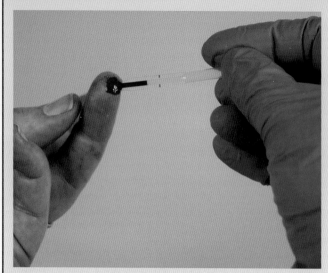

B, Collecting capillary blood to the black line on the disposable capillary tube.

Equipment and Supplies (Figures A and D)—Preanalytical
QuickVue+ mononucleosis test kit containing the following:
- Developer
- Individually wrapped reaction units
- Capillary tubes (for capillary specimens) and pipettes (for venous specimens)
- Capillary puncture supplies or venipuncture supplies
- Positive and negative liquid external control
- NOTE: the package insert is seen in Figure D.

Procedure—Analytical
1. Sanitize the hands and apply gloves.
2. Remove the test device from its protective pouch and label it with the patient's identification.
3. Draw a capillary sample to the line marked on the capillary tube (Figure B).
    - If using whole blood from a venous specimen, use the pipette provided in the kit.
    - Use separate pipettes and devices for each specimen and the controls.
4. Dispense all the blood from the capillary tube into the "Add" well or transfer a large drop from the venous whole blood specimen with the pipette.
5. Add 5 drops of developer to the "Add" well. Hold the bottle vertically above the well and allow drops to fall freely.
6. Read the results at 5 minutes (Figure C). The "Test Complete" line must be visible by 10 minutes.
7. Interpretation of results; see Figure D:
    - Positive result: A vertical line in any shade of blue forms a plus sign in the "Read Result" window along with a blue "Test Complete" line. Even a faint blue vertical line should be reported as a positive.
    - Negative result: No blue vertical line appears, leaving a minus sign in the "Read Result" window along with a blue "Test Complete" line.
    - Invalid result: After 10 minutes, no line is observed in the "Test Complete" window, or a blue color fills the "Read Result" window. If either of these

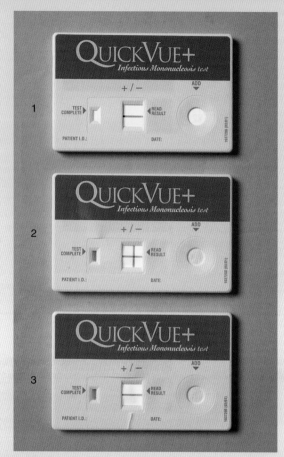

C, Results of mononucleosis test. *1*, Reaction unit before testing; *2*, positive result and "test complete" result; *3*, negative result and "test complete" result.

occurs, the test must be repeated with a new reaction unit. If the problem continues, request technical support.

Follow-Up—Postanalytical
8. Properly dispose of biohazard waste material and disinfect the work area.
9. Remove personal protective equipment and sanitize the hands.
10. Document patient and control results on the lab logs and the patient's chart.

Quality Control Procedures
The internal control occurs in the "Test Complete" window built into each reaction unit. External positive and negative liquid controls are provided with each new kit. Each new operator of the test should perform liquid positive and negative external controls once to confirm that his or her testing technique is correct. Chart the control results in the control log with the operator's initials. Also, external controls should be tested and charted when a new kit is used.

PROCEDURE 7.2 QuickVue+ Mononucleosis Test Procedure—cont'd

TEST PROCEDURE – SERUM, PLASMA, WHOLE BLOOD
Read all of the procedural instructions before running patient samples.

Remove the Reaction Unit from the pouch and place it on a well-lit and level surface.

The "Read Result" window contains a horizontal blue line pre-printed on the membrane.

Hanging Drop Procedure
Add 2 hanging drops of fingertip blood directly to the center of the "Add" Well.

OR

Capillary Tube Procedure
For fingertip blood, fill the Capillary Tube (50 µL) to line.
Dispense all blood into the "Add" well.

OR

Venipuncture, Serum or Plasma Procedure
For serum, plasma or whole blood samples in Tubes, use the Sample Pipette provided. **Place one drop of sample in the "Add" well.**

When adding drops, hold the Developer bottle vertically so that a complete drop forms. **Add 5 drops of Developer to the "Add" well.**

Read test result when ANY blue color appears in the Test Complete window (approximately 5 minutes).

Do not read test result after 10 minutes.

Refer to Interpretation of Results section for further information.

INTERPRETATION OF RESULTS
FOR PATIENT SAMPLES, POSITIVE AND NEGATIVE CONTROLS

Positive Result:
Any shade of a blue vertical line forming a (+) sign in the "Read Result" window along with the blue "Test Complete" line, is a positive result. **Even a faint blue vertical line should be reported as a positive.**

Negative Result:
No blue vertical line in the "Read Result" window along with the blue "Test Complete" line is a negative result.

Invalid Result:
Test result is invalid if after 10 minutes no blue color is observed in the "Test Complete" window.

An invalid result indicates either the test was not performed correctly or the reagents are not working properly.

Should an invalid result occur, re-test the sample using a new Reaction Unit.

If the problem continues, contact Technical Support (in the U.S.) at 800.874.1517. Outside the U.S., contact your local representative.

LIMITATIONS
- As is the case of any other diagnostic procedure, the results obtained by this kit yield data that must be used in addition to other information available to the physician.
- QuickVue+ Mononucleosis Test is a qualitative test for the detection of IM heterophile antibodies.
- A negative result may be obtained from patients at the onset of the disease due to antibody concentration below the sensitivity of this test kit. If symptoms persist or increase in intensity, the test should be repeated.
- Some segments of the population who contract Infectious Mononucleosis do not produce measurable levels of heterophile antibodies. Approximately 50% of children under 4 years of age who have IM may test as IM heterophile antibody negative.[4]

D, Package insert showing instructions for QuickVue+ test and how to interpret results. (Courtesy of and modified from Quidel Corporation, San Diego, Calif.)

PROCEDURE 7.3   QuickVue *Helicobacter pylori* gII Test (CLIA-Waived) Procedure

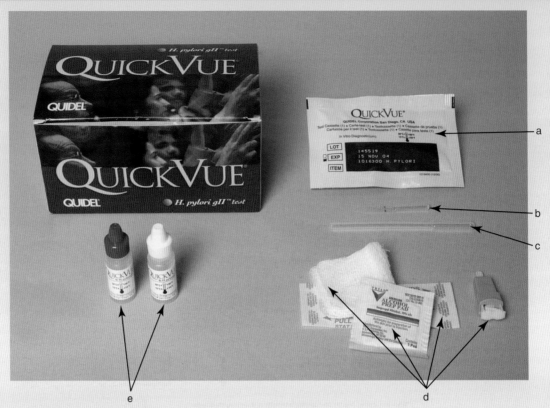

A, QuickVue *Helicobacter pylori* test kit. *a,* Test cassette; *b,* capillary tube for obtaining capillary puncture blood specimen; *c,* transfer pipette for venous blood specimens; *d,* capillary puncture supplies; *e,* positive and negative external liquid controls.

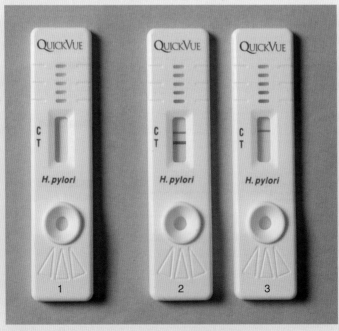

B, *Helicobacter pylori* test results. *1,* Test cassette before adding specimen; *2,* positive result: pink band in test area and blue internal control band; *3,* negative result: no band in test area and blue internal control band.

PROCEDURE 7.3 QuickVue *Helicobacter pylori* gII Test (CLIA-Waived) Procedure—cont'd

Equipment and Supplies (Figure A)—Preanalytical
- Foil-wrapped test cassette
- Capillary tube for capillary puncture blood
- Transfer pipette for venous blood
- Capillary puncture supplies
- Positive and negative external liquid controls
- Gloves and OSHA disposal equipment *(not pictured)*

Procedure—Analytical
1. Sanitize the hands and apply gloves.
2. Add 1 drop of venous whole blood (using disposable dropper in the kit), 1 capillary tube (from kit) of whole blood from a capillary puncture (see Procedure 7.2) or 2 hanging drops of whole blood from a fingerstick to the round sample well on the test cassette.
3. Do not move the test cassette until the assay is complete. Read and record the results of the test after 10 minutes or less (Figure B).
   - Positive result: A pink line appears next to the letter *T* and a blue line next to the letter *C*.

- Negative result: Only a blue line forms next to the letter *C*. The blue line is the internal control indicating that the capillary flow occurred and the functional integrity of the strip was maintained. If the blue line does not show, the test results are invalid and should not be reported.
4. Discard all the test materials in the appropriate biohazard containers.
5. Remove and discard gloves in the biohazard container and sanitize the hands.

Follow-Up—Postanalytical
6. Disinfect the work area.
7. Chart the patient and control results on the lab logs and the patient chart.

Quality Control Procedure
The external positive and negative controls should be performed when a new kit is used and with each new operator of the test method. The procedure is done by adding 2 drops of the positive control to a test well and reading and recording the results after 5 minutes. The same procedure is done with the negative control.

OSHA, Occupational Safety and Health Administration.

PROCEDURE 7.4 Uni-Gold Recombigen HIV Blood Test

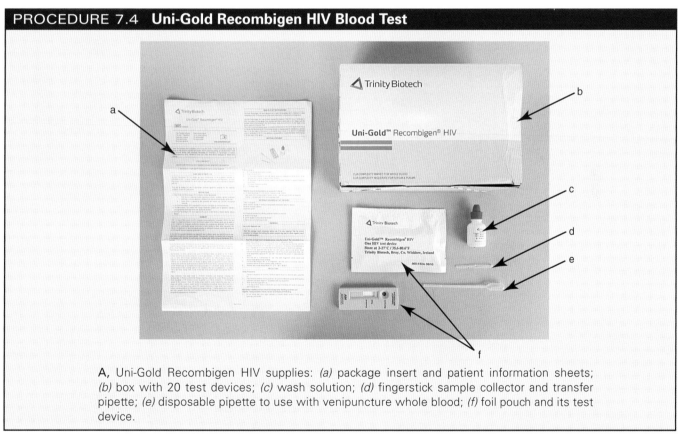

A, Uni-Gold Recombigen HIV supplies: *(a)* package insert and patient information sheets; *(b)* box with 20 test devices; *(c)* wash solution; *(d)* fingerstick sample collector and transfer pipette; *(e)* disposable pipette to use with venipuncture whole blood; *(f)* foil pouch and its test device.

Continued

PROCEDURE 7.4   Uni-Gold Recombigen HIV Blood Test—cont'd

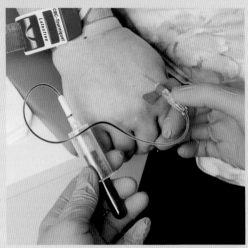

B, Collect a venipuncture whole blood specimen using a lavender blood collection tube containing ethylenediaminetetraacetic acid (EDTA), or an acid citrate dextran (ACD) tube, or a green heparin anticoagulant tube. Then draw up a sample from the vacutainer tube using the pipette provided in the test kit (seen in Fig. D, below).

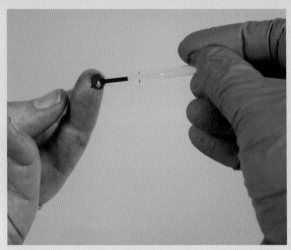

C, Alternatively, collect the whole blood sample from a fingerstick using the smaller sample transfer pipette. NOTE: It is important to hold the pipette gently in a horizontal position and allow the blood to fill to the mark on the pipette without squeezing the bulb.

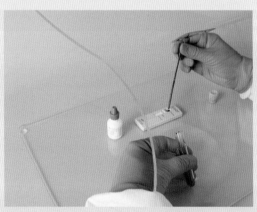

D, Use appropriate personal protective equipment (PPE), including a face shield. Deliver 1 drop of venipuncture blood from the pipette provided in the kit. Hold the pipette vertically over the test port. Then carefully dispose the pipette into a biohazard container.

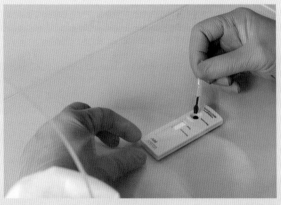

E, Alternatively, after collecting the blood from a fingerstick, immediately squeeze the bulb on the pipette until the blood is fully discharged into the sample port while using PPE, including a face shield. Discard the empty pipette into a biohazard container.

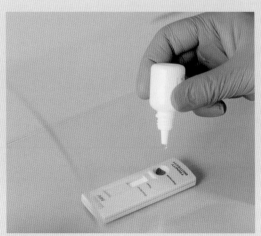

F, After the blood is in the port, hold the wash bottle vertically over the port and deliver 4 drops. Then set the timer for 10 minutes. Read results after 10 minutes but not more than 12 minutes of incubation time.

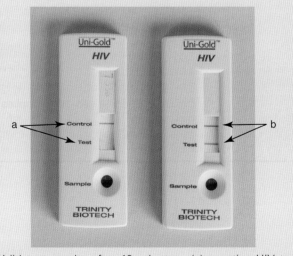

G, Valid test results after 10 minutes: *(a)* negative HIV test result showing no line in the test area and a line in the control area; *(b)* preliminary positive HIV test result showing lines in both the test and control areas.

PROCEDURE 7.4 Uni-Gold Recombigen HIV Blood Test—cont'd

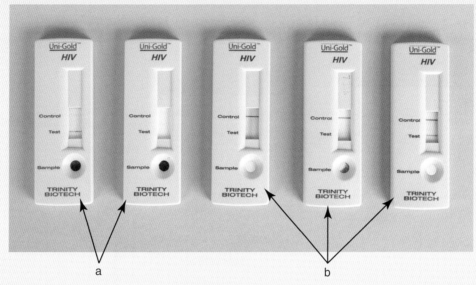

a   b

H, Invalid test results that cannot be reported because of the following: *(a)* these two tests do not show a reaction in the control area; *(b)* these three tests do not show a full red area in the sample port.

Equipment and Supplies—Preanalytical

Uni-Gold Recombigen HIV supplies (Figure A):

* Package insert and patient information sheets (NOTE: Read these thoroughly before testing.)
* Box with 20 test devices
* Wash solution
* Fingerstick pipette for sample collection and transfer
* Disposable pipette to transfer venipuncture whole blood
* Foil pouch and test device
* Other supplies *(not pictured)*
* Positive and negative external liquid controls
* PPE to include gloves, face protection, gown, and OSHA disposal equipment
* Blood collection supplies for capillary or venipuncture samples (e.g., lancets, gauze, alcohol swab, appropriate Vacutainer tube, bandages)

Procedure—Analytical

1. Sanitize the hands and apply PPE.
2. Document that information sheet has been given to the patient and that patient has read it.
3. Allow the unopened foil packet and wash solution to come to room temperature. **Only perform one test at a time.**
4. Open kit and lay the testing device on a clean, flat surface.
5. Label the device with the appropriate patient information.
6. Collect the sample via venipuncture using EDTA (lavender-top tube) or heparin (green-top tube) (Figure B). Alternatively, collect the sample from a fingerstick using the appropriate transfer pipette until the blood reaches the mark as seen in Figure C. Note that it is important to hold the pipette gently in a horizontal position and allow the blood to fill to the mark on the pipette.
7. Add 1 free-flowing drop of the venous whole blood to the sample port (using the proper disposable transfer pipette in the kit; see Figure D. Alternatively, immediately dispense all the blood in the capillary pipette from the fingerstick into the sample port as seen in Figure E. NOTE: Both of the aforementioned procedures should be done with a barrier shield or a full face mask to protect the operator from possible blood exposure to the mucous membranes.

8. Discard the pipette in biohazard waste.
9. Hold the dropper bottle of wash solution above the sample port in a vertical position, and add 4 free-flowing drops of the wash solution to the sample port as seen in Figure F.
10. Do not move the test cassette until the assay is complete. Read and record the results of the test after 10 minutes but not more than 12 minutes (Figure G).
    a. Negative result: Only one red line forms next to the letter *C*. The pink/red line is the internal control indicating that the capillary flow occurred and the functional integrity of the test was maintained. Report as "Negative."
    b. Positive result: A pink/red line appears next to the letter *T* and next to the letter *C*. Report as "Preliminary Positive."
    c. Invalid results: For a test to be valid, a pink/red control line must be present, and the sample port must show a full red color. See Figure H for examples of five possible invalid results. If any of these results appear, do not report the patient result. The test must be repeated with a new testing device.
11. Discard all the test materials in the appropriate biohazard containers.
12. Remove and discard gloves in the biohazard container and sanitize the hands.

Follow-Up—Postanalytical

13. Properly dispose of biohazard waste material and disinfect the work area with 10% bleach or proper decontaminant.
14. Document the results on the lab log and the patient's chart.

Quality Control Procedure

The external positive and negative controls should be performed when a new kit is used and with each new operator of the test method. The procedure is done by adding 1 drop of the positive control to the test device using the venipuncture pipette followed by 4 drops of the wash solution and reading and recording the results after 10 minutes. The same procedure is done with the negative control.

OSHA, Occupational Safety and Health Administration.

PROCEDURE 7.5 HIV OraQuick Test

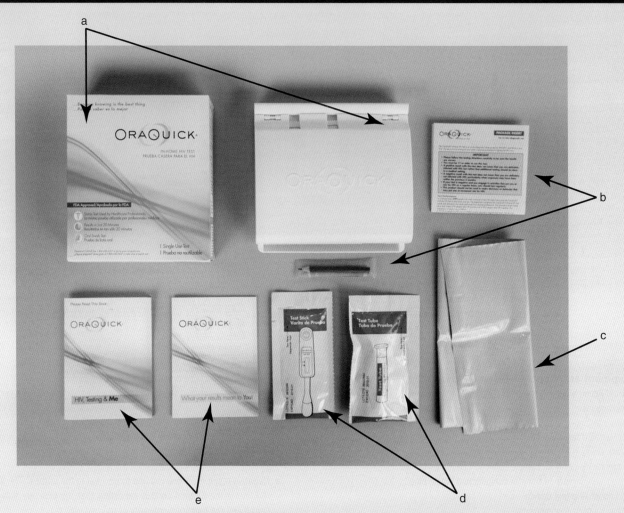

A, OraQuick HIV self-test kit contents. *(a)* Box and plastic test kit containing the flip chart directions and the following displayed items; *(b)* required manufacturer's insert and pencil for writing start and finish times; *(c)* plastic bag for disposal of the test supplies when finished; *(d)* foil-wrapped test stick and test tube; *(e)* two booklets labeled as follows: "Please Read This Book First—HIV, Testing" and "Me and What Your Results Mean to You!"

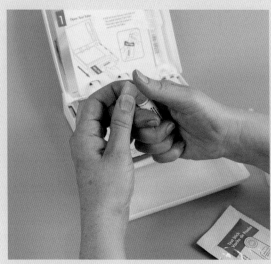

B, Test instructions: Steps 1 and 2—Gently pop off the test tube's cap. Then hold the test tube upright and place it in the holder located on the right side of the plastic lid of the kit.

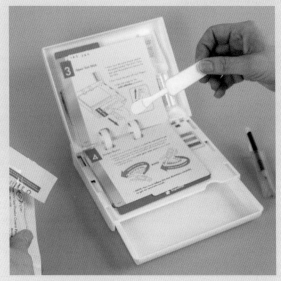

C, Step 3—Open foil wrap and remove the test stick; do not touch the pad with your fingers.

PROCEDURE 7.5 HIV OraQuick Test—cont'd

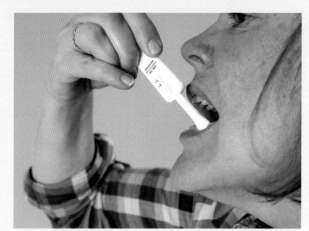

D, Step 4—Gently swipe the pad along your upper gums once and then your lower gums once.

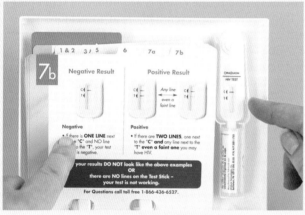

F, Steps 6 and 7—After 20 minutes, read the results by comparing the swab stick results (on the right) with the three keys (on the left) indicating negative and positive results. This test on the right shows a Negative Result.

Equipment, Supplies, and Patient Preparation—Preanalytical
OraQuick HIV self-test kit contents (Figure A):
  (a) Box and its white plastic test kit containing the flip chart directions and the following displayed items located in the pull-out drawer:
  (b) Required manufacturer's insert and pencil for writing start and finish times
  (c) Plastic bag for disposal of the test supplies when finished
  (d) Foil-wrapped test stick and test tube
  (e) Two booklets labeled "Please Read This Book First—HIV, Testing" and "Me and What Your Results Mean to You!"
  Additional items (when performing the HIV OraQuick test in the office):
• Positive and negative external liquid controls
• PPE to include gloves, face protection, gown, and OSHA-disposal equipment

Patient Preparation
1. Most people feel anxious when taking an HIV test. If the patient feels very anxious about taking the self-test, the patient may want to wait until he or she is calmer or get tested by the physician at a local clinic.

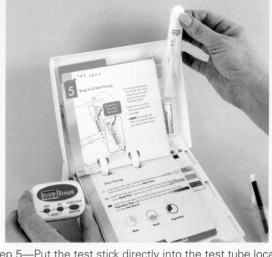

E, Step 5—Put the test stick directly into the test tube located on the right of the plastic lid of the kit. And start the timer for 20 minutes.

2. It is important not to eat, drink, or use oral care products (e.g., mouthwash, toothpaste, or whitening strips) 30 minutes before starting the test.
3. Remove dental products, such as dentures or any other products that cover the gums.
4. Find a quiet, well-lit place where you can be for at least 20 minutes.
5. You must follow the test directions carefully to obtain an accurate result.
6. Make sure you have a timer, watch, or any device that can time 20 to 40 minutes.

Procedure—Analytical
7. Sanitize the hands and apply PPE.
8. Ensure that the pretest booklet, "Read This First," has been given to the patient and that the patient has read it.
9. Open kit drawer and arrange all the supplies as seen in Figure A.
10. With the white plastic lid in the open position, proceed by following the directions and demonstrations on each of the numbered flip charts:
  • Step 1: Open test tube—Find the packet labeled "Test Tube" and open the packet to remove the test tube.
  • Step 2: Setup—Be careful! There is liquid at the bottom of the tube. Hold the tube upright. Then gently pop off the test tube's cap—do not twist (Figure B). Then put the test tube in the holder labeled "Test Tube Holder" located on the right side of the plastic lid that is opened and upright.
  • Step 3: Open test stick—Locate the packet labeled "Test Stick." Tear open the packet and remove the test stick, being careful not to touch the pad with your fingers (Figure C).
  • Step 4: Swipe gums—Make sure the timer is ready and set for 20 minutes but do not start it yet. Gently swipe the pad along the upper gums once and then the lower gums once (Figure D). Make sure you swipe the pad between the gum and lips from one side all the way to the other on both the upper and lower gums.
  • Step 5: Drop in and start timing—Put the test stick pad directly into the test tube located on the right side of the plastic lid and start the timer for 20 minutes as seen in Figure E. NOTE: The kit also provides a pencil and a place to enter the start time, the time after 20 minutes, and the time after 40 minutes.

Continued

PROCEDURE 7.5 HIV OraQuick Test—cont'd

- **Step 6: Wait 20 minutes**—The test kit provides a flap to cover the test area on the stick. The area will turn pink for a few minutes. This is normal. Do not read the results before 20 minutes (this may give a wrong result). Read the results between 20 and 40 minutes. After 40 minutes, the test will no longer be accurate. While waiting for the results, the patient should read the second booklet, "What Your Results Mean to You!"
- **Step 7: Reading your results**—Move the flap that covered the test area to see the results. Compare the test stick with the pictures on the flip chart as in Figure F. If the results *do not* look like the examples on the flip chart *or* there

are *no* lines on the test stick, the test is not working. For questions, call toll free: 866-436-6527. NOTE: A positive result with this test does not mean the person tested is definitely infected with HIV but rather that additional testing should be done in a medical setting. Also, a negative result with this test does not mean that the person is definitely not infected with HIV, particularly when exposure may have been within the previous 3 months.
- **Step 8: Dispose**—Remove the test stick, put the cap on the test tube, place all the contents in the disposal bag provided in the test kit, and dispose of the bag.

OSHA, Occupational Safety and Health Administration; *PPE,* personal protective equipment.

❖ ADVANCED CONCEPTS

Agglutination Reactions (Non–CLIA-Waived Tests)

Agglutination is the visible clumping of blood cells or other particulate matter, such as latex beads. Agglutination is caused by antibodies adhering to their antigens. This type of antibody is referred to as an *agglutinin.* An antibody–antigen reaction produces a visible, latticelike network or large clumps of cells or beads that have agglutinated and fallen out of solution. The agglutination reaction can be seen on a slide or in a test tube and becomes visible to the naked eye as the slide or tube is tilted or centrifuged. Agglutination reactions require interpretation that is beyond the scope of CLIA-waived testing. They are therefore usually performed in hospital and reference laboratories.

Immunohematology

The most common antibody–antigen agglutination reactions are seen in immunohematology laboratories (also referred to as *blood banks*). Immunohematology uses agglutination testing to determine blood types and compatibility tests for transfusions, paternity determinations, mother–baby blood compatibility, and forensic investigations.

ABO Blood Typing

The reasons for determining blood type are to provide safe blood transfusions, to prevent hemolytic disease in the newborn, to identify parentage, and for forensic (criminal) reasons. More than 300 types of inherited blood antigens are found on RBCs. The ABO and Rh blood types are most important because of their intense antigenic responses when transfused or transmitted into incompatible recipients.

Karl Landsteiner discovered the ABO blood groups in the early 1900s. He determined that two inherited antigens are present on the surface of RBCs: A and B. The presence or absence of each antigen produces the four blood types: A, B, AB, and O. Landsteiner also determined that individuals produce a natural antibody against any antigen absent on their RBC surface. Therefore, a type A person has A antigens on his or her RBCs and produces anti-B antibodies in the plasma. A type B person has B antigens on his or her RBCs and anti-A antibodies in the plasma. A type AB person has both A and B antigens on his or her RBCs and no antibodies

in the plasma. A type O person has neither A nor B antigens on his or her RBCs and has both anti-A and anti-B antibodies in the plasma. Table 7.2 provides a summary of these characteristics.

In the immunohematology department, agglutination testing is performed to determine blood types and the compatibility between the donor's blood and the recipient's blood. If a blood antigen comes in contact with its corresponding antibody, the result is agglutination (clumping) of the RBCs, which may eventually lead to hemolysis (breakdown) of the RBCs. These dangerous reactions occur when the wrong type of blood is administered to a patient during a blood transfusion. For example, if a type A person is given type B blood, the recipient's blood, containing anti-B antibodies, would agglutinate the donor's RBCs containing the B antigen. The clumped RBCs would be unable to pass through the kidneys, which might lead to kidney failure. The universal ABO donor is type O because *no antigens* are present on the donor's RBCs, and the universal ABO recipient is AB because *no antibodies* are present in the recipient's plasma. (NOTE: The ideal transfusion is a perfect match. Universal donor and recipient transfusions are used only in "medical emergencies.")

Rh System

The Rh or D antigen is also found on the surface of RBCs. A person with the Rh antigen is referred to as *Rh positive (D+ or Rh+).* All the previously discussed blood types (A, B, AB, and O) will be either Rh+ or Rh− independent of their ABO type.

TABLE 7.2 Summary of ABO Blood Types

Blood Type	Antigens on Cells	Antibodies in Plasma	Transfusion Compatibility
A	A antigens	Anti-B antibodies	Can receive A or O
B	B antigens	Anti-A antibodies	Can receive B or O
AB	A and B antigens	No antibodies	Can receive A, B, AB, and O; Universal recipient
O	No antigens	Anti-A and anti-B	Can receive only O; Universal donor

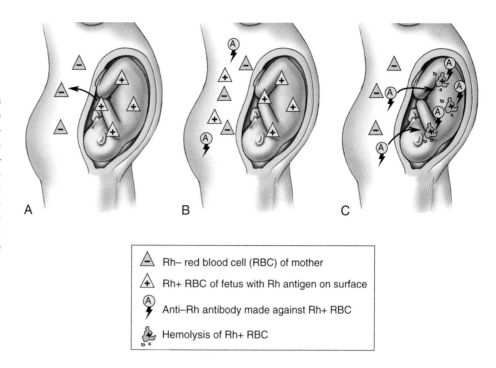

FIG. 7.7 A, *Rh negative* mother is carrying a *Rh positive* baby. **B,** The baby's *Rh-positive* cells have entered the mother's blood stream causing the mother to produce *Anti-Rh antibodies* made to hemolyze the foreign *Rh-positive* RBCs. **C,** The *Anti-Rh Antibodies* enter the baby's blood stream and hemolyze the baby's *Rh-positive RBCs.* (From Herlihy B: *The human body in health and illness,* ed 5, St. Louis, 2015, Elsevier.)

⊖	Rh− red blood cell (RBC) of mother
⊕	Rh+ RBC of fetus with Rh antigen on surface
Ⓐ	Anti−Rh antibody made against Rh+ RBC
	Hemolysis of Rh+ RBC

In the United States, 85% of the population is Rh positive (Rh+). The remaining 15% of the population does not have the Rh antigen and are referred to as *Rh negative* (Rh− or D−). An *Rh-negative* person has no naturally occurring anti-D *(Rh)* antibodies as in the ABO blood types. However, anti-D *(Rh)* antibody production may be induced *after* an *Rh-negative* person is mistakenly transfused with *Rh-positive* blood or after an *Rh-negative* mother has carried an *Rh-positive* baby. In both cases, the exposure to *Rh-positive* cells has a strong antigenic effect in the *Rh-negative* recipient. The *Rh-negative* recipient starts producing anti-D (Rh) antibodies that hemolyze and destroy *Rh-positive* cells. Also, the recipient's IgM levels rise and then switch to IgG

Hemolytic disease of the newborn and RhoGAM. Hemolytic disease of the newborn (HDN), or erythroblastosis fetalis, is a hemolytic anemia in newborns resulting from maternal–fetal blood group incompatibility. Figure 7.7 illustrates the way an *Rh-negative* mother becomes sensitized to her first baby's *Rh-positive* blood cells before or after delivery (see Figures 7.7A–B). Subsequent pregnancies with *Rh-positive* babies activate the mother's anti-Rh antibody response. The anti-Rh antibodies can cross the placenta and cause the destruction of the baby's *Rh-positive* blood cells (see Figure 7.7C). The clinical manifestations in the *Rh-positive* newborn include severe anemia, jaundice, and enlargement of the liver and spleen. These can lead to cardiac failure, respiratory distress, and death.

Hemolytic disease of the newborn can be prevented by the injection of anti-Rh gamma globulin (RhoGAM) during and after the pregnancy of an *Rh-negative* mother. RhoGAM prevents the mother from becoming sensitized, thereby preventing the production of Rh antibodies that would have destroyed the baby's Rh-positive blood cells.

Enzyme-Linked Immunosorbent Assay: Quantitative Analysis

The term immunosorbent pertains to the attachment of an antigen or antibody to a solid surface such as latex beads, wells in plastic dishes, or plastic cartridges (devices capable of absorbing the antigen or antibody). In the ELISA method, an antigen is fixed to a well in a plastic dish. A serum specimen is added to the well to test for a particular antibody. The well is then rinsed to remove anything that did not bind. Next, an enzyme–antibody complex is added that will further bind to the human antibody, if present, and the well is rinsed again to remove any enzyme or antibody that was not bound. The final step uses an enzyme color developer that reacts with the enzyme, if present, and produces a color change. If the serum contained the antibody specific to the antigen, a color change occurs. The more antibody present, the darker the color produced. This quantitative method of indirectly measuring antibodies is a non–CLIA-waived test and is performed in reference and hospital laboratories. (NOTE: This is an "in vitro" lab testing method that is often used in allergy testing.)

Antibody Titers

Reference and hospital laboratories perform both agglutination and ELISA tests with moderately complex equipment to determine the quantity of antibodies present in a specimen. Another quantitative method to determine the amount of a specific antibody in the blood is the titer (a quantitative test that measures the amount of antibody that reacts with a specific antigen). Quantitative antibody information can provide the physician with additional information regarding the extent of acquired immunity. For example, a physician might order a series of Rh titers to measure the level of anti-Rh antibodies in an Rh-negative pregnant woman's serum. The Rh antibody titers could then be used to monitor the degree of sensitivity the mother might be developing against her Rh-positive baby's cells during the pregnancy.

Summary of Immunologic Tests

The ability to detect specific antibodies and antigens associated with disease has made immunology a rapidly growing biomedical science. Table 7.3 describes CLIA-waived and non–CLIA-waived immunology tests commonly ordered for diagnosing bacterial, viral, and other immune-related disorders.

TABLE 7.3   Common Immunology Tests

Tests	Clinical Significance
BACTERIAL INFECTIONS	
Group A *Streptococcus* (strep throat, fever)	The CLIA-waived rapid screening test detects the presence of group A *Streptococcus* antigens in a throat-swabbed specimen.
Helicobacter pylori (ulcers)	The CLIA-waived screening test detects the antibodies specific for *H. pylori* in the blood of an infected individual with ulcers.
Syphilis	Syphilis is a sexually transmitted disease. Three immunology tests for syphilis are rapid plasmin reagin, fluorescent treponemal antibody, and the Venereal Disease Research Laboratory (VDRL) test.
Chlamydia	*Chlamydia trachomatis* is the most common cause of sexually transmitted venereal infection in the world. Rapid lateral flow immunoassays are available for the qualitative detection of Chlamydia directly from endocervical swab and cytology brush specimens.
Gardnerella vaginalis (vaginal infection)	This enzyme activity test is used to detect *G. vaginalis* in vaginal fluid specimens from patients suspected of having bacterial vaginosis, the most common vaginal infection.
Borrelia burgdorferi (Lyme disease)	Lyme disease is transmitted by ticks infected with *B. burgdorferi*. The immunology tests used are either the ELISA or the indirect fluorescent antibody test. If either of these test results is positive or uncertain, it is followed by the Western immunoblot.
VIRAL INFECTIONS	
Respiratory syncytial virus (RSV)	RSV is a highly contagious virus that causes acute respiratory illness. It is the most important cause of bronchiolitis and pneumonia in infants.
Epstein-Barr virus (EBV) (mononucleosis)	The CLIA-waived mononucleosis test detects the heterophile antibody associated with EBV infections.
Influenza A and B	The CLIA-waived rapid screening test detects the presence of influenza A and B in nasal-swabbed or nasal wash specimens.
HIV/AIDS	The CLIA-waived test detects antibodies in blood or oral cells that are specific for HIV-1.
Rubella (German measles)	The test is given to evaluate whether a woman is immune to rubella (as a result of childhood exposure or immunization) or presently infected with the disease. If a woman is not immune and becomes infected during pregnancy (first trimester), the rubella virus could cause birth defects in the fetus.
Hepatitis C (bloodborne pathogen)	The "silent killer," hepatitis C is a growing public health concern. An at-home test provides a confidential hepatitis C result.
Varicella-zoster (chickenpox and shingles)	Immunofluorescence is a diagnostic technique used to identify antibodies to a specific virus. In the case of herpes zoster, ultraviolet rays are applied to a preparation composed of cells taken from the herpes blisters. The specific characteristics of the ultraviolet light as seen through a microscope identify the presence of the antibodies. This test is less expensive and more accurate than a culture, and the results are faster.
OTHER ANTIGENIC SUBSTANCES	
hCG hormone (pregnancy test)	hCG is produced by the placenta during pregnancy.
CA 125 (ovarian cancer)	This test detects the ovarian cancer antigen.
Prostate-specific antigen (PSA) (prostate cancer)	The PSA and percent-free PSA blood tests aid in the detection and treatment of prostate cancer.
Bladder tumor–associated antigen (BTA)	The BTA stat test was the first tumor marker test to be placed in the CLIA-waived category by the CDC. The test detects BTA in the urine of persons being monitored for recurrent bladder cancer.
Rheumatoid factor (arthritis)	Rheumatoid arthritis is a chronic inflammatory disease that affects the connective tissue of the body and leads to crippling deformities. Most patients with this disease develop an antibody called *rheumatoid factor* that can be detected immunologically.
Fecal occult blood (screening for colon cancer)	The iFOB test is highly sensitive to blood on the feces. If the result is positive, the patient will be evaluated as to what is causing the bleeding in the colon.

AIDS, Acquired immunodeficiency syndrome; *CDC,* Centers for Disease Control and Prevention; *ELISA,* enzyme-linked immunosorbent assay; *hCG,* human chorionic gonadotropin; *HIV,* human immunodeficiency virus.

REVIEW QUESTIONS*

1. Which of the following is the causative agent of infectious mononucleosis?
   a. Variola major
   b. Epstein-Barr virus
   c. Cytomegalovirus
   d. Human immunodeficiency virus

2. Which of the following types of immunology tests involve the visible clumping of blood cells or latex beads caused by antibodies adhering to their antigens?
   a. Titer
   b. Lateral flow immunoassay
   c. Agglutination
   d. All the above

3. hCG is produced by the developing placenta during pregnancy with the levels peaking
   a. between the 20th and 80th days of pregnancy.
   b. between the 30th and 70th days of pregnancy.
   c. between the 10th and 60th days of pregnancy.
   d. between the 50th and 80th days of pregnancy.

4. Which of the following cells differentiate into plasma cells and memory cells, with the subsequent production of antibodies produced by the plasma cells?
   a. B cells
   b. T cells
   c. Natural killer cells
   d. All the above

5. Which of the following nonspecific immunity mechanisms involves the process of certain cells engulfing and destroying microorganisms and cellular debris?
   a. Normal flora
   b. Phagocytosis
   c. Intact skin and mucous membranes
   d. Inflammation

6. Which of the five types of antibodies are elevated in acute allergic reactions and subsequent encounters?
   a. IgE
   b. IgM
   c. IgG
   d. IgA

7. Which antibody protects mucous membranes from bacterial and viral infections?
   a. IgG
   b. IgM
   c. IgE
   d. IgA

8. Type A blood consists of
   a. B antigens and anti-B antibodies.
   b. A antigens and anti-B antibodies.
   c. B antigens and anti-A antibodies.
   d. A antigens and anti-A antibodies.

9. Which of the following pregnancy scenarios could be a problem for the baby?
   a. Mother Rh positive and fetus Rh positive
   b. Mother Rh negative and fetus Rh negative
   c. Mother Rh positive and fetus Rh negative
   d. Mother Rh negative and fetus Rh positive

10. Name the antigens present in a B-positive individual.

11. Name two specimens that are used in HIV CLIA-waived tests.

*Answers to these Review Questions are located in the Appendix on p. 279.

WEBSITES

The National Primary Immunodeficiency Resource Center (NPI) is the central resource and clearinghouse on primary immunodeficiency, serving researchers, scientists, physicians, government, industry, patients, and their families. Click "related links" on the home page for access to additional sites related to the immune system and immunology:
www.info4pi.org/index.cfm?CFID=8903943&;CFTOKEN=22787603

Link to laboratory that performs IgA, IgG, and IgE testing for food and inhalant allergies:
www.usbiotek.com

Quidel-sponsored video on how to perform and read Quidel's CLIA-waived influenza test:
www.flutest.com/flu-facts/animation2b.htm

Links to all Quidel point-of-care test kits, including chlamydia, streptococcus A, *H. pylori* gII, influenza A and B, OneStep hCG urine, and infectious mononucleosis:
www.quidel.com/products/

Links to all Thermo BioStar kits for waived and moderately complex testing. The waived tests available are for hCG, streptococcus A, and mononucleosis:
www.pointofcare.net/vendors/thermobiostar.htm

Primary Care rapid diagnostic test products available from Beckman Coulter:
www.beckmancoulter.com/wsrportal/wsr/diagnostics/clinical-products/rapid-diagnostics/index.htm

Microbiology

OBJECTIVES

After completing this chapter, you should be able to do the following:

1. Define and match key terms in this chapter.

Fundamental Concepts

2. Classify microorganisms into the categories of virus, bacteria, fungi, and parasites and describe the general characteristics of each category.
3. Describe the proper collection and transportation procedures for various microbiological specimens.
4. Explain the importance of Gram staining in microbiology and recognize gram-positive and gram-negative bacteria, along with describing their morphologic characteristics.
5. Perform or describe the following microbiological procedures according to the stated task, conditions, and standards listed in the Learning Outcome Evaluation in the student workbook:
   - Throat swab specimen collection procedure
   - Gram stain on a bacterial smear
   - Acid-fast stain, wet mount, and potassium hydroxide (KOH) preparation
   - Cellulose tape procedure for the identification of pinworms

CLIA-Waived Microbiology Tests

6. Describe the diseases caused by group A *Streptococci* and by influenza A and B; and perform or describe a rapid group A *Streptococcus* test and a rapid influenza A and B test according to the stated task, conditions, and standards listed in the Learning Outcome Evaluation in the student workbook.

Advanced Concepts

7. List and describe the following microbiology supplies and procedures found in microbiology labs:
   - Culture media and their uses
   - Inoculating equipment
   - Incinerating equipment used in microbiology laboratories
   - Culture plate streaking methods for colony isolation and colony counting
   - Sensitivity testing
8. List pathogenic bacteria, fungi, and parasites frequently seen in the physician's office laboratory.
9. List some of the emerging infectious diseases and discuss some of the organisms that could be used in bioterrorism.

KEY TERMS

aerobic: requires oxygen for growth

aerosols: fine particles suspended in air

agar: gelatinous substance obtained from seaweed that is liquid when heated and becomes solid when cooled; used in culture media

anaerobic: able to grow and function in the absence of oxygen

binary fission: asexual reproduction in which the cell splits in half producing two identical cells

colonies: visible masses of bacteria formed on a culture medium by one bacterium growing and multiplying

culture: the reproduction of microorganisms in a laboratory culture medium under controlled laboratory conditions

eukaryotic: pertaining to organisms that possess a true nucleus with a nuclear membrane and organelles

expectoration: coughing up of sputum and mucus from the trachea and lungs

fastidious: requires specific nutrients in media for growth

gram-negative: displaying the pink/red color of the counterstain used in Gram's method of staining microorganisms

gram-positive: displaying the purple color of the primary stain used in Gram's method of staining microorganisms

Gram stain: differential method of staining microorganisms that serves as a primary means of identifying and classifying bacteria into two groups, Gram positive or Gram negative

hyphae: tube-like filaments seen in fungal organisms

infection: disease that occurs when pathogenic microorganisms invade the body and overcome its natural defense mechanisms

inoculation: process of transferring microorganisms into or on a culture medium for growth

malaise: feeling of weakness, distress, or discomfort

media (singular: medium): liquid, semisolid, or solid substances containing nutrients needed to grow microorganisms

microbiology: study of microorganisms, including bacteria, fungi, protozoa, and viruses

microorganism: any tiny, usually microscopic, entity capable of carrying on living processes

molds: a fungal growth consisting of Mycelium and hyphae giving it a fuzzy appearance when cultured

morbidity: the rate at which an illness occurs

mortality: the rate of deaths

myalgia: diffuse muscle pain

mycelium: mass of hyphae that some fungi produce

peptidoglycan: component made of polysaccharides and peptides that gives rigidity to the bacterial cell wall

Petri dish: dish containing medium in which to grow microorganisms

prokaryotic: pertaining to unicellular organisms that do not have a true nucleus with a nuclear membrane nor organelles.

purulent: containing pus

sensitivity test: identification of the antibiotic of choice to treat an infection

sputum: mucus expelled from the lungs

yeast: a fungal growth consisting of single cells that reproduce by budding

❖ FUNDAMENTAL CONCEPTS

Overview of Microbiology

Microbiology is the study of microorganisms, including bacteria, fungi, protozoa, and viruses. A microorganism is "any tiny, usually microscopic entity capable of carrying on living processes." Microorganisms were first discovered in 1676, when a Dutch linen merchant and self-made microbiologist named Anthony van Leeuwenhoek created a magnifying glass through which they could be observed.

Microorganisms are found everywhere—in the air, soil, and water. Some microorganisms are involved in the decomposition of waste and the natural recycling process of life and death. Microorganisms that are normally found in and on the human body are referred to as *normal flora* or *normal biota*. Normal flora assist in preventing the growth and spread of disease-causing microorganisms. An example of protective normal flora is the bacteria *Lactobacillus,* which creates an acidic environment in the female vagina. Certain antibiotics destroy *Lactobacillus,* thereby allowing opportunistic infections such as candidiasis (caused by the yeast *Candida albicans*) to take hold.

Research has determined that fewer than 1% of all microorganisms are pathogens. When pathogenic microorganisms invade the body and overcome its natural defense mechanisms, as discussed in Chapter 7, an infection occurs. Some infections are contagious, which means they can spread from person to person.

The role that pathogenic microorganisms play in causing disease should be understood, as well as the means to prevent the spread of these organisms. Table 8.1 shows a timeline of efforts to control infectious diseases throughout history.

When a patient contracts an infection, the first step is to identify the pathogenic organism that is causing the problem; then find the appropriate treatment to control the infection. The following is an overview of the ways in which microorganisms are classified.

Classification of Microorganisms

Although the more complex microorganism identification procedures are not performed in all laboratories, it is important to have a general knowledge of the classification, nomenclature, structure, and growth requirements of pathogenic microorganisms. Microorganisms are categorized as viruses, bacteria, fungi, or parasites.

Viruses. Viruses are the smallest microorganisms, consisting of either ribonucleic acid (RNA) or deoxyribonucleic acid (DNA) molecules. They are so small they can be seen only under a very high magnification using an electron microscope. They need to live in a host cell and use the host cell's metabolic machinery to multiply. Therefore, unlike bacteria and other microorganisms, viruses must be grown inside tissue cells rather than on typical culture media (liquid, semisolid, or solid substances containing nutrients needed to grow microorganisms).

Bacteria. Bacteria are classified as prokaryotic, which means they are unicellular organisms that do not have a true nucleus with a nuclear membrane nor specialized organelles. Bacteria do have a cell membrane and a cell wall. They reproduce by binary fission, asexual reproduction in which the cell splits in half, producing two identical cells. Bacteria can reproduce very rapidly on the culture media containing nutrients for their growth. They are able to form colonies (visible masses of bacteria formed on a culture medium by one bacterium growing and replicating itself). Culture is the reproduction of microorganisms in a predetermined laboratory culture medium under controlled laboratory conditions. Bacteria are cultured (grown) to isolate a pure culture of the organism in question, which is then used to test for identification.

Fungi. Fungi (singular: fungus) are eukaryotic, which means they possess a true nucleus with a nuclear membrane. They lack chlorophyll, can be grown on culture media, and are generally classified as molds or yeasts or a combination. Yeasts are single cells that reproduce by budding, the most common mode of growth. A new cell forms on the surface of the yeast cell, grows, pinches off, and becomes a separate cell. They form visible colonies on culture media, that look smooth and creamy. In contrast, molds are made up of mycelium, which have tube-like structures called hyphae. Molds have a fuzzy or woolly appearance when cultured.

Parasites. Parasites are organisms that live in or on a host and derive nourishment from the host. They can be one-celled protozoa (e.g., amoeba) or many-celled organisms such as helminths (roundworms, tapeworms, and flukes).

Nomenclature of Microorganisms

More than 250 years ago, Carl von Linné, a Swedish botanist, created a nomenclature system for all living things. In this system, each plant and animal has a name with two taxonomic parts: genus (group) and species (kind). The standard rule is to capitalize the genus name and write the species name in lowercase. The genus and species names are always underlined or italicized, as in *Staphylococcus aureus.*

Structural Characteristics of Bacteria

Bacteria are classified and identified according to their shapes and growing patterns. Figure 8.1 illustrates three growing patterns of

TABLE 8.1 History of Infection Control

1300s	Quarantine practices began. Passengers on ships were not allowed to disembark for 40 days after anchoring to protect coastal cities from epidemics of plague. The Latin word *quaresma*, from which "quarantine" is derived, means 40.
1600s	Bubonic plague killed half the population of Europe. Latin as a spoken language disappeared as a result. During this period, infectious diseases were believed to be caused by poisonous vapors, sin, God, and foreigners.
1800s	The germ theory and Koch's postulates proved that microorganisms caused many diseases. Industrialization and immigration in the United States caused overcrowding in many cities. Inadequate waste disposal systems and unsafe drinking water led to outbreaks of diseases such as cholera, dysentery, tuberculosis, typhoid fever, yellow fever, and malaria. In 1878, after a yellow fever epidemic, the U.S. Congress passed the Federal Quarantine Legislation, which called for federal involvement in quarantine activities. In the late 1800s, patients with infectious disease were isolated by disease in wards or floors. Although nursing books from this period discuss aseptic techniques, approximately 40% of maternal deaths were caused by pregnancy complications that occurred because aseptic procedures were not practiced.
1900s	In 1910, a cubicle system of isolation was introduced, consisting of multiple-bed wards, the practice of nurses changing gowns between patients, use of antiseptic hand-washing techniques, and disinfection of objects that patients had touched. In 1928, Alexander Fleming discovered penicillin. This antibiotic was first used in the 1940s by the U.S. military to treat sick and wounded soldiers. A 33-year-old woman was the first civilian to be treated with penicillin when her temperature rose to 107°F after she was hospitalized for more than a month with a streptococcal infection. She recovered from the infection, later met Sir Alexander Fleming, and died at 90 years of age.
1950s	Staphylococcus infections acquired in the hospital were still causing the loss of limbs and death. Hospitals for infectious diseases began closing, except for tuberculosis sanatoriums.
1960s	Tuberculosis sanatoriums began to close.
1970s	In 1970, seven isolation categories for grouping patients with infectious diseases were developed by the CDC. In 1975, hospitals across the nation developed infection-control manuals.
1980s	New nosocomial (HCAI) infections arose, such as those caused by multidrug-resistant organisms and new pathogens. In 1985, the HIV epidemic began, and Universal Precautions were introduced.
1990s	Multidrug resistance, increase in the number of tuberculosis cases, shorter hospital stays, overuse of antibiotics, and new diseases such as those caused by *Hantavirus* and Ebola virus were some of the medical issues of this decade. In 1991, the OSHA Bloodborne Pathogens Standard was instituted. In 1997, the CDC revised isolation guidelines and introduced Standard Precautions (a combination of Universal Precautions and Body Substance Isolation and Transmission-Based Precautions).
2000s	The CDC has stated that airplanes have replaced ships as the dominant vehicles for the international transmission of diseases. Emerging infectious diseases include: • Bird flu (H5N1) • Swine flu (influenza A, H1N1) • Hepatitis C (HCV) • MRSA • *Clostridium difficile* (intestinal bacterial infection) • MERS-CoV (respiratory coronavirus similar to SARS) Hospitals were alerted to strongly enforce infection control (Standard Precautions) requiring vigilant hand sanitization and wearing of scrubs by physicians. High numbers of patients were contracting HAIs (Healthcare Acquired Infections) in health care facilities.
2013	HIV infection controlled using early detection and antiretroviral medication to prevent replication of virus reduced the spread of HIV and progression to AIDS (but still no cure for HIV)
2014 to 2016	HCV infection was now highest in "Baby Boomers" who were born between 1945 and 1965, causing liver cancer to become the leading cause of cancer deaths. Ebola reappeared worldwide. New rigorous PPE procedure was recommended when dealing with patients with Ebola.
2016	Zika virus, a bloodborne pathogen transmitted by mosquitos, required the same rigorous bloodborne pathogen standards.

CDC, Centers for Disease Control and Prevention; *HCAI*, health care–acquired infection; *HCV*, hepatitis C virus; *HIV*, human immunodeficiency virus; *MERS-CoV*, Middle East Respiratory Syndrome-Coronavirus; *MRSA*, methicillin-resistant *Staphylococcus aureus*; *OSHA*, Occupational Safety and Health Administration; *PPE*, personal protective equipment; *SARS*, severe acute respiratory syndrome.

the circular cocci (diplococci, streptococci, and staphylococci), as well as rod-shaped bacilli and spiral-shaped spirilla.

Coccus. The coccus (plural: cocci) is a round bacterium that grows in a variety of formations, depending on the division pattern of the cocci and whether the cocci remain attached afterwards. Cocci are arranged in singles, in pairs (diplococci), in patterns of four (tetrads), in chains (e.g., *Streptococcus*), and in clusters (e.g., *Staphylococcus*, seen as grapelike clusters).

The most common species of *Staphylococcus* are *epidermidis* and *aureus*. *Staphylococcus epidermidis* is found normally on the surface of the skin and the mucous membrane of the mouth. *S. aureus*, on the other hand, is commonly associated

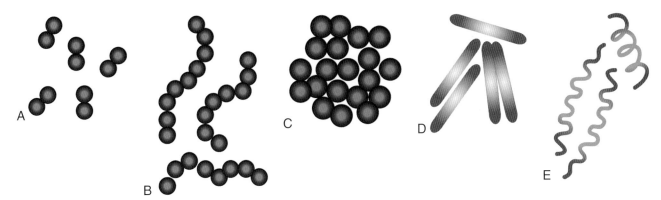

FIG. 8.1 Classification of bacteria based on their shapes and groupings. **A**, Diplococci—pairs of circular cocci. **B**, Streptococci—chains of circular cocci. **C**, Staphylococci—clusters of circular cocci. **D**, Bacilli—rod-shaped bacteria. **E**, Spirilla—spiral-shaped bacteria.

with pathogenic conditions such as boils, carbuncles, pimples, impetigo, abscesses, wound infections, and even food poisoning.

Streptococci are cocci arranged in chains. Although some *Streptococci* are part of normal flora, some cause pathogenic conditions such as strep throat, scarlet fever, and rheumatic fever, which are discussed later in this chapter. In addition, *Streptococcus* can cause carbuncles, impetigo, pneumonia, puerperal sepsis (infection after childbirth), and erysipelas (infectious skin disease).

Bacillus. The bacillus (plural: bacilli) is rod shaped and can also be described as coccobacillus when it appears as a combination of cocci and bacilli (rod shaped but rounded on the ends) or diplobacillus (when it is arranged in pairs) (see Figure 8.1D).

Bacilli cause diseases such as urinary tract infections, botulism, tetanus, gas gangrene, gastroenteritis, typhoid fever, pertussis (whooping cough), bacillary dysentery, diphtheria, tuberculosis (TB), leprosy, and the plague.

Spirillum. Spirillum (plural: spirilla) is a spiral-shaped microorganism that can be a gently curved rod or look more like a corkscrew or a spring. Some spiral bacteria are *Treponema pallidum*, which causes syphilis, and *Vibrio cholerae*, which causes cholera.

Other bacterial structures. Some bacteria have the following additional structures:

- *Flagella* are projections that resemble whips and allow the organism to be motile. Flagella can be seen with the aid of certain stains.
- Some bacteria have *capsules* that surround the cell wall. A capsule is a virulence factor that helps the organisms evade engulfment or phagocytosis by macrophages, thereby enhancing the ability of the organisms to cause disease.
- Some bacteria produce *endospores* when conditions become unfavorable for growth. Endospores are resistant to heat, cold, chemicals, and certain conditions. They reactivate back to a vegetative state when conditions improve. Some endospores survive for many years. Examples of bacteria that can produce endospores are *Clostridium tetani* (causes tetanus, or lockjaw), *Clostridium botulinum* (causes botulism), and *Bacillus anthracis* (causes anthrax).

Collecting, Transporting, and Processing Microbiology Specimens

Collection of microbiological specimens requires the use of infection-control techniques and precautions to prevent infecting yourself or others. The following precautions should be observed at all times:

- Wear the appropriate personal protection devices.
- Disinfect specimen containers after collection.
- Put the specimens in transport bags after collection.
- Wash the hands after specimen collection.

As with all specimen collections, the results are only as good as the specimen collected. The ideal time to collect a microbiological specimen is *before* antibiotics have been administered because the antibiotics will kill the microbes that are needed to be grown and identified.

Specific containers are used to transport a variety of specimens, such as blood cultures, body fluids, skin scrapings, exudates from deep wounds or abscesses, sputum from the lungs, and feces and urine specimens (Figure 8.2). The specific directions for collecting these specimens are discussed later in the chapter.

Collecting a microbiological specimen from the following sites generally involves applying a swab to the infected area: eyes, rectum, urogenital areas, throat, nose, and wounds. The microbiology specimens must be processed as soon as possible. Transport systems provide the conditions microorganisms need to survive during the transport to the laboratory. These specimen collection and transport systems contain transport media that maintains the viability of the organisms. Two examples of transport systems are shown in Figure 8.3. The system at the top of the figure includes two blue-handled Dacron swabs on plastic sticks. When the specimen is obtained, the swabs are put into the holder, and the bottom of the tube is squeezed, releasing the transport media onto the swab to maintain the organisms. The two swabs with the purple handle, at the bottom of the figure, each contain dried nutrient media. The transport system to be used will depend on the type of specimen collected or the specific organisms for which the culture was ordered.

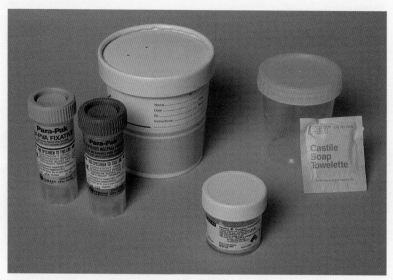

FIG. 8.2 Specimen containers from *left to right:* ova and parasite containers (blue and red), sputum cup, skin scraping/biopsy container, and sterile urine cup and towelette.

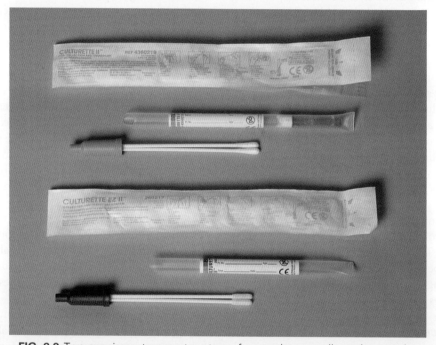

FIG. 8.3 Two specimen transport systems for specimens collected on swabs.

Collecting a Throat Specimen

The swabbed throat specimen collection is one of the most common microbiology procedures performed in the physician's office laboratory (POL). The specimen may be tested for several different pathogens but is most commonly used to test for streptococcal infections.

The **Collecting a Throat Specimen** procedure check sheet is provided in the workbook and is demonstrated in Procedure 8.1, located at the end of this section.

Collecting a Nasal Specimen

Nasal specimens are most commonly collected when testing for influenza A and B. It is important to insert a sterile

Dacron or nylon swab, or foam swab at the base of the nostril as seen in Figure 8.4. The swab is then directly inserted along the base of the nostril at least 1 inch and is gently rotated while rocking it back and forth. More information is provided in Procedure 8.6: OSOM Influenza A and B Test Procedure.

Collecting a Blood Culture Specimen

Blood cultures are collected in containers such as BACTEC bottles (Becton Dickinson, Franklin Lakes, NJ) seen in Figure 8.5. Approximately 10 mL of blood is required for each bottle when collecting blood from an adult. NOTE: The aerobic bottle grows oxygen-dependent bacteria and must be collected first when

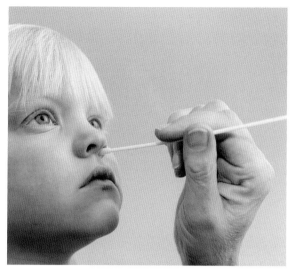

FIG. 8.4 Nasal swab specimen. Note the proper angle to insert the foam swab when collecting a nasal specimen. The swab is inserted at least 1 inch along the base of the nostril on the side that has the most discharge. When inside, the swab is rotated and rocked back and forth gently for 5 seconds to obtain a good specimen. (Photo by Zack Bent.)

using the butterfly method of draw. The anaerobic bottle grows bacteria that thrive best in the absence of oxygen. (It is drawn second when using a butterfly system.) Also displayed are the blood collection tubes with their light yellow caps. Pediatric patients generally need 1 to 3 mL collected into one aerobic bottle or culture tube. When a patient has a fever of unknown origin, the physician often orders a blood culture to determine whether microorganisms are present in the blood. A specific aseptic preparation of the puncture site and the equipment is required when drawing blood cultures. The anaerobic bottle is filled first unless the butterfly method is used, in which case the aerobic bottle is filled first because of the air in the tubing.

Collecting a Urine Culture Specimen

When a urinary tract infection is present, the physician will typically order a urine culture and sensitivity test to determine the type of pathogen causing the infection and the antibiotic that will most effectively treat the infection. The patient is instructed to collect a clean-catch midstream urine into a sterile specimen container, as described in Chapter 3. If the urine specimen must be transported to the microbiology lab, the urine can be transferred into a sterile Vacutainer tube with the appropriate preservatives, as seen in Figure 8.6.

Collecting a Chlamydia Specimen

Chlamydia is a sexually transmitted disease caused by *Chlamydia trachomatis,* a tiny gram-negative (having the pink/red color of the counterstain used in Gram's method of staining microorganisms) intracellular bacterium that requires a host cell for growth. Women with this disease may have no symptoms or may have any of the following: dysuria; itching; irritation of the genital area; and an odorless, yellowish vaginal discharge. Left untreated, chlamydia can cause pelvic inflammatory disease and infertility. The symptoms in men are mild dysuria and a thin, watery discharge from the penis. If not treated in men, the disease can cause epididymitis, which could result in infertility. Using a sterile swab, the physician collects a specimen from the previously cleansed female endocervical canal or the male urethra. The collection swab is placed in a tube containing a transport medium to preserve the specimen during transport and is sent to a reference laboratory for testing. NOTE: The Centers for Disease Control and Prevention–recommended testing for *Chlamydia* is now done using a nucleic acid amplification test (NAAT), which uses a DNA probe (the test is based on DNA detection) (Figure 8.7).

Collecting a Gonorrhea Specimen

The JEMBEC transport system (Becton Dickinson) (Figure 8.8) consists of a JEMBEC plate, a small white pill, and a plastic bag.

FIG. 8.5 Blood culture equipment. *(a)* Aerobic bottle that grows oxygen-dependent bacteria is drawn first when using the butterfly method of draw. *(b)* Butterfly needle attached to a Vacutainer holder with yellow Vacutainer tube for blood culture testing. *(c)* Anaerobic bottle that grows bacteria in the absence of oxygen is collected second when using a butterfly needle system. *(d)* Blood culture Vacutainer tubes that have a light yellow stopper for pediatric patients. (Photo by Zack Bent.)

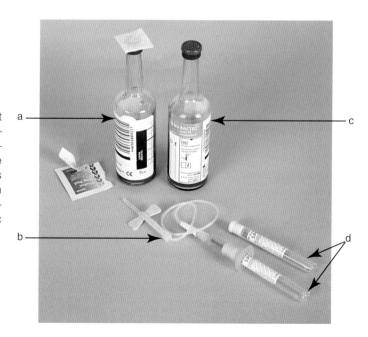

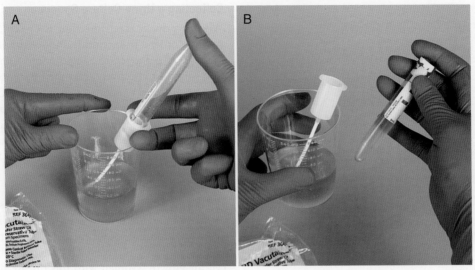

FIG. 8.6 Preparing a clean-catch midstream urine specimen for transport. **A,** The white sterile "straw" and Vacutainer holder with a needle inside are inserted into the urine. The Vacutainer tube is pushed into the needle, causing the urine to fill the tube. **B,** The filled Vacutainer tube is then labeled and sent to the lab. (Photo by Zack Bent.)

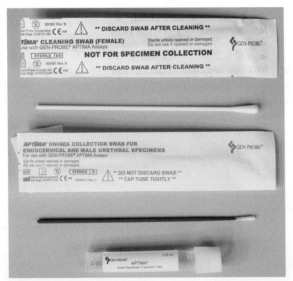

FIG. 8.7 DNA-probe Test Kit. *Top to bottom:* sterile swab for cleansing, the sterile DNA probe, and its tube containing transport media for sending to the lab. (Photo by Zack Bent.)

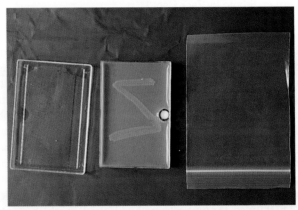

FIG. 8.8 JEMBEC transport system for growing *Neisseria gonorrhoeae* that causes gonorrhea (a sexually transmitted disease). (From Mahon CR, Manuselis G: *Textbook of diagnostic microbiology,* ed 4, St. Louis, 2011, Saunders.)

It is used for transporting and growing *Neisseria gonorrhoeae,* the gram-negative diplococcus that causes gonorrhea. When activated, the pill creates a 10% carbon dioxide atmosphere that this organism needs for growth. Gonorrhea is a sexually transmitted disease of the genitourinary tract. Women either show no symptoms or have dysuria and a yellow discharge. If untreated, the infection can result in pelvic inflammatory disease, which could lead to infertility. Men infected with gonorrhea have dysuria and may have a whitish discharge from the penis that may become thick and creamy. Epididymitis may occur in untreated men, which can lead to infertility. Similar to *Chlamydia, N. gonorrhoeae* can be diagnosed with NAAT testing using a DNA probe, which tests for the presence of the

gonorrhea DNA. The collection procedure is the same as that for *Chlamydia* (see Figure 8.7).

Collecting a Fecal Specimen for Ova, Parasites, and Bacteria

Collection kits for transporting fecal ova and parasite specimens are available and consist of two vials—one with formalin and one with polyvinyl alcohol (Figure 8.9). The vials must be filled to the designated line with a fecal specimen. The kit is used for the preservation of fecal ova (eggs) and or their parasites. A third vial (with Carey Blair preservative) is often ordered to detect a possible bacterial infection that causes similar gastrointestinal (GI) symptoms.

Transporting Specimens by Mail

When specimens are transported by mail, they must be packed in the correct container (Figure 8.10). The specimen is placed

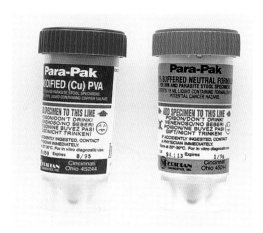

FIG. 8.9 Ova and parasite collection kit for fecal specimens. (From Proctor D, Adams A: *Kinn's the medical assistant: an applied learning approach,* ed 12, St. Louis, 2014, Saunders. Courtesy of Meridan Bioscience, Inc.)

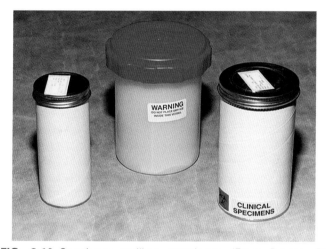

FIG. 8.10 Specimen mailing containers. (From Proctor D, Adams A: *Kinn's the medical assistant: an applied learning approach,* ed 12, St. Louis, 2014, Saunders.)

in a container, which is then placed inside a mailing container. A biohazard emblem must be affixed to every container, including the outside one.

Microbiology Smears, Stains, and Wet Mounts

After the microbiology specimen is collected, the next step is to examine the infectious microorganism microscopically. A portion of the specimen is generally smeared directly onto a slide or mixed into a solution on a slide. The smeared specimen is then dried and fixed to the slide followed by staining it to demonstrate its characteristics.

Gram Stain

More than 100 years have passed since the Gram stain was developed by Dr. Hans Christian Gram. The Gram stain is a "method of staining microorganisms as a primary means of identifying and classifying bacteria." The Gram stain reaction is still used today to distinguish between gram-positive organisms that retain a purple color and **gram-negative** organisms that retain a pink/red color. Table 8.2 lists the four reagents used in Gram staining and the positive (dark purple) and negative (pink/red) results that can occur.

Medical assistants should be able to perform a Gram stain on a specimen that has been smeared and fixed on a slide. Although medical assistants do not interpret Gram stains, it is important that they understand why the identification of bacterial shapes and growth patterns is important, as well as understand the significance of whether an organism is gram positive (purple) or gram negative (pink/red). (See Tables 8.4 and 8.5 for the lists of pathogenic bacilli and cocci, with their Gram reactions in column 3 of the tables.)

Smear Preparation

The bacterial specimen must be smeared onto a glass slide, fixed, and then stained to identify it as gram positive or gram negative. The specimen is obtained from the following three possible sources:

1. A direct smear is made by rolling a specimen swab onto a glass slide after the culture plates have been inoculated. All areas of the swab must touch the slide.

TABLE 8.2	**Gram Stain Reactions**				
Stain Step	**Staining Reagent**	**Color of Gram-Positive Organism**	**Example Gram-Positive Cocci**	**Color of Gram-Negative Organism**	**Example Gram-Negative Bacilli**
1. Primary stain	Crystal violet	Purple	● ● ●	Purple	⬮ ⬮
2. Mordant	Gram's iodine	Purple	● ● ●	Purple	⬮ ⬮
3. Decolorizer	Acetone or ethyl alcohol	Purple	● ○ ●	Colorless	⬯ ⬯
4. Counterstain	Safranin	Purple	● ● ●	Pink/red	⬮ ⬮

2. A colony of bacteria growing on a culture plate is transferred to a glass slide. This is done by taking a colony and rubbing it into a drop of normal saline on the glass slide.

3. A smear may be made from a liquid media culture. Either a sterile swab or a sterilized inoculating needle is dipped in the culture broth and then rolled or placed on the glass slide.

The smear is allowed to dry and is then heat fixed either by running it through a natural gas Bunsen burner or by placing the slide on an electric incinerator for a few seconds. (Do not overheat because this could cause distortion of the bacterial cells.) Heat fixing kills the microorganisms and causes the swabbed material to stick to the slide during the staining procedure. The methanol fixative, used in blood smears, may also be used to affix the smear to the slide.

The Gram stain procedure consists of the four basic steps seen in Table 8.2 on the previous page. First, crystal violet is applied to the slide, and then it is rinsed off. Second, Gram's iodine is applied and then rinsed off. Third, a decolorizer is used and then rinsed off. Fourth, a counterstain, safranin, is applied and then rinsed off.

The most critical step in the Gram stain procedure is the decolorizing step. If the decolorizing is not done for a sufficient length of time, all the bacteria will be purple, and, conversely, if decolorizing is done for too long a duration, all the bacteria will be pink/red.

Gram-positive organisms stain purple because they have a large **peptidoglycan** layer present in their cell walls that holds the crystal violet stain. Peptidoglycan is a component that gives rigidity to the bacteria's cell walls. Gram-negative organisms, on the other hand, have a small layer of peptidoglycan. In addition, they have an outer layer that is soluble in the decolorizing solution. When the decolorizer is applied, it dissolves the lipid portion of the gram-negative outer layer, allowing the crystal violet to leach out. A counterstain of red safranin stains all the material that is not stained by the crystal violet. At the end of the staining procedure, the gram-positive organisms are purple, and the gram-negative organisms are pink/red.

The Gram reaction and shape of the pathogen give the microbiologist the necessary information to help identify the bacteria that are causing the infection in question. For example, gram-positive cocci (GPC) are seen as purple, circular bacteria (Figure 8.11), and gram-negative bacilli (GNB) are seen as pink/red, rod-shaped bacteria (Figure 8.12).

The Gram stain procedure check sheet is provided in the workbook and is demonstrated in Procedure 8.2, located at the end of this section.

Acid-Fast Stains

Acid-fast bacilli (AFB) such as *Mycobacteria* resist staining by the Gram stain method because of the large amount of lipid material and mycolic acid in their cell walls. The acid-fast stain is a differential stain used to identify acid-fast microorganisms such as the *Mycobacterium* genus that resist decolorization with acid alcohol. *Mycobacterium tuberculosis* causes TB, a lung infection in which tubercles (nodules) are formed. Symptoms include night sweats, pulmonary hemorrhage, and **expectoration** (coughing up of sputum

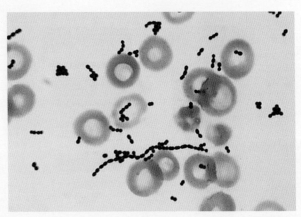

FIG. 8.11 Purple stained gram-positive cocci in chains (streptococci) seen with red blood cells. (From Proctor D, Adams A: *Kinn's the medical assistant: an applied learning approach,* ed 12, St. Louis, 2014, Saunders.)

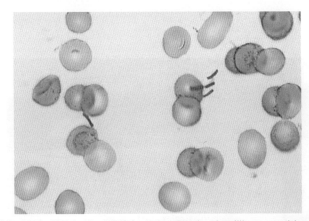

FIG. 8.12 Pink/red stained gram-negative bacilli seen with red blood cells. (From Proctor D, Adams A: *Kinn's the medical assistant: an applied learning approach,* ed 12, St. Louis, 2014, Saunders.)

and mucus from the trachea and lungs) containing **purulent** (pus filled) sputum. Another pathogen, *Mycobacterium avium* complex, disseminates throughout the body in patients with acquired immunodeficiency syndrome (AIDS). Both mycobacterial diseases have been on the increase with the spread of AIDS.

Although AFB staining is not done in a POL, medical assistants should understand how the stain is done and recognize the appearance of the stained AFB organism. Two methods of AFB staining break down the wax in the AFB cell wall: the Ziehl-Neelsen stain, which uses heat, and Kinyoun, a cold stain that mixes a detergent with the dye. Both methods use carbolfuchsin solutions for the primary stain, decolorize with acid alcohol, and counterstain with methylene blue. When the stain is complete, the acid-fast organisms appear as red beaded rods. The slide is observed under the microscope using the oil immersion objective.

Fluorescent staining is another method used to identify pathogens. Auramine or auramine-rhodamine fluorochrome stain is used. It is viewed under a fluorescence microscope equipped with the appropriate filter system for this type of stained smear. The stain may be screened at a lower magnification, which allows more fields to be examined in a shorter period of time. Higher magnification is needed for final identification. TB organisms appear as bright yellow-orange bacilli against a dark background.

Wet Mounts

Wet mounts are rapid microscopic techniques that are done to view organisms in their living state. They allow for the examination of motility, shape, and other identifying features of microorganisms such as *Trichomonas vaginalis*. This organism is a pear-shaped protozoa with four flagella that give it a characteristic jerky movement. *T. vaginalis* is one of the most common sexually transmitted diseases. Approximately 70% of infected people exhibit no signs or symptoms. In women, the infection is located primarily in the vagina, where it can cause itching and a frothy, creamy discharge. Men may also notice irritation or itching in the inside of the penis, a burning sensation after urination or ejaculation, and discharge from the penis. The organism is found in urine or vaginal specimens in women and in urine or prostatic sections in men.

Wet mounts are also done to detect the presence of "clue cells," which are vaginal epithelial cells covered with *Gardnerella vaginalis*, a gram-negative coccobacillus, or other anaerobic bacteria that can cause bacterial vaginosis. Demonstration of clue cells on a wet mount is considered to be the most specific diagnostic criterion. Women infected with *G. vaginosis* produce a watery discharge that lacks white blood cells and usually has a fishy odor.

The **Wet Mount** procedure check sheet is provided in the workbook and is demonstrated in Procedure 8.3, located at the end of this section.

KOH Preparation

Another type of microbiology slide identification is the KOH (potassium hydroxide) preparation. KOH is a strong alkaline solution that breaks down protein material and clears the tissues. This allows any fungus that may be present in skin scrapings, vaginal specimens, or mucus to be seen under the microscope. A KOH preparation shows fungal hyphae from skin dermatophyte infections, as well as yeast such as *Candida albicans*. Although the KOH preparation may be done by a medical assistant, it is interpreted by a trained laboratorian or physician.

The **KOH Preparation** procedure check sheet is provided in the workbook and is demonstrated in Procedure 8.4, located at the end of this section.

Pinworm Specimen Collection and Microscopic Results

Enterobius vermicularis is a tiny, thin, white roundworm commonly known as *pinworm*. The female pinworm normally lays her eggs during the nighttime hours in the anal area of the human host. This causes itching, and the host scratches this area, contaminating the hands and fingernails. Autoinfection occurs because of poor hygiene, inadequate hand washing, and nail biting. The eggs can be ingested or inhaled (anus-to-mouth transmission). Pinworm infections are common among young children in preschools (or day care centers). Infectious transfer occurs by touching contaminated surfaces such as toys and bathroom fixtures, that are contaminated with pinworm eggs.

The identification test is performed by using either swabs coated with petroleum jelly or cellulose tape or seeing the actual adult worm on the anus or on the outside of the feces. The *cellulose tape test* consists of placing cellulose tape (sticky side) over the patient's anal area and then placing the tape sticky side down on a glass slide (Figure 8.13). A physician or trained laboratorian examines the tape microscopically for *E. vermicularis* eggs.

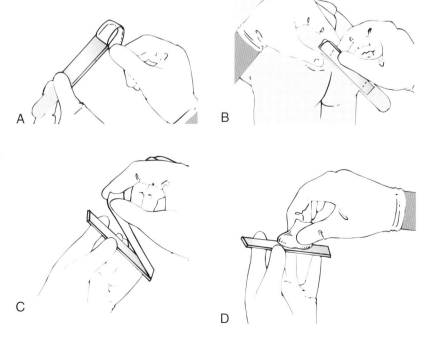

FIG. 8.13 A to **D,** Cellulose tape procedure for collecting pinworm eggs. (From Proctor D, Adams A: *Kinn's the medical assistant: an applied learning approach,* ed 12, St. Louis, 2014, Saunders.)

PROCEDURE 8.1   **Procedure for Collecting a Throat Specimen**

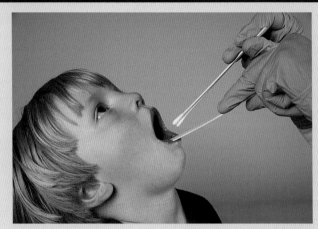

A, Have the patient sit with head back. Use a sterile tongue depressor to hold down the tip of the tongue and have the patient say, "Ahh" while inserting the two sterile swabs to the back of the throat. (Photo by Zack Bent.)

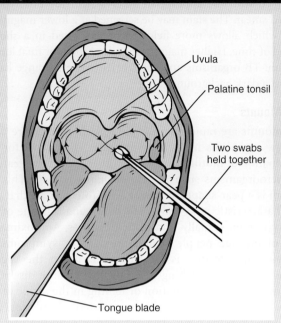

B, Figure-eight technique for obtaining a throat specimen. (From Stepp CA, Woods M: *Laboratory procedures for medical office personnel,* Philadelphia, 1998, Saunders.)

Equipment and Supplies
- Gloves
- Sterile Dacron swabs (not cotton because it inhibits *Streptococcus* growth)
- Swab container
- Tongue depressor

Procedure
1. Sanitize the hands and apply gloves.
2. Aseptically (following techniques that prevent contamination) remove the sterile swab from the package, holding it by the tip.
3. Have the patient sit with the head back. Use a sterile tongue depressor to hold down the tip of the tongue and have the patient say, "Ahh" (Figure A).

4. Rotate the swab on the back of the throat (Figure B) in a circular motion or figure-eight pattern and place it in the appropriate container. Do not touch the teeth or the back of the tongue because these areas have normal flora. Two swabs may be used at the same time, as seen in Figure A.
5. Depending on the microbiology requisition, one swab may be used for a Rapid Strep test, and the other will be placed in a sterile culture transportation tube as seen in Figure 8.3.
6. Remove gloves (unless the rapid test is done immediately after specimen collection), sanitize the hands, and document the collection procedure.

PROCEDURE 8.2   **Gram Stain Procedure**

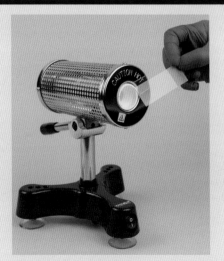

A, The specimen must first be "fixed" onto a slide. Before staining, the specimen from the collecting swab is smeared onto a slide and allowed to dry completely. Then the specimen is "fixed" to the slide using 1. the methanol method (as seen in Procedure 5.1 Diff-Quick step A when the blood smear was fixed onto the slide by dipping the slide into the methanol) or 2. the slide is heated on the back side of the smear using a Bunsen burner or a microbiology "incinerator" as seen in this figure.

PROCEDURE 8.2 Gram Stain Procedure—cont'd

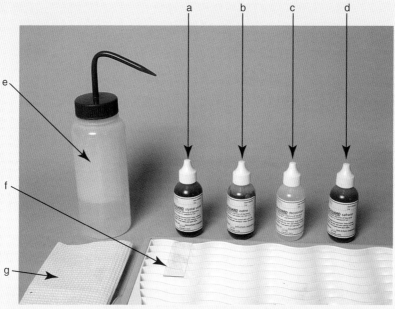

B, Gram stain equipment. *a,* Crystal violet; *b,* Gram's iodine; *c,* decolorizer; *d,* safranin; *e,* rinse water; *f,* staining rack; *g,* bibulous paper.

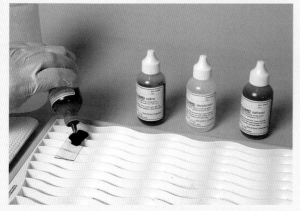

C, Apply crystal violet onto the smeared fixed slide and time for 1 minute.

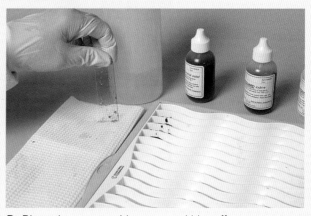

D, Rinse the smear with water and blot off excess water.

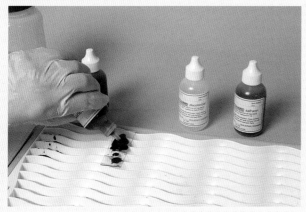

E, Apply Gram's iodine and time for 1 minute then rinse and blot.

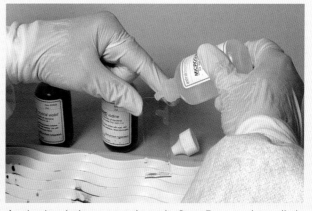

F, Apply decolorizer approximately 3 to 5 seconds until the unbound purple dye is removed (seen at the bottom of the slide when the purple run-off becomes clear).

Continued

PROCEDURE 8.2   Gram Stain Procedure—cont'd

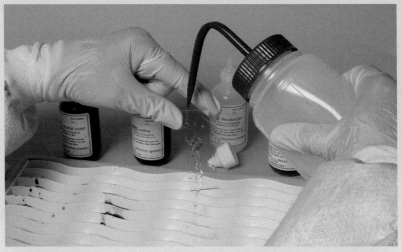

G, Immediately rinse with water to stop the decolorizing reaction.

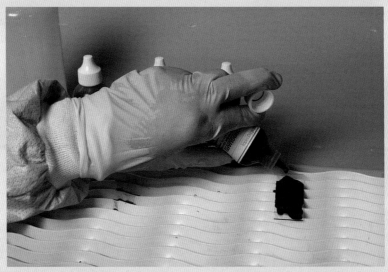

H, Apply the safranin counterstain for 1 minute; then rinse and blot dry.

Equipment and Supplies for the Gram Stain (Figure B)

Gram stain reagents:

- Crystal violet
- Gram's iodine
- Decolorizer
- Safranin
- Rinse water
- Staining rack
- Bibulous (highly absorbent) paper
- Gloves *(not pictured)*

Procedure

1. Sanitize the hands and apply gloves.
2. Pour crystal violet over the smeared and fixed slide and leave it on for 1 minute (Figure C). Using the rinse water bottle, flood the slide with water. Then use gloved fingers or forceps to tip the slide and blot the end of the slide onto the absorbent paper to remove water (Figure D). At this stage, both gram-positive and gram-negative organisms are purple.
3. Pour Gram's iodine over the slide (Figure E) and leave it on for 1 minute. Rinse the slide with water. Again, at this stage, both gram-positive and gram-negative organisms are purple. Iodine acts as a mordant to hold the crystal violet dye in gram-positive organisms.
4. Holding the slide vertically, pour decolorizer, which consists of alcohol or acetone, over the slide, and allow it to run off the slide (Figure F). Watch carefully to note when the purple dye stops flowing (3 to 5 seconds). Rinse the slide immediately with the water to stop the reaction (Figure G). The crystal violet is removed from gram-negative organisms during this step and they become colorless.
5. Apply the red dye, safranin (Figure H). This dye acts as a counterstain and should be left on for 1 minute. Rinse the slide with water. The safranin stains everything red that was no longer stained purple.
6. Blot the slide dry with bibulous paper. Gram-negative organisms are pink/red, and gram-positive organisms are purple at this end stage of Gram staining.
7. Position the slide under the microscope for the physician to view.
8. Remove gloves, sanitize the hands, and document the procedure.

PROCEDURE 8.3 Wet Mount Procedure

Equipment and Supplies
- Glass slide or slide with a well carved into it
- Coverslip
- Gloves
- Drop of saline or water
- Specimen

Procedure
1. Sanitize the hands and apply gloves.
2. Place a small amount of the specimen on the slide or in the slide well.

3. Place a drop of water or saline (normal, 0.9%) on the specimen and a coverslip over the specimen.
4. Position the slide under the microscope just before the physician will view the slide to prevent it from drying out.
5. Remove gloves, sanitize the hands, and document the procedure.

PROCEDURE 8.4 KOH Preparation Procedure

Equipment and Supplies
- Glass slide
- Coverslip
- KOH
- Scalpel
- Swabs
- Specimen
- Gloves

Procedure
1. Sanitize the hands and apply gloves.
2. Clean the specimen area with 70% alcohol.

3. The sample of hair, skin, or nail is scraped with a scalpel by the physician. A vaginal swab specimen may also be obtained by the physician for yeast determination.
4. Place a drop of 10% KOH on the glass slide.
5. Position the specimen in the KOH on the slide.
6. Place a coverslip on the specimen and let it sit for 30 minutes. The 10% KOH will dissolve all protein material, leaving any fungal organisms to be seen microscopically.
7. Position the slide under the microscope just before the physician views the slide to prevent it from drying out.
8. Remove gloves, sanitize the hands, and document the procedure.

❖ CLIA-WAIVED MICROBIOLOGY TESTS

Streptococcus Group A Testing

Streptococcus species are GPC in chains. Some streptococci are capable of producing hemolytic toxins, which hemolyze red blood cells (RBCs) when grown on blood agar. Part of the identification of *Streptococcus* depends on which of the following types of hemolytic reactions (breaking down RBCs) occur on blood agar:

- Alpha hemolysis, incomplete hemolysis of RBCs, is seen as a green color around the colonies.
- Beta hemolysis, complete hemolysis of RBCs, is seen as a cleared area where the colonies have hemolyzed the blood. *Streptococcus pyogenes,* the bacteria that cause strep throat, demonstrates beta hemolysis as seen on the left side of (Figure 8.14).
- Gamma hemolysis occurs when no toxin is present and therefore no hemolysis is seen around the colonies, as seen on the right side of Figure 8.14.

Streptococcus species can also be divided into groups A through O according to the antigenic properties (the ability to induce the formation of specific antibodies) in their cell walls. This system of classification is named after Dr. Rebecca Lancefield, who identified the various groups. *S. pyogenes* is beta hemolytic and serologically types in group A. This organism, which is often called group A *strep,* causes strep throat, a contagious disease passed from one person to another through droplets of saliva or nasal secretions. The symptoms of strep throat are a very sore throat, a bright red pharynx, white patches on the tonsils, swollen glands in the neck, a tired feeling, and muscular aches.

Some complications of strep throat that may occur if inadequately treated are scarlet fever, rheumatic fever, and

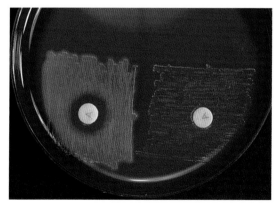

FIG. 8.14 Bacitracin group A test. Notice how the beta hemolysis is on the left side but not present around the bacitracin disk. The absence of bacterial growth around the bacitracin disk (zone of inhibition) is a positive test for group A *Streptococcus.* The bacterial growth on the right shows no beta hemolysis and is not inhibited by the bacitracin disk: this is a negative result for group A *Streptococcus.* (From Mahon CR, Manuselis G: *Textbook of diagnostic microbiology,* ed 4, St. Louis, 2011, Saunders.)

glomerulonephritis. Scarlet fever is a contagious disease characterized by symptoms such as sore throat, fever, enlarged lymph nodes in the neck, flushing of the face, strawberry tongue, and a bright red rash. Acute rheumatic fever is an inflammatory disease (that can be a progression of inadequately treated scarlet fever). It may result in inflammation of the brain, heart, joints, skin, or subcutaneous tissues. This disease usually occurs in children ages 5 to 15 years old. Rheumatic fever can cause permanent damage to the heart that is referred to as rheumatic heart disease. Poststreptococcal glomerulonephritis is an inflammation of the glomerulus of the kidney characterized by decreased urine production, edema, and protein and blood in the urine.

Rapid Strep Testing (CLIA Waived)

There are many CLIA-waived group A strep kits that test directly for the extracted *Streptococcus* A antigen using a throat swab specimen. An example is the Acceava kit (Thermo Electron Corp.).

The **Acceava Strep A Test** procedure check sheet is provided in the workbook and is demonstrated in Procedure 8.5, located at the end of this section.

Bacitracin Method

If the Rapid Strep test result is negative, a culture (with a bacitracin disk) is usually to be done at a reference lab. The specimen might not have contained enough organisms to be detected by the Rapid Strep test. Preparing the culture consists of swabbing a blood agar culture plate with the throat specimen. The agar is streaked for isolation. A disk impregnated with a specified amount of the antibiotic bacitracin ("A" disk) is then placed on the initial swabbed area. The plate is incubated overnight at 37°C. After 24 hours, the plate is observed for *S. pyogenes* group A, which will cause beta hemolysis (clearing of the RBCs) on the blood agar plate. It will also show a zone of no growth or beta hemolysis around the bacitracin disk because strep A is sensitive to the antibiotic. In Figure 8.14, the positive of inhibited growth around the bacitracin disk is seen on the left, and the negative of no inhibited growth around the disk is on the right. A positive bacitracin result indicates presumptive diagnosis of group A streptococcus, and no further testing is required.

Influenza

Influenza is commonly known as the flu. It is caused by a virus that affects the respiratory tract. Symptoms, which last 1 to 2 weeks, are fever (100° to 103°F or higher in children), cough, sore throat, runny or stuffy nose, headache, muscle aches, and fatigue. GI symptoms are rare.

Some individuals with the flu develop complications such as pneumonia. The elderly and people with chronic health problems are at greater risk for complications. Three types of human influenza exist: A, B, and C. Types A and B cause the winter epidemics that occur almost every year. Type C influenza is milder.

Influenza viruses have the capacity to mutate. One type of mutation is called *antigenic drift*, which refers to a gradual change in the virus strain. Antigenic drift occurs in viruses from one season to another. Another type of mutation, *antigenic shift*, involves an abrupt change in the antigenic properties of the virus. When an antigenic shift occurs, it causes a pandemic, in which large numbers of people contract the disease. The following are examples of past influenza pandemics:

- From 1918 to 1919, the "swine flu," also known as *Spanish flu* H1N1 because Spain was one of the countries most seriously affected, killed 675,000 people in the United States and 50 million worldwide. This was probably the most devastating epidemic ever to affect the human race.
- In 1957, the "Asian flu" H2N2 caused 70,000 deaths in the United States.
- In 2005, the "avian flu" became widespread in humans and affected 50 countries in Asia, Europe, and Africa.
- In 2009, the "swine flu," which was referred to as *H1N1,* was considered pandemic and it now circulates seasonally worldwide as a regular human influenza virus.
- In 2013, the World Health Organization identified a serious threat of H7N9 bird flu based on 126 cases diagnosed in China with a 20% fatality rate.

Influenza Testing (CLIA Waved)

The OSOM influenza A and B test (Genzyme Corp.) is a qualitative lateral flow immunoassay. The kit detects the presence of influenza types A and B (direct immunoassay test).

A nasal swab specimen is collected by inserting a soft foam swab approximately 1 inch into the nose (or until resistance is felt). The swab can then be placed in a dry, closed container for up to 8 hours. Refer to Figure 8.4 for proper angle of swab when collecting nasal specimens.

The **OSOM Influenza A and B Test** procedure check sheet is provided in the workbook and is demonstrated in Procedure 8.6.

PROCEDURE 8.5 Acceava Strep A Test Procedure

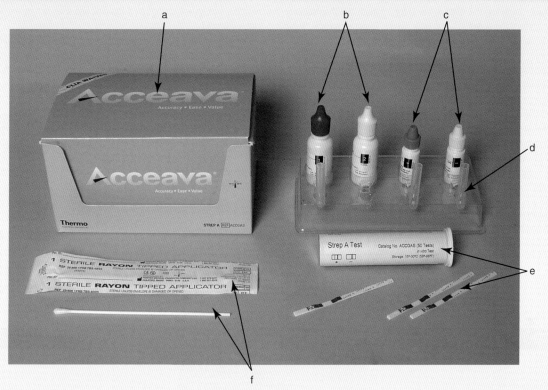

A, Acceava group A strep kit. *(a)* Acceava test kit box; *(b)* reagents 1 and 2; *(c)* positive and negative liquid external controls; *(d)* testing tubes; *(e)* test sticks and their air-tight container; *(f)* sterile swab.

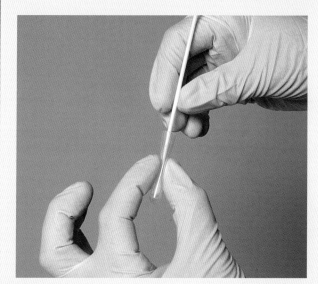

B, Place the throat specimen in the tube with extraction fluid.

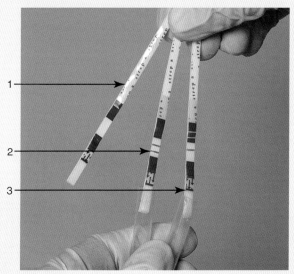

C, Reading results. *1,* Strip before testing; *2,* positive result; *3,* negative result.

Equipment and Supplies (Figure A)
- Acceava group A *Streptococcus* test kit box
- Reagents 1 and 2
- Liquid external controls, positive and negative
- Soft plastic testing tubes
- Test sticks and their container
- Sterile rayon swab taken from wrapper (NOTE: Cotton swabs may inhibit *Streptococcus* growth.)
- Personal protective equipment—gloves and face mask

Procedure
1. Sanitize the hands and apply gloves.
2. Just before testing, add 4 drops of reagent 1 and 4 drops of reagent 2 into a test tube. (The solution should turn light yellow. If it does not, do not proceed with the test.) Immediately put the rayon swab (from the test kit) containing the patient's specimen in the extract solution.
3. Vigorously mix the solution by rotating the swab forcefully against the side of the tube at least 10 times. The best results are obtained when the specimen is vigorously extracted in the solution.

Continued

PROCEDURE 8.5 Acceava Strep A Test Procedure—cont'd

4. Allow the tube containing the swab to stand for 1 minute and then squeeze the swab against the sides of the tube while withdrawing the swab (Figure B). Discard the swab in a biohazard container.

5. Remove a test stick from the container and recap immediately. Place the absorbent end of the test stick into the extracted sample in the tube.

6. After 5 minutes, read and record the results (Figure C). A positive test result shows as a blue line indicating the presence of *Streptococcus pyogenes* antigen. A pink line indicates that the specimen flowed up the entire strip and activated the internal control. A negative test result shows no blue line in the test area. The pink line indicates that the internal control worked.

7. Discard all the test materials in the appropriate biohazard containers.

8. Remove and discard gloves in a biohazard container, sanitize the hands, and document the procedure.

Quality Control Procedures

Internal controls are built into each test strip. The appearance of the pink line indicates that the extracted solution passed through the test area and reacted with the pink antigenic control. If the pink line does not appear, the test is considered invalid.

External positive and negative liquid controls must be performed when a new kit is used. In addition, each operator of the test kit should perform a positive and negative control once with each test kit method to confirm that the testing technique is correct. The controls should be documented.

The liquid control procedure is performed in the same way as the patient procedure, except for the step in which the patient swab is added to the extract solution. Instead of the patient swab, add 1 drop of well-mixed positive control to the plastic tube along with a sterile swab. Follow the directions in the patient procedure, starting with step 3. Observe and record the results in 5 minutes. Repeat the procedure with a drop of well-mixed negative control.

PROCEDURE 8.6 OSOM Influenza A and B Test Procedure

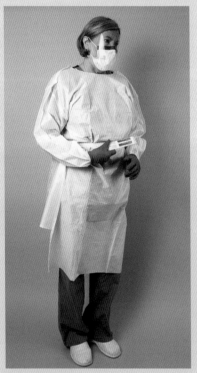

A, Personal protective equipment for highly infectious diseases. NOTE: When collecting the nasal specimen and testing the specimen, it is essential to wear a disposable gown, gloves, and a disposable full face protection mask to protect all the facial mucus membranes from potential exposure.

PROCEDURE 8.6 OSOM Influenza A and B Test Procedure—cont'd

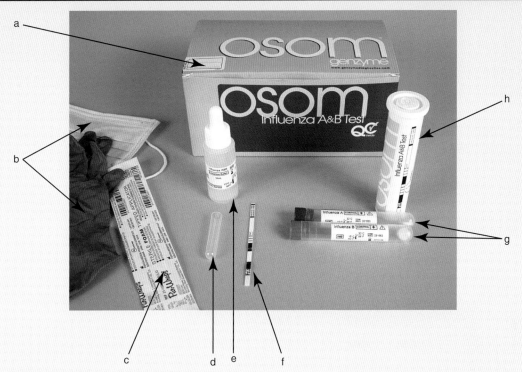

B, OSOM influenza A and B test kit supplies. *(a)* OSOM kit; *(b)* gloves and face mask; *(c),* foam swab; *(d)* plastic test tube; *(e),* extract solution; *(f)* test strip; *(g),* control swabs; *(h)* air-tight strip container with key to results.

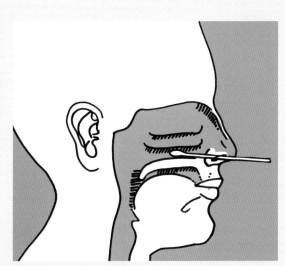

C, Collect the nasal specimen by inserting the foam swab 1 inch into the nostril displaying the most discharge and gently rotate while rocking it back and forth for 5 seconds.

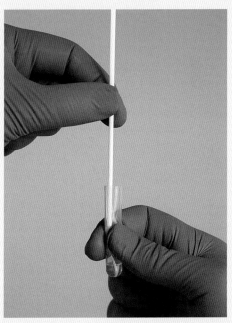

D, After mixing the nasal swab in the buffer extract solution, extract all the solution from the swab by squeezing the swab with the plastic tube while removing it from the tube.

Continued

PROCEDURE 8.6   OSOM Influenza A and B Test Procedure—cont'd

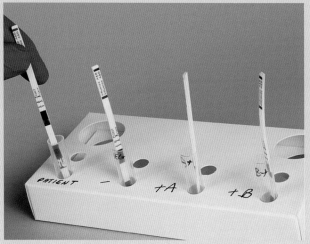

E, Place the testing strip into the extracted fluid in the patient's tube and wait 10 minutes. NOTE: The tubes to the right of the patient's test are the negative and positive controls.

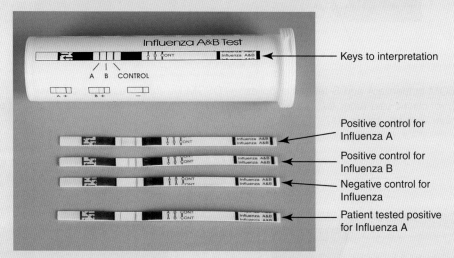

Keys to interpretation

Positive control for Influenza A

Positive control for Influenza B

Negative control for Influenza

Patient tested positive for Influenza A

F, Using the interpretation key on the container and the control results, determine the patient's reaction.

Equipment and Supplies (Figure B)

OSOM influenza A and B PPE and test kit supplies:

- OSOM kit containing all supplies
- Personal protective equipment (face mask and gloves)
- Sterile foam swab provided in kit to collect nasal specimen
- Plastic testing tube provided in kit
- Extract solution provided in kit
- Testing strip provided in kit
- Control swabs for influenza A and B
- Air-tight container of testing strips with diagram showing how to interpret results

Procedure

1. Sanitize the hands and apply gloves and face mask.
2. Before running the first patient test from a new test kit, run a negative control test and both of the positive A and the positive B controls to see whether they react correctly. If they are correct, then proceed with the patient testing.
3. Insert the foam swab provided in the test kit into the patient's nostril displaying the most secretion. Using a gentle rotation, push the swab until resistance is met at the level of the turbinates (at least 1 inch into the nostril; see Figure C). Rotate the swab a few times against the nasal wall and gently rock it back and forth. Hold the swab in place for 5 seconds to ensure maximum absorbency.
4. Place the nasal swab into the plastic tube containing the designated amount of extraction buffer solution and vigorously twist the swab against the sides and bottom of the tube at least 10 times. This disrupts the virus particles and releases the internal viral nucleoproteins into the solution.
5. Extract all the solution from the swab by squeezing the plastic tube against the swab while removing it from the tube, as seen in Figure D. Dispose of swab properly.
6. Dip the influenza test strip into the tube with the extraction buffer solution with the arrows on the strip pointing down, as seen in Figure E. It takes 10 minutes for the sample to be absorbed by the strip. During this time, the liquid sample migrates across the test areas and control area of the strip, and the colored reactions develop. The nucleoproteins from the virus will react with the reagents on the test strip.
7. Read the test results for influenza A and B (Figure F). A positive test result is shown by a pink or purple line in the "A" or "B" test area and a pink line in

PROCEDURE 8.6 OSOM Influenza A and B Test Procedure—cont'd

the internal control area. A negative test result shows no color change in the test area and a pink line in the internal control area.

8. Discard all the test materials in the appropriate biohazard containers.

9. Remove and discard gloves, mask, and gown in the biohazard container; sanitize the hands; and chart the results.

Quality Control Procedure

Internal quality controls are built into each strip. The appearance of a pink line in the control area of the strip is the positive control demonstrating that sufficient flow has occurred and the functional integrity of the test strip has been maintained. If the pink line does not appear, the test is considered invalid. A clearing of the background color is the negative internal control and verifies that the test was correctly performed. If background color appears, it will interfere with test interpretation and render the test results invalid.

External quality controls include one influenza A positive control swab and one influenza B positive control swab. The control swabs supplied in the kit are tested following the swab procedure described previously. See Figure F for the three external control results.

- The presence of a light pink to purple line in the "A" test line position and at the "Control" line position when the influenza A positive control swab is tested indicates that the influenza antigen binding property of the test stick is functional.
- The presence of a light pink to purple line in the "B" test line position and at the "Control" line position when the influenza B positive control swab is tested indicates that the influenza antigen binding property of the test stick is functional.
- The influenza A control swab acts as a negative control for the influenza B antigen, and, conversely, the influenza B control swab acts as a negative control for the influenza B antigen.

External positive and negative liquid controls must be performed when a new kit is used. In addition, each operator of the test kit should perform a positive and negative control once with each test kit method to confirm that the testing technique is correct. The control results should be documented.

❖ ADVANCED CONCEPTS

When a microbiology specimen is sent to a reference laboratory, various steps are followed in the growth, identification, and sensitivity testing of the microorganisms.

Growth Requirements of Bacteria

Identification of bacteria is made on the basis of their growth requirements, particularly their need for oxygen, carbon dioxide, and specific nutrients.

Oxygen Requirements

Of the three gases that are needed for growth—oxygen, carbon dioxide, and nitrogen—oxygen has the greatest impact on an organism's ability to adapt. Organisms can be classified into the following two types:

- Aerobic organisms require oxygen for growth. *M. tuberculosis* is an example of an aerobe.
- Anaerobic organisms can grow and function in the absence of oxygen. *Clostridium tetani* is an anaerobe found in soil. If this organism penetrates a wound deep in the tissue, it will grow and produce a deadly neurotoxin that causes tetanus or lockjaw. Therefore, all patients with a puncture wound, cuts especially when wound area is contaminated with dirt, and even animal bites should be assessed and receive a tetanus booster if they have not had one within the past 10 years.

Nutrient Requirements

In general, the nutrients that most pathogenic bacteria require outside the body are beef or yeast extracts; peptone (a nitrogen compound); mineral salts made of sodium, calcium, potassium, magnesium, chlorine, and phosphorus. These are provided in enriched media. Some organisms are fastidious, which means they require specific nutrients and conditions for growth. An example of a fastidious pathogen is *N. gonorrhoeae*, which requires blood serum, X and V factors (in chocolate agar), some amino acids, vitamins, and 10% carbon dioxide. (NOTE: There are different types of media with different types of nutrients to support the growth of different pathogens that would be cultured from different areas of the body.)

Media Used for Growing Bacteria

Bacteria are grown and isolated on culture media for identification purposes. Media contain essential nutritious substances that allow microorganisms to grow and multiply. Media can be solid, semisolid, or liquid. Solid media contain agar, a gelatinous substance obtained from seaweed that is liquid when heated and becomes solid when cooled in a Petri dish (Figure 8.15). When a bacterium is placed on a solid medium, it will grow and replicate until it forms a visible mass of bacteria, or a colony. Liquid media such as thioglycolate broth are used to grow most bacteria, including anaerobes. Increased turbidity in liquid media indicates growth of the organisms. Location of growth in liquid media indicates oxygen requirements.

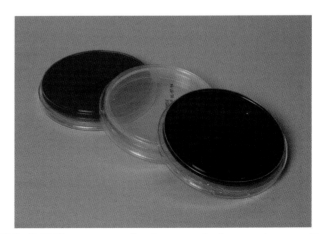

FIG. 8.15 Three types of culture media for growing specific bacteria based on their nutrient requirements.

Microbiology Equipment

Several types of equipment used in a microbiology laboratory are very large and are not usually found in a POL.

Larger equipment commonly used in a microbiology laboratory includes the following:

- Incubator (37°C)—used for growing cultures at body temperature
- Safety hood—built-in area with a fan to pull the airflow away from the operator
- Autoclave—destroys microorganisms by applying steam under pressure
- Refrigerator—for storage of culture plates and supplies and some specimens
- Microscopes—used to identify microorganisms

Equipment Used to Inoculate Culture Plates

The most common equipment used to transfer microorganisms from specimens to various culture media are inoculation loops and needles. The inoculating loop has a bubble wand at the end that varies in size. One type of inoculating loop is a reusable wire type that is sterilized before and after each use. Another type is a sterile disposable loop (Figure 8.16). Loops can be calibrated to collect a precise amount of specimen. An example is the urine culture loop, made of platinum, which is calibrated to collect either 0.01 or 0.001 mL of urine for culturing. The inoculating needle is straight at the end and is used to collect colonies of bacteria.

Equipment Used for Incineration

The incineration equipment used to fix microbiology smears, and sterilize loops and needles are Bunsen burners and electric incinerators (Figure 8.17). Bunsen burners produce a flame by igniting natural gas that is connected to the burner. This method is dangerous because of the fire hazard and because the organisms could splatter as they are heated. The electric incinerator is much safer because it prevents splattering.

Culturing Methods
Inoculation of Media

If a patient's clinical signs and symptoms indicate that a bacterial infection is present, the physician orders a "culture and sensitivity" to determine what bacteria are present (culture) and what antibiotics will kill them (sensitivity).

After microbiology specimens are collected, they are placed on the correct media according to the source of the specimen. If the specimen is sent to the laboratory on a swab or a sterile swab is dipped into the specimen (e.g., sputum), the swab is rolled in the upper quadrant of a solid-medium Petri dish so that all sides of the swab touch the medium. If the specimen is liquid, an inoculating loop or sterile swab is used. The loop must be sterilized first by placing it in a Bunsen burner or incinerator until it is red and then allowing it to cool. The sterilized loop or sterile swab is placed in the liquid specimen and applied to the upper quadrant of the solid culture medium.

The following two techniques are used for spreading a specimen:

- The isolation technique, or *quadrant technique*, consists of using the sterilized loop to spread the specimen over four areas of the plate to establish isolated colonies of bacteria that can be used for identification (Figure 8.18). Better isolation is achieved if the streak lines are kept close together and the loop is sterilized between quadrants.
- The *colony count*, or *lawn technique*, involves streaking the entire plate (Figure 8.19). The lawn method is used for

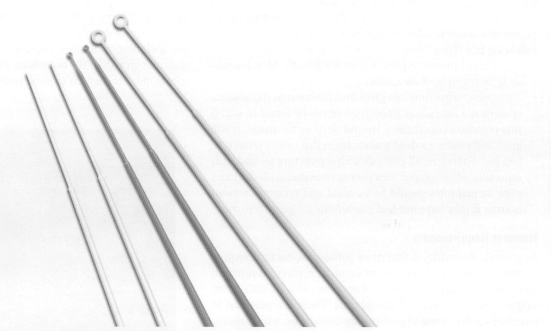

FIG. 8.16 Disposable inoculating loops for transferring liquids to culture plates. (From Proctor D, Adams A: *Kinn's the medical assistant: an applied learning approach,* ed 12, St. Louis, 2014, Saunders. Courtesy Simport Scientific Inc., Beloeil, Quebec.)

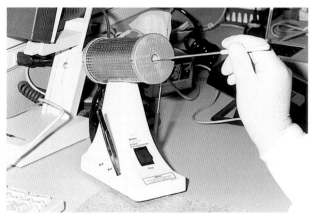

FIG. 8.17 Reusable metal loops (for transferring liquids and inoculating culture plates) being "sterilized" using the electronically heated incinerator. (From Stepp CA, Woods M: *Laboratory procedures for medical office personnel,* Philadelphia, 1998, Saunders.)

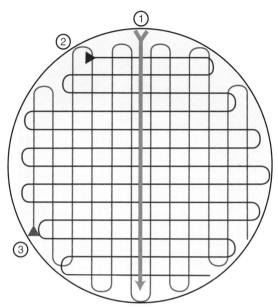

FIG. 8.19 Lawn spread or colony count streaking used when testing a pure bacterial culture for antibiotic sensitivity testing or for counting colonies that form when applying a urine specimen using a calibrated loop.

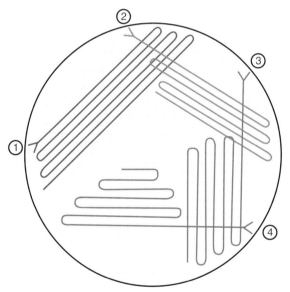

FIG. 8.18 Quadrant streaking method used for inoculating a swab specimen on a culture plate to establish isolated colonies for further identification and testing of the pathogenic organism.

antibiotic sensitivity testing and consists of using a swab that has been dipped in a broth containing only one kind of organism (pure culture) and swabbing the entire plate (see the following section titled Sensitivity Testing). In the urine colony count method, the whole plate is streaked with a calibrated loop so that the colonies that grow on the plate can be counted.

After the specimens are streaked onto the appropriate media plates, the plates are placed in an incubator with the correct amount of atmospheric gases to grow the organisms. The temperature of the incubator is usually 37°C, which is body temperature.

Sensitivity Testing

Physicians often order sensitivity tests to determine the type of antibiotics that would be most effective at treating patients' bacterial infections. One of the methods used for sensitivity testing is the Kirby-Bauer method. A liquid nutrient broth is inoculated with a pure culture of the bacteria grown to a specific turbidity, or cloudiness. The bacteria are then spread over the whole plate (lawn method) of the appropriate media. The Kirby-Bauer apparatus fits over the media plate and drops disks, with each disk containing a specific amount of antibiotic on the bacteria. After the plates are incubated overnight, each disk on the plate is checked for zones of inhibition. The zones are measured in millimeters, compared with the manufacturer's values, and recorded as *S* (sensitive), *I* (intermediate), or *R* (resistant) (Figure 8.20).

For a physician, the best antibiotic is the one that meets the following criteria:

- It is the most sensitive, showing no growth of bacteria (clear) around the white disk.
- It should also be the least toxic to the patient and the patient's normal flora.
- It should be the most cost-effective.

NOTE: Automated antimicrobial sensitivity testing systems are available as well.

Urine Culture

A urine culture is commonly ordered to evaluate urinary tract infections. It involves sending the urine to the laboratory to perform a colony count as described previously. The urine must be collected by the midstream clean-catch method and should be the first morning specimen.

There are also rapid urine culture tests that may be performed in the medical office. See Procedure 8.7 at the end of

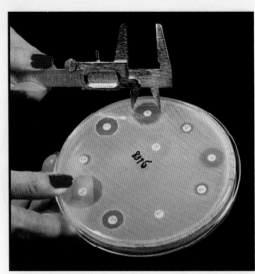

FIG. 8.20 Reading a Kirby-Bauer sensitivity test using calipers to measure whether the bacteria is *S* (sensitive), *I* (intermediate), or *R* (resistant) to the antibiotic by measuring the cleared areas surrounding each of the antibiotic disks. (Modified from Mahon CR, Manuselis G: *Textbook of diagnostic microbiology,* ed 4, St. Louis, 2011, Saunders.)

this advanced concepts section and in the workbook for the Uricult rapid screening for urine culture.

Pathogenic Organisms Seen Frequently in Physician Office Laboratories

Medical assistants should understand some of the common causes of diseases frequently seen in patients in physicians' offices.

Pathogenic Bacteria

The following are bacterial infections most commonly seen in POLs:

- Strep throat—*Streptococcus pyogenes group A,* GPC in chains
- Urinary tract infections—*Escherichia coli, Proteus* spp., Klebsiella spp., *Pseudomonas aeruginosa,* all gram-negative bacilli
- Pneumonia—*Streptococcus pneumoniae,* gram-positive diplococci
- Wound infections—*S. aureus,* GPC in clusters
  NOTE: Because of the danger of methicillin-resistant *S. aureus* (MRSA), strict aseptic technique is necessary for all cultures to prevent nosocomial infections.
- Gonorrhea—*N. gonorrhoeae,* gram-negative diplococci (kidney-bean shape, facing each other)
- Chlamydia—*C. trachomatis,* gram-negative group of bacteria that can reproduce only in a cell

Pathogenic Fungi

The following are fungal infections commonly seen in POLs:

- Yeast infections—*C. albicans,* oval-shaped organisms that absorb crystal violet and can be seen budding
- Dermatophyte infections (athlete's foot, jock itch, ringworm)—*Trichophyton* spp., *Microsporum* spp., and others

Parasites and Protozoa

The following are pathogenic parasites frequently seen in POLs:

- Pinworm—*E. vermicularis*
- Giardiasis—*Giardia lamblia,* protozoan flagellate that causes GI symptoms
- Trichomonas—*T. vaginalis*
- Lice—*Pediculus humanus* (body louse) *Phthirus pubis* (crab louse, or crab)

Emerging Infectious Diseases

The relation between microorganisms and known diseases is not static. New infectious diseases may emerge suddenly, but others seem to disappear and then reemerge. According to most experts, the rate at which infectious diseases emerge and reemerge has risen in recent years. Some of the most important reasons for this trend are the growth of human populations, the increase in international travel, and the effect of environmental changes. Table 8.3 lists some emerging diseases and the microorganisms that cause them (causative agents).

Bioterrorism

As a result of the bioterrorism threats that occurred in the aftermath of 9/11, all laboratories (including POLs) should perform a risk assessment. Laboratories must identify procedures and methods that have the potential to produce aerosols (fine particles suspended in the air). The use of biosafety cabinets or hoods when performing tasks is one way to avoid exposure to aerosols. The Centers for Disease Control and Prevention recommends referring any suspicious organisms or substances to the proper authorities and practicing the proper biosafety techniques at all times.

Most of the bacteria, viruses, and toxins used as bioterrorism agents can be spread by an aerosol route, which is very stable. They also produce high morbidity (rate of illness) and mortality (rate of deaths). Other bioterrorism agents are transmitted person to person, and some are difficult to treat.

Agents Used in Viral Bioterrorism

Smallpox. Some historians believe that smallpox has killed more people than any other disease (300 million deaths in the 20th century). *Variola major* is the most virulent strain and causes severe blistering and high fever that kills approximately half of those affected. *Variola minor* is a milder form, with a death rate of less than 1%. As of 1980, smallpox was declared eradicated, thanks to vaccination programs around the world. This victory over smallpox could be in jeopardy if it were to be used as a weapon of bioterrorism.

Viral hemorrhagic fever. Viral hemorrhagic fever is thought by some to be the most lethal disease known to humans. The Ebola virus is one of the causes of the fever and is spread by direct contact with infected blood or body parts. The disease is characterized by high fever, extensive bleeding, and destruction of internal organs.

Biological Toxin Used in Bioterrorism

Botulism. *Clostridium botulinum* produces a neurotoxin, botulinum, which is the most poisonous natural substance

TABLE 8.3 Some Emerging Infectious Diseases

Disease	Causative Agent	Description
HIV/AIDS	HIV	HIV, first discovered in 1981, is the cause of AIDS. Early detection and antiretroviral medication prevents replication of virus and lowers the chance of infecting others (but does not eliminate the viral infection).
Hemolytic uremic syndrome	*Escherichia coli* 0157:H7	First detected in 1982, hemolytic uremic syndrome is a life-threatening condition characterized by severe anemia caused by RBC destruction and kidney failure.
Influenza—avian	Influenza A (H5N1)c	In 1997, a novel strain of flu virus was discovered in poultry in South Asia and China. In 2005, more human cases were reported, including those in 50 countries in Asia, Europe, and Africa. The majority of human infections have been attributed to direct or indirect contact with poultry that are infected or dead. Human-to-human transmission is rare and not sustainable. There is currently no test to confirm human to human transmission.
SARS	Coronavirus	From November 2002 through July 2003, a total of 8098 people worldwide became sick with SARS, which was accompanied by either pneumonia or respiratory distress syndrome (probable cases), according to the WHO.
MRSA		In 2005, the CDC reported more deaths attributed to MRSA than to AIDS. This superbug caused nosocomial wound infections such as toxic shock syndrome, scalded skin syndrome, scarlet fever, erysipelas, impetigo, and pneumonia. The antibiotic-resistant staphylococcus also emerged in the community, causing skin infections, such as pimples and boils, to occur in otherwise healthy people.
Influenza—swine	Influenza A (H1N1)	On June 11, 2009, the WHO signaled that a pandemic of 2009 H1N1 flu was under way. The virus had mutated genes from former flu viruses that normally circulated in pigs in Europe and Asia and in bird (avian) genes and human genes.
Clostridium difficile colitis	*C. difficile*	Major cause of colitis and antibiotic-induced diarrhea. It produces two toxins, which cause inflammation of the intestinal wall (colitis) along with diarrhea, abdominal pain, and fever. It is one of the most common hospital (nosocomial) infections in the world. As of 2009, it was becoming resistant to most antibiotics.
Hepatitis C	HCV (bloodborne virus)	HCV infects up to 3% of the world's population. It was identified in 1989. In 2013, 80% of cases were the "Baby Boomers" born between 1945 and 1965.
MERS-CoV	New corona respiratory virus	This deadly respiratory virus (similar to SARS) was discovered in India in 2013.
Hemorrhagic disease	Ebola virus in infected blood	Ebola was first discovered in 1976 after two simultaneous outbreaks in Africa (Sudan and Congo). It causes fever, extensive bleeding, and destruction of internal organs. In 2016, there were outbreaks in Africa, Europe, and the United States.
Microencephaly and other neurologic disorders	Zika virus transmitted by mosquitos and blood	First discovered in a monkey in 1947. Before 2007, at least 14 human cases were reported. From January 2014 to 2016, there were outbreaks in the United States (Florida and Texas). In February 2016, the WHO declared Zika a public health emergency of international concern.

AIDS, Acquired immunodeficiency syndrome; *CDC,* Centers for Disease Control and Prevention; *HCV,* hepatitis C virus; *HIV,* human immunodeficiency virus; *MERS-CoV,* Middle East Respiratory Syndrome-Coronavirus; *MRSA,* methicillin-resistant *Staphylococcus aureus*; *RBC,* red blood cell; *SARS,* severe acute respiratory syndrome; *WHO,* World Health Organization

known. It causes dry mouth, dilated pupils, and a progressive muscle weakness that leads to respiratory failure and death. There are seven types of botulism toxin, but types A, B, and E are most commonly associated with human disease. Toxin A is the most potent.

Agents Used in Bacterial Bioterrorism

Plague. In the Middle Ages between a quarter and a third of the population of Europe was killed by the plague. In 1891, approximately 6 million people died as a result of the plague in India. Currently, only a dozen cases are reported in the United States each year. The plague is known as the "black death" because in its later stages, in untreated patients, the blood vessels are destroyed, and subcutaneous bleeding leads to black spots on the skin.

Yersinia pestis is the causative agent of the plague. The disease primarily affects rodents, but it is transferred to human beings by flea bites. Two forms of the plague are the following:

- Bubonic plague results from flea bites.
- Pneumonic plague is spread person to person by respiratory droplets. If the disease is not treated, the death rate is 100%.

Tularemia. Tularemia is caused by *Francisella tularensis*, a gram-negative bacillus. Human beings are usually infected after being bitten by ticks or deer flies, skin contact with infected animals (skinning animals), ingestion of contaminated water, or inhalation of aerosols. The disease is characterized by fever and flulike symptoms. The patient may develop ulcerated skin lesions with localized lymph node enlargement as the result of direct contact.

Pneumonic tularemia may result from exposure to aerosols. The incubation period is 3 to 5 days, with the abrupt onset of chills, fever, headache, myalgia, and nonproductive cough. The death rate is 30% if the disease is untreated and less than 10% if treated.

Anthrax. Anthrax, caused by *Bacillus anthracis,* is a very old disease—the fifth plague of the Bible. The bacterial spores are found in soil, animal feces, and carcasses. It is a disease of livestock, which become infected after feeding on plants contaminated with the organism. Human beings contract the disease mostly through contact with infected animals or animal products. The organism is a gram-positive bacillus. Endospores can live for 40 years. The endospores must be ground into a very fine powder before they can penetrate deep into the lungs and cause infection.

Three forms of anthrax can be contracted in human beings: cutaneous, inhalation (or pulmonary), and GI.

- *Cutaneous anthrax*—Blisters form and develop into blackened craters, called *eschars* (Figure 8.21). These may heal spontaneously or be treated with penicillin; this form is seldom fatal. However, if the anthrax organism spreads to the blood, the toxins released cause swelling, internal bleeding, and tissue death. Therefore, early treatment is important.
- *Inhalation or pulmonary anthrax*—Naturally occurring pulmonary anthrax is rare. In September and October 2001, pulmonary anthrax was spread through letters in the mail. The cutaneous form developed in a number of people, and at least 10 people contracted the inhalation form. Six of those 10 survived, probably because they were treated early with combinations of antibiotics—ciprofloxacin or doxycycline along with one or more other antibiotics effective against anthrax.
- *GI anthrax*—Intestinal eschars, similar to those produced by cutaneous anthrax, are characteristic of this disease. It can progress to generalized toxemia. With proper medical treatment, the survival rate is 60%.

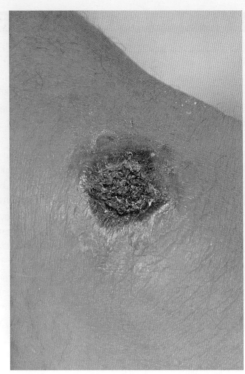

FIG. 8.21 Cutaneous anthrax eschar. (Courtesy of the Centers for Disease Control and Prevention.)

Reference Tables for Common Infectious Diseases Categorized

The following tables are an excellent resource for locating information on the most common infectious diseases, with descriptions of the organisms that cause each disease, ways the disease is transmitted, symptoms of the disease, test specimens required for diagnosis of the disease, and actions that will help prevent infection (Tables 8.4 to 8.9).

TABLE 8.4 Common Diseases Caused by Bacilli

Disease	Organisms	Description	Transmission	Symptoms	Tests or Specimens	Prevention and Immunization
Tuberculosis	*Mycobacterium tuberculosis*	Acid-fast branching bacilli, anaerobic	Inhalation	Pulmonary: cough, hemoptysis, sweats, weight loss; may affect other systems	Sputum for culture, radiographs, skin tests	BCG vaccine (not routinely given in United States)
Urinary tract infections	*Escherichia coli, Proteus* spp., *Klebsiella* spp., *Pseudomonas aeruginosa*	Gram-negative bacilli, many flagellated	Ascends urethra; catheterization	Cystitis: frequency, burning, blood in urine Pyelonephritis: flank pain, fever	Clean-catch urine for culture and analysis	Good personal hygiene (always wipe from front to back)
Clostridium difficile infection	*C. difficile*	Spore-forming, gram-positive, anaerobic bacilli	Nosocomial: direct contact with contaminated equipment and hands; patients receiving antibiotic therapy are susceptible	Diarrhea, fever, nausea, belly pain, colitis	Stool culture and toxin confirmation followed by endoscopy	Antibiotics taken only as prescribed; proper washing of hands and equipment after bowel movements

TABLE 8.4 Common Diseases Caused by Bacilli—cont'd

Disease	Organisms	Description	Transmission	Symptoms	Tests or Specimens	Prevention and Immunization
Legionnaires disease	Legionella pneumophila	Gram-negative bacillus (stains poorly with usual methods)	Grows freely in water (air-conditioning systems)	Pneumonia-like symptoms	Sputum, blood	Isolation
Tetanus (lockjaw)	Clostridium tetani	Gram-positive spore-forming bacilli; anaerobic	Open wounds, fractures, punctures	Toxin affects motor nerves; muscle spasms, convulsions, rigidity	Blood	DPT vaccine in childhood; T or Td vaccine every 10 years
Gas gangrene	Clostridium perfringens	Gram-positive spore-forming bacilli; anaerobic	Wounds	Gas and watery exudate in infected wound	Swab, aspirate of wound for culture	Proper wound care
Botulism	Clostridium botulinum	Gram-positive spore-forming bacilli; anaerobic	Improperly cooked canned foods	Neurotoxin affects speech, swallowing, vision; paralysis of respiratory muscles; death	Contaminated food, blood	Botulinum antitoxin; canned goods boiled for 20 minutes before tasting or eating
Diphtheria respiratory secretions	Corynebacterium diphtheriae	Gram-positive bacilli; club shaped		Sore throat, fever, headache, gray membrane in throat	Swabs; Gram stain, culture; Schick test for immunity	DPT in childhood
Whooping cough	Bordetella pertussis	Gram-negative bacilli	Respiratory tract secretions	Upper respiratory tract symptoms; high-pitched crowing "whoop"	Swabs for culture	DPT in childhood
Plague	Yersinia pestis	Gram-negative bacilli	Flea bite from infected rodents	Fever and chills, delirium; enlarged, painful lymph nodes	Sputum for culture, blood	Vaccine, rodent control

BCG, Bacille Calmette-Guérin vaccine; DPT, diphtheria-pertussis-tetanus vaccine; T, tetanus (toxoid); Td, tetanus and diphtheria (toxoids).
Modified from Proctor D, Adams A: Kinn's the medical assistant: an applied learning approach, ed 12, St. Louis, 2014, Saunders.

TABLE 8.5 Common Diseases Caused by Cocci

Disease	Organism	Description	Transmission	Symptoms	Specimens	Tests	Prevention
Pneumonia	Streptococcus pneumoniae	Gram-positive encapsulated cocci in pairs	Direct contact, droplets	Productive cough, fever, chest pain	Sputum, bronchoscopy secretions	Culture, Gram stain	Vaccine
Strep throat	Streptococcus pyogenes (group A strep)	Gram-positive cocci in chains	Direct contact, droplets, fomites	Severe sore throat, fever, malaise	Direct swab	Rapid Strep test, throat culture	None
Wound infection, abscesses, boils	Staphylococcus aureus and MRSA	Gram-positive cocci in clusters	Direct contact, fomites, carriers; poor hand washing	Area red, warm, swollen; pus; pain; ulceration or sinus formation	Deep swab, aspirate of drainage	Culture and sensitivity (aerobic and anaerobic)	None
Staphylococcal food poisoning	S. aureus	Gram-positive cocci in clusters	Poor hygiene and improper refrigeration of foods	Vomiting, abdominal cramps, diarrhea	Suspected food, stool	Culture of food (organism is not found in stool)	Properly refrigerated food to prevent toxin production
Toxic shock	S. aureus	Gram-positive cocci in clusters	Use of absorbent pack materials (e.g., tampons, nasal packs)	Fever, headache, nausea, vomiting, delirium, low blood pressure	Swab, blood	Culture and serology	Frequent changing of tampons, packing material

Continued

TABLE 8.5   Common Diseases Caused by Cocci—cont'd

Disease	Organism	Description	Transmission	Symptoms	Specimens	Tests	Prevention
Gonorrhea	*Neisseria gonor-rhoeae*	Gram-negative cocci in pairs; intracellular in white blood cells	Sexually transmitted	Women: pelvic pain, discharge; may be asymptomatic. Men: urethral drip, pain on urination	Swab of cervix, urethra; rectal and pharyngeal swabs in homosexuals	Gram stain, culture	Avoidance of unprotected sex
Meningococcal meningitis	*Neisseria meningitidis*	Gram-negative diplococci	Respiratory tract secretions	High fever, headache, projectile vomiting, delirium, neck and back rigidity, convulsions, petechial rash	Nasopharyngeal swabs, CSF, blood	Gram stain, culture, cell counts and chemistries	Vaccine, prophylactic antibiotics

CSF, Cerebrospinal fluid; *MRSA,* methicillin-resistant *Staphylococcus aureus.*
Modified from Proctor D, Adams A: *Kinn's the medical assistant: an applied learning approach,* ed 12, St. Louis, 2014, Saunders.

TABLE 8.6   Common Diseases Caused by Spirilla

Disease	Organism	Description	Transmission	Symptoms	Tests or Specimens	Prevention and Immunization
Syphilis	*Treponema pallidum*	Spirochete	Sexually, congenitally	Primary: painless sore (chancre). Secondary: generalized rash involving palms and soles of feet. Congenital: birth defects	Blood for serologic tests: VDRL, RPR, FTA-ABS	Avoidance of unprotected sex
Lyme disease	*Borrelia burgdorferi*	Spirochete	Tick bite	Fever, joint pain, red bull's-eye rash	Swab for culture	Avoidance of tick-infested areas
Pyloric ulcers	*Helicobacter pylori*	Gram-negative, spiral-shaped	Unknown; possibly food and water	Burning pain in stomach, especially between meals	Stomach biopsy for staining; urea breath test, stool for EIA Ag testing	Unknown
Food poisoning (most common cause in United States)	*Campylobacter jejuni*	Paired gram-negative curved rods forming a seagull shape	Contaminated food, water, and milk	Bloody or watery diarrhea	Stool culture; microaerophilic conditions at 42°C	Sanitary food preparation and control of water and milk supplies

EIA, Enzyme immunoassay(s); *FTA-ABS,* fluorescent treponemal antibody absorption (test); *RPR,* rapid plasma reagin (test); *VDRL,* Venereal Disease Research Laboratory.
From Proctor D, Adams A: *Kinn's the medical assistant: an applied learning approach,* ed 12, St. Louis, 2014, Saunders.

TABLE 8.7 Diseases Caused by *Rickettsia, Chlamydia,* and *Mycoplasma*

Disease	Organism	Transmission	Symptoms	Tests or Specimens
Rocky Mountain spotted fever	*Rickettsia rickettsiae*	Tick bite	Headache, chills, fever, characteristic rash on extremities and trunk	Blood for serological tests, skin biopsy for direct fluorescent microscopy
Typhus	*Rickettsia prowazekii*	Tick bite	Fever, rash, confusion	Blood for serological tests
Atypical (walking) pneumonia	*Mycoplasma pneumoniae*	Respiratory tract secretions	Fever, cough, chest pain	Molecular testing
Nongonococcal urethritis and vaginitis	*Chlamydia trachomatis*	Sexual	May be asymptomatic	Swabs for NAAT testing
Inclusion conjunctivitis, pneumonia		Congenital	Severe conjunctivitis in newborns; afebrile pneumonia in newborns	Swab conjunctiva of eyelids of neonate, Giemsa stain

NAAT, Nucleic acid amplification test.
From Proctor D, Adams A: *Kinn's the medical assistant: an applied learning approach,* ed 12, St. Louis, 2014, Saunders.

TABLE 8.8 Common Diseases Caused by Fungi

Disease	Organism	Predisposing Conditions and Transmission	Symptoms	Tests or Specimens
Thrush (oral yeast), vulvovaginal candidiasis, or *Monilia* (vaginal yeast)	*Candida* spp. (yeast)	Oral: during birth Other: after antibiotic therapy, oral birth control, severe diabetes	White, cheesy growth	Swab for KOH prep, culture
Athlete's foot, jock itch, ringworm (tinea)	*Trichophyton* spp., *Microsporum* spp., and others (skin fungi)	Opportunistic; direct contact; clothing; prolonged exposure to moist environment	Hair loss, thickening of skin, nails; itching; red, scaly patches	Skin scraping for KOH prep; skin, hair for culture
Histoplasmosis	*Histoplasma capsulatum*	Inhalation of dust contaminated with bird or bat droppings	Mild, flulike to systemic	Serologic, culture of biopsy material
Cryptococcosis	*Cryptococcus neoformans*	Contact with poultry droppings	Cough, fever, malaise; can become systemic	Sputum culture; blood and CSF for fungal culture; cryptococcal Ag test
Sporotrichosis	*Sporothrix schenckii*	Farmers, florists, people exposed to soil	Skin lesions that spread along lymphatics; can become systemic	Fungal culture, skin culture India ink direct examination, scrapings, serologic KOH (potassium hydroxide)
Pneumocystis pneumonia	*Pneumocystis jirovecii*	Widely prevalent in animals; occurs in debilitated persons, immunosuppressed; common in patients with AIDS	Pneumonia-like	Sputum, bronchoalveolar lavage or biopsy; PCR testing

AIDS, Acquired immunodeficiency syndrome; *CSF,* cerebrospinal fluid; *KOH,* potassium hydroxide; *PCR,* polymerase chain reaction.
From Proctor D, Adams A: *Kinn's the medical assistant: an applied learning approach,* ed 12, St. Louis, 2014, Saunders.

TABLE 8.9 Common Protozoan and Parasitic Diseases

Disease	Organism	Transmission	Symptoms	Tests or Specimens
Malaria	*Plasmodium* spp. (protozoa)	Bite of *Anopheles* mosquito	Chills, fever (cyclic)	Blood: examination of stained blood for parasites
Toxoplasmosis	*Toxoplasma gondii* (protozoa)	Fecal contamination (cat litter), congenital	Febrile illness, rash; congenital: jaundice, enlarged liver and spleen, brain abnormalities	Serologic testing, molecular tests
Amoebic dysentery	*Entamoeba histolytica* (protozoa)	Fecal contamination of food and water	Bloody diarrhea, cramping, fever	Stool for O&P

Continued

TABLE 8.9 Common Protozoan and Parasitic Diseases—cont'd

Disease	Organism	Transmission	Symptoms	Tests or Specimens
Giardiasis	*Giardia lamblia* (protozoa)	Common in intestinal tract, opportunistic; contaminated surface water	Asymptomatic to severe diarrhea and abdominal discomfort	Stool for O&P, intestinal biopsy, string test
Trichinosis or trichinellosis	*Trichinella spiralis* (roundworm)	Ingestion of undercooked pork or bear meat	Nausea, fever, diarrhea, muscle pain and swelling, edema of face	Biopsy, Ab blood tests
Tapeworm	*Taenia* spp., *Diphyllobothrium latum*	Undercooked meats (beef and pork); undercooked fish; common among Norwegians and Japanese	Abdominal discomfort, diarrhea, weight loss; as above, may become anemia	Stool for O&P
Pinworm	*Enterobius vermicularis* (roundworm)	Fecal–oral	Severe rectal itching, restlessness, insomnia	Adhesive tape applied to perianal region for ova
Scabies	Itch mite: *Sarcoptes scabiei*	Direct contact, clothing, bedding	Nocturnal itching, skin burrows	Skin scrapings for parasites
Lice	*Pediculus humanus*, *Pthirus pubis* (crabs)	Direct contact, clothing, bedding, furniture (can transmit other diseases by bite)	Intense itching, skin lesions	Finding adult lice or eggs (nits) on body or hair

O&P, Ova and parasites.

PROCEDURE 8.7 Rapid Urine Culture Test

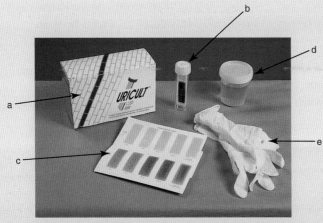

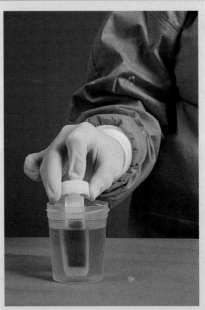

A, Uricult testing supplies. *(a)* Uricult box kit containing the following: *(b)* vial with agar-coated slide attached to plastic screw top; *(c)* reference chart to compare growth results after 18 to 24 hours; *(d),* midstream clean-catch urine specimen (preferably first morning specimen); *(e)* gloves. (From Bonewit-West K: *Clinical procedures for medical assistants,* ed 10, St. Louis, 2018, Elsevier.)

B, After unscrewing the agar-coated slide from the vial, dip the slide into the urine specimen, making sure all the surfaces have made contact with the urine, and then replace the slide into the vial and screw cap loosely. (From Bonewit-West K: *Clinical procedures for medical assistants,* ed 10, St. Louis, 2018, Elsevier.)

PROCEDURE 8.7 Rapid Urine Culture Test—cont'd

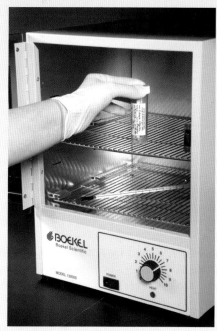

C, Incubate specimen vial for 18 to 24 hours at a temperature of 93° to 100°F (35° to 38°C). (From Bonewit-West K: *Clinical procedures for medical assistants,* ed 10, St. Louis, 2018, Elsevier.)

Purpose
Testing for bacterial growth in a urine specimen

Equipment and Supplies
- Clinical incubator
- Uricult kit containing vial with agar-coated slide and reference chart (Figure A)
- Gloves

Procedure
1. Sanitize and glove your hands and assemble the equipment. Check the expiration date on the reagent kit.
2. Into the appropriate sterile container, have the patient produce a freshly voided clean-catch midstream urine specimen that has been in the bladder for a minimum of 4 to 6 hours. Be sure to mix the urine sample thoroughly before testing.

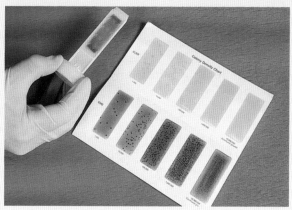

D, Read and record the color results on the slide using the reference chart from the kit. (From Bonewit-West K: *Clinical procedures for medical assistants,* ed 10, St. Louis, 2018, Elsevier.)

3. After you unscrew the agar-coated slide from the vial, do not touch the agar.
4. Make sure the agar on both sides of the slide is completely immersed into the urine but do not immerse more than several seconds (Figure B). (NOTE: If the urine volume in the cup is too small to dip, the urine may be poured over the agar surfaces.)
5. Place the urine-dipped specimen back into the vial and screw the cap on loosely. Label the vial with the patient's name, date, time, and your initials. Then place in the incubator (Figure C).
6. Read the results using the reference chart supplied with the kit after 18 to 24 hours of incubation (do not exceed 24 hours) (Figure D). Results are interpreted as follows:
   - *Normal:* Color that reads as less than 10,000 bacteria/mL of urine indicates the absence of infection.
   - *Borderline:* Color that reads 10,000 to 100,000 bacteria/mL of urine may indicate a chronic or relapsing infection, and it is recommended that the test be repeated.
   - *Positive:* More than 100,000 bacteria/mL of urine indicates complete coverage of the agar surface with bacterial colonies.
7. Replace the agar slide in the vial and discard in a biohazard bag.
8. Remove the gloves and sanitize your hands.
9. Document the procedure, indicating the results, the brand name of the test used, the date, the time, and the name of the person testing and charting (or record results on the preprinted requisition or report).

REVIEW QUESTIONS*

1. Which of the following statements is incorrect (false)?
   a. The most important step in the Gram stain procedure is the decolorizer step.
   b. If too much decolorizer has been applied, at the end of the Gram stain procedure, all the organisms will be pink/red.
   c. At the end of the decolorizer step, the gram-positive organisms are purple, and the gram-negative organisms are colorless.
   d. If too little decolorizer has been applied, at the end of the Gram stain procedure, all the organisms will be pink/red.

2. Which of the following organisms is gram positive? (HINT: Check "Pathogenic Bacteria" or Tables 8.4 and 8.5.)
   a. *Escherichia coli*
   b. *Proteus* spp.
   c. *Staphylococcus* spp.
   d. *Pseudomonas* spp.

3. Which of the following statements about *Neisseria gonorrhoeae* is incorrect (false)?
   a. *N. gonorrhoeae* is a sexually transmitted disease.
   b. *N. gonorrhoeae* requires 10% carbon dioxide for growth.
   c. *N. gonorrhoeae* organisms are gram-positive cocci in pairs.
   d. The JEMBEC transportation system is used to transport and grow *N. gonorrhoeae*.

4. Which of the following statements about normal flora is incorrect (false)?
   a. Normal flora inhabit parts of the body.
   b. Normal flora are never pathogenic.
   c. Normal flora assist in preventing the colonization of pathogens.
   d. If normal flora are destroyed in a part of the body, opportunistic pathogens can invade the area.

5. When collecting a throat specimen for a Rapid Strep test, which of the following steps is incorrect (false)?
   a. Use a cotton swab.
   b. Have the patient sit with the head back.
   c. Use a sterile tongue depressor to hold down the tongue and have the patient say, "Ahh."
   d. Rotate the swab on the back of throat in a circular motion or figure-of-eight pattern.

6. In the aftermath of the 9/11 bioterrorism threats, all laboratories (including POLs) should do which of the following?
   a. Identify procedures and methods that have the potential to produce aerosols.
   b. Refer any suspicious organisms or substances to the proper authorities.
   c. Use proper biosafety techniques at all times.
   d. All of the above are true.

7. Which of the following statements about pinworm testing is incorrect (false)?
   a. The female pinworm normally lays her eggs during the night in the anal area of the human host.
   b. The cellulose tape test consists of pressing cellulose tape (sticky side) over the patient's anal area.
   c. The tape is placed with the tape sticky side down on a glass slide.
   d. A physician or trained laboratorian microscopically examines the tape for *Giardia lamblia* eggs.

8. Which of the following statements concerning bioterrorism organisms is incorrect (false)?
   a. Anthrax has three forms: cutaneous, pulmonary, and gastrointestinal.
   b. The causative agent of plague is *Yersinia pestis*.
   c. Bioterrorism smallpox is caused by the bacteria *Variola minor*.
   d. Tularemia is caused by *Francisella tularensis*, a gram-negative bacillus.

9. Name the three sources from which smears on slides are made.

10. Which of the following associations is incorrect (false)?
    a. Eukaryotic/contains a nucleus
    b. Aerobe/oxygen
    c. Aerosols/particles suspended in air
    d. Morbidity/rate of deaths

*Answers to these Review Questions are located in the Appendix on p. 279.

WEBSITES

The Public Health Image Library is a great site for microbiology pictures. Click "continue" to enter the PHIL directory and search for microbiology pictures:
http://phil.cdc.gov/Phil/home.asp
American Society for Microbiology:
www.asm.org/
Great slideshow on MRSA:
www.medicinenet.com/mrsa_picture_slideshow/article.htm

Information on swine flu (H1N1):
www.cdc.gov/h1n1flu/qa.htm
World Health Organization:
www.who.int/en/
World Health Organization info on Ebola:
http://www.who.int/mediacentre/factsheets/fs103/en/
World Health Organization info on Zika virus:
http://www.who.int/mediacentre/factsheets/zika/en/

CHAPTER 9

Toxicology

OBJECTIVES

After completing this chapter, you should be able to do the following:
1. Define and match key terms in this chapter.

Fundamental Concepts
2. List the most common illicit drugs used in the United States and describe the most widely used and abused legal drug, ethanol (alcohol).
3. Identify the types of specimens commonly used for drug testing and explain why urine specimens are very useful and convenient for drug screening tests.
4. Describe or perform proper collection of urine and blood specimens used for drug testing and monitoring.

CLIA-Waived Drug Screening Tests
5. Describe or perform urine drug screening and monitoring testing for addictive drugs of abuse and explain a positive drug test result seen in a urine specimen.

Advanced Concepts
6. Define and elaborate on therapeutic drug monitoring and list examples of therapeutic drugs that may require monitoring.
7. Describe the five steps in pharmacokinetics and discuss the meaning of "drug half-life."
8. List the most common poisonous metals and cite a source for each.

KEY TERMS

absorption: the movement of a substance through a surface of the body into body fluids and tissues

buprenorphine: a Food and Drug Administration–approved drug for treating opioid drug addiction

cannabinoid: the primary psychoactive compound in marijuana (cannabis)

distribution: the transport of a drug through the body by the blood

idiosyncrasy: an abnormal susceptibility to a drug or other agent that is peculiar to the individual

liberation: when a prescribed drug has entered the body and has released the active component from its dosage

metabolism: the chemical processes that occur within a living organism

metabolite: a substance produced by the metabolic break down of a drug in the body

opioids: drugs (such as morphine and methadone) containing or derived from opium, or that have morphinelike effects

pharmacokinetics: the movement of drugs through the body from the time of introduction to elimination

qualitative drug screening: a measurement that determines if a substance is present or absent

quantitative drug screening: a precise measurement of the amount of a substance present in a specimen

toxicity: the level at which a drug becomes poisonous in the body

❖ FUNDAMENTAL CONCEPTS

Overview of Toxicology

The toxicology department in the medical laboratory tests the levels of both therapeutic drugs and drugs of abuse to determine their presence and their harmful or "toxic" effect on the body. These departments may also test for other poisons, such as lead. In the toxicology laboratory, tests are generally performed using blood or urine specimens and sometimes saliva, sweat, or stomach contents. A toxicology test may be used to denote the presence of 1 specific drug or more than 20 drugs.

Drugs may be accidentally or deliberately injected, inhaled, swallowed, or absorbed through the skin or mucous membranes. Toxicity is the level at which a drug becomes poisonous in the body.

Medical assistants may be responsible for collecting urine or blood specimens, which are then sent to the toxicology lab, also for testing the specimen for screening or monitoring purposes. The following are common reasons for performing drug screening tests:

- To determine the cause of bizarre behavior, unconsciousness, or life-threatening symptoms in an emergency situation when drug overdose may be a possibility
- To test for drug use in the workplace or in schools, particularly among bus and truck drivers, childcare workers, and public safety workers. These professions generally require a urine or blood drug test as part of the application process and may also require employees to undergo periodic drug testing (especially after an accident that occurred during work activities).
- To test athletes for drugs that enhance their athletic ability

The Fundamental Concepts section of this chapter includes an overview of the common drugs of abuse that can become toxic or addictive (or both) when taken incorrectly. It then describes proper collection of urine and blood specimens used for drug testing. When testing for drugs of abuse, the medical assistant must ensure that collection of the specimen adheres to the legal "chain of custody" guidelines certifying that the collection of the specimen was witnessed and there was no opportunity for the specimen to be tampered with in any way.

The CLIA-Waived Drug Screening Tests part of this chapter presents in-office drug screening tests and the procedure for monitoring patients on buprenorphine (a Food and Drug Administration [FDA]–approved drug for treating drug addiction).

The Advanced Concepts section presents the principles of therapeutic drug monitoring and collecting a blood specimen for lead poisoning.

Drugs of Abuse

Thousands of drugs are available worldwide. Over-the-counter (OTC) drugs fill the shelves of pharmacies and are useful for many minor medical conditions. Unfortunately, these drugs may have toxic effects on the body if taken incorrectly. Three causes of drug toxicity with OTCs are overdosage, interactions with other drugs, or idiosyncrasy (an abnormal susceptibility to a drug or other agent that is peculiar to the individual). The medical assistant should be mindful of these possibilities and faithfully record any OTC drugs that are being taken.

Any drug can be abused, but "drugs of abuse" are considered to be those that are illegally obtained for recreational purposes or to satisfy an addiction. Some therapeutic drugs may be misused or become addictive over time.

Each of the drugs produces a specific metabolite, the substance produced by the metabolism (breaking down) of the drug in the body. The metabolite is then excreted in the urine. A qualitative drug screening test of the drug is performed to see if the metabolite is present in the same way that the urine dipstick tested for various analytes (e.g., glucose, protein). Urine is the specimen of choice for screening drugs of abuse and is the only testing method approved for federally mandated urine drug testing. Urine is easily obtained, and it is relatively simple to perform multiple drug tests at the same time. Testing of urine detects drugs used in the previous 24 to 72 hours. Specific drugs or panels of drugs can be ordered for testing. Urine samples are also tested to determine if the specimen has been subjected to alteration methods. For example, laboratories test for Na^+, Cl^-, creatinine, pH level, and specific gravity (to determine if the individual had water loaded before voiding), oxidant identification, and urine fingerprinting. Table 9.1 lists the time intervals for detecting various drugs in urine (also see Procedure 9.1 located at the end of this section).

If a quantitative drug screening test is necessary to determine the amount of the drug that is in the patient, a whole blood specimen is collected. The blood specimen is the most common test ordered for medical alcohol tests by law enforcement officials who arrest a person for alcohol intoxication. Legal testing requires a strict chain of custody.

TABLE 9.1 Typical Time Intervals for Detecting Drugs in Urine

Drug	Time Found in Urine
Alcohol	Urine: 2–12 hr (NOTE: also found in serum/plasma: 1–12 hr)
Amphetamines	Up to 2 days
Barbiturates	Short acting: 2 days Long-acting: 1–3 weeks (based on half-life)
Benzodiazepines	Short-term therapeutic use: 3 days Long-term chronic use: 4–6 weeks
Marijuana, cannabinoids	Single use: 2–7 days Prolonged, chronic use: 1–2 months or longer
Cocaine	Urine test: up to 4 days
Codeine	2 days
LSD	1–4 days
MDMA (Ecstasy)	Up to 2 days
Methadone	3 days
Methamphetamine	Up to 2 days
Opiates (heroin)	2 days
PCP	Casual use: 8–14 days Chronic use: up to 30 days
Tricyclic antidepressants	2–7 days

LSD, Lysergic acid diethylamide; *MDMA*, 3,4-methylenedioxy methamphetamine; *PCP*, phencyclidine.
Adapted from Anderson, L. (2017). Drug testing FAQS. Retrieved from https://www.drugs.com/article/drug-testing.html.

The most common legal drug of abuse in the United States is ethanol, also known as grain alcohol. It is found in beer, wine, and distilled liquors. Table 9.2 lists the approximate ethanol content in alcoholic beverages. Ethanol depresses the central nervous system and may lead to coma, progressing to death at the following "panic" (possibly lethal) levels: greater than 2000 µg/mL in the blood or greater than 1600 µg/mL in the urine.

Alcohol is one of the few drugs that has a direct correlation between blood levels and impaired driving ability. Drug alcohol

TABLE 9.2 Approximate Ethanol Content in Alcoholic Beverages

Beverage	Ethanol Content (%)
Beer	3–10
Ciders	4–5
Wines	8–12
Sherry, madeira, port	18–20
Whiskey, gin	40
Vodka	40
Brandy	40
Rum	40

From National Institute on Alcohol Abuse and Alcoholism. (n.d). What is a standard drink? Retrieved from https://www.niaaa.nih.gov/alcohol-health/overview-alcohol-consumption/what-standard-drink.

testing for prosecution of an accused drunk driver is strictly regulated by law (Procedure 9.2).

It is important to note that screening for illicit drugs or alcohol requires the consent of the patient. The patient has the right to refuse. Blood drawn for other tests cannot be used for drug screening or alcohol testing unless the patient gives consent. If a patient is unconscious and unable to give consent, the emergency exception to consent applies. If these tests are performed, they become a part of the medical records just like any other test needing to be performed in an emergency situation as needed.

PROCEDURE 9.1 Assisting with Urine Collection for Drug Screening

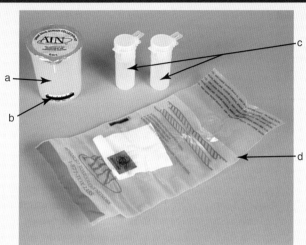

A, (a) Urine drug screening collection kit specimen cup; (b) temperature indicator on collection cup; (c) urine specimen containers to be sent to the lab; (d) plastic sealable pouch for the two urine specimen containers and the chain of custody documents.

Equipment and Supplies for Collecting and Processing Urine Specimen (Figure A)
- Urine drug screening collection kit specimen cup
- Temperature indicator on collection cup
- Urine specimen containers to be sent to the laboratory
- Plastic sealable pouch for the two urine specimen containers and the chain of custody documents

Procedure
1. Prepare the bathroom before the patient collects urine by turning off the water and adding blue dye to the toilet bowl.

2. Call in the patient and explain the purpose of the test and the procedure to be followed for a midstream clean-catch specimen collection (see Chapter 3). Also explain that no personal belongings may be taken into the bathroom and that patient may lock belongings in a provided locker.
3. Sanitize hands and apply gloves.
4. Obtain a signed consent form from the patient.
5. A trained professional must witness the actual voiding of at least 50 mL of urine into the specimen cup provided in the urine collection drug kit.
6. Originate the chain of custody document at the time of the sample collection. The person who witnessed the voiding must sign the document, as must every other person who handles the sample.
7. After the collection, verify the temperature of the urine as seen on the indicator at the bottom of the cup and document it. NOTE: If the temperature of the urine specimen is out of range (too cold), a second specimen must be collected. If the donor refuses to provide the second specimen under direct observation, the collection would be considered "refusal to test."
8. Transfer the specimen to the two containers that must be labeled with the following information:
   - Full name of the patient
   - Date and time of collection
   - Your initials
   - Initials of the witnessing officer
9. Place the two sample containers into the sealed plastic pouch, mark it with a notary-style seal or with tamper-proof tape to protect the integrity of the sample, and send the specimen to the toxicology laboratory.
10. If you are trained and qualified to do the testing, proceed with the testing according to laboratory and state regulations.
11. After both the initial and the confirmatory testing are complete, mark the urine sample, reseal it, and securely store it for a minimum of 30 days or for the length of time specified by laboratory protocols.
12. Clean or discard all equipment and supplies according to safety guidelines.
13. Remove gloves and wash hands.

PROCEDURE 9.2 Assisting with Blood Collection for Alcohol Testing

Equipment and Supplies
- Gray-topped Vacutainer tubes
- Venipuncture needle and holder (or syringe and transfer device)
- Nonvolatile disinfectant (e.g., benzalkonium [Zephiran] or aqueous thimerosal [Merthiolate])
- Gauze
- Tourniquet
- Gloves
- Legally authorized transportation envelope, container, or plastic pouch

Patient Preparation
1. An officer of the law will be present to act as a witness to the procedure.
2. The patient will probably still be under the influence of alcohol, so explain what you will be doing in a brief and concise manner. NOTE: Do not allow yourself to become irritated by the speech or mannerisms of the patient. Treat the patient with the respect and dignity with which you treat all your patients.

Blood Collection Procedure
NOTE: The Department of Justice for each state has established uniform standards for the collection, handling, and preservation of blood samples used for alcohol testing. If you are authorized to obtain specimens for forensic analysis, check your laboratory's procedure manual so that you perform the collection exactly as required by the uniform standards established for your state.
3. Sanitize hands and apply gloves.
4. Prepare the draw site using Zephiran, aqueous Merthiolate, or another aqueous disinfectant. Do not use alcohol or other volatile organic disinfectants to clean the skin site.

Continued

PROCEDURE 9.2   Assisting with Blood Collection for Alcohol Testing—cont'd

5. Complete the blood draw, filling both tubes with sufficient blood to permit duplicate blood alcohol determinations (see Chapter 4).
6. Label the two gray-stoppered tubes with the following information:
   - Full name of the patient
   - Date and time of collection
   - Your initials
   - Initials of the witnessing officer
7. Give the labeled blood samples to the witnessing officer, who will immediately complete the required information on the transportation envelope, container, or plastic pouch. The officer will then seal it securely. Information on the envelope or container should include the following:
   - Full name of the patient
   - Whether the patient is alive or dead

- The submitting agency
- The geographical location where the blood was drawn (e.g., hospital, clinic, jail)
- The name of the person drawing the blood sample
- The date and time the blood sample was drawn
- The signature of the witnessing officer

8. After the envelope or container is sealed, it must not be opened, except for analysis. Each person who is subsequently in possession of the sealed sample must sign his or her name in the space provided on the envelope or container (chain of custody). The integrity of the sample *must* be safeguarded.
9. Remove gloves and wash hands.

❖ CLIA-WAIVED DRUG SCREENING TESTS

Some offices may perform drug screening tests for companies as part of pre-employment physical examinations or as a requirement for insurance or government mandates (e.g., the federally mandated testing of transportation workers, after a workplace accident).

Although plasma samples may be used in drug testing, they are not used as often as urine samples. Blood samples provide information on drugs or alcohol present in the blood at the time of collection and do not measure drug residues that are present as the drug is metabolized. Urine drug testing provides information on drugs taken within 24 to 72 hours. CLIA-waived urine test kits are available to provide an *initial screening* for the presence of a variety of drugs, including amphetamines, marijuana (cannabinoid), cocaine, and opioids (e.g., methadone and morphine). The urine drug testing kits generally contain a rapid drug screening device and a wide-mouth collection container. Be sure to read the step-by-step instructions on the package inserts. Generally, the instructions require that the operator dip the testing device into the urine and observe the qualitative reactions in a specified time. The results are reported as positive, negative, or inconclusive (which requires an additional confirmation test using the same urine sample). Be sure to follow the shipping instructions if the screening device indicates the presence of drugs in the sample or if the results are inconclusive.

CLIA-waived saliva alcohol tests are also available for facilities that screen clients or patients for alcohol. These qualitative tests generally consist of a test strip that turns shades of green or blue if alcohol is present in the subject's saliva.

A growing number of drug screening products are also FDA approved for home use. (For a list of the drugs that may be detected in urine, saliva, hair, and breath, see the website at the end of the chapter.) Schools, employers, and the Department of Transportation (DOT) may also use these products to randomly monitor their students and employees. NOTE: If performing drug testing for the DOT in the office, the physician must be a certified Medical Review Officer (MRO). As an MRO, the licensed physician is responsible for receiving laboratory results and interpreting and evaluating an individual's positive test result.

Most rapid urine drug tests are immunoassay tests based on the principle of competitive binding of the antibody and antigen. Drugs that may be present in the urine specimen compete against their respective drugs for binding sites with their specific antibody. During testing, the urine specimen migrates upward on the test strip by capillary action. If the drug in question has a sufficiently high concentration, it will saturate all the binding sites of the test antibody so that it will *not* react in the test area of the strip. Therefore, if the drug is present in the urine in an amount that is equal to or exceeds the cutoff of the test device, the test area will show no reaction. (NOTE: The immunoassay results discussed in Chapter 7 showed an opposite positive reaction.) Conversely, if the drug is not present, it will not saturate the antibody sites, and the antibody will then react in the test area, causing a colored line to appear. The control area *(C)* of the strip indicates that the proper volume of urine migrated through the test area and that the color change was caused by antibody conjugation. (NOTE: The colored line in the internal control area does not represent a positive reaction, as in other immunoassays because a positive reaction in this method inhibits the formation of a colored band.) See Figure D in Procedure 9.3, which demonstrates drug screening test results.

Physicians who treat patients with opioid addiction using buprenorphine must monitor their patients using CLIA-waived urine drug screening test kits. These physicians are authorized by the FDA and the Substance Abuse and Mental Health Services Association (SAMHSA) to treat and monitor up to 30 patients. (For more information on buprenorphine treatment, see the websites at the end of this chapter.) The urine test cassettes detect the presence of nine addictive drugs, in addition to the therapeutic buprenorphine and assist the physician in monitoring the patient's drug use and treatment progress. NOTE: The presence of buprenorphine ensures that the patient is taking the therapeutic drug and not selling it. Table 9.1 lists each drug with its three- or four-digit testing code along with the drug's street name, source, method of administration, medical use, side effects, and overdose information. Table 9.2 shows the time intervals for detecting various drugs in urine.

PROCEDURE 9.3   Urine Drug Panel Testing Procedure

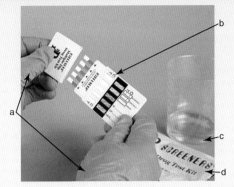

A, *(a)* Gloves; *(b)* test card with multiple test strips (five tests are on each side of the card); *(c)* fresh urine specimen or specimen that has been stored at 2° to 8°C (refrigerated) for up to 48 hours and then brought to room temperature; *(d)* metal pouch that stored the card at 2° to 30°C (refrigerator or room temperature).

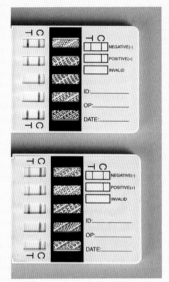

C, Results after 5 minutes from both sides of the card showing six negative results (testing area shows two colored bands) and four positive results (the testing areas have only one colored band in the control area).

Equipment and Supplies (Figure A)

- Gloves
- Test card with multiple test strips (five tests are on each side of the card)
- Fresh urine specimen or specimen that has been stored at 2° to 8°C for up to 48 hours and then brought to room temperature
- Metal pouch that has been stored at 2° to 30°C also brought to room temperature (check expiration date)

Procedure

1. Sanitize the hands and apply gloves.
2. Remove the test device from its protective pouch and label it with the patient's identification. NOTE: If the specimen has been stored in the refrigerator, bring it to room temperature before opening to prevent condensation.
3. Remove the cap from the end of the test card (Figure A).
4. With the arrows pointing toward the urine specimen, immerse the strips of the test card vertically into the urine specimen for at least 10 to 15 seconds. Immerse the strips to at least the level of the wavy lines on the strips but not above the arrows on the test card (Figure B).

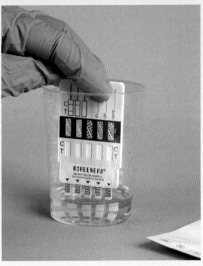

B, Immerse the strips to at least the level of the wavy lines on the strips but not above the arrows on the test card for 10 to 15 seconds.

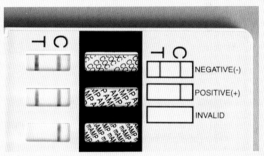

D, Close-up on first three drug results: *COC* = cocaine is negative; *AMP* = amphetamine is negative; *mAMP* = methamphetamine is positive.

5. Place the test card on a nonabsorbent surface and wait for the colored lines to appear.
6. At 5 minutes, read and record the results (Figure C).
   - Positive test result: One distinct pink band appears in the control region *(C)* and no line in the test region *(T)*.
   - Negative test result: Two pink bands appear, one pink band in the control region *(C)* and one pink band in the patient test region *(T)*.
   - Invalid: Pink bands are absent from the control region; repeat the test with a new device; if the problem persists, call for technical assistance.
7. See Figure D for close-up results on the following three drugs:
   - COC = Cocaine is negative.
   - AMP = Amphetamine is negative.
   - mAMP = Methamphetamine is positive.
8. See Table 9.3.

Quality Control Procedure

In addition to the internal control region built into the test device, external positive and negative liquid controls should be performed when a new kit is used. Also, each operator of the test should perform a positive and negative control once with each testing method to confirm that his or her testing technique is correct. The results of the control tests should be logged in the drug screening control log.

The positive liquid control procedure is performed in the same way as the patient procedure, with a new testing card. Observe and record the results within 5 minutes. Repeat the procedure with a drop of well-mixed negative control.

TABLE 9.3 Common Drugs of Abuse Detected on Multiple Drug Urine Screening Tests*

Drug (Test Code)*	Street Name Examples	Source	Route	Medical Use	Brand Names	Side Effects and Risks	Overdose
1. Cocaine (COC)	Rock, crack, coke, blow, nose nachos, hooter, yeyo	Refined coca bush leaves	Nasal administration, smoked	Topical anesthetic, natural stimulant, anesthetic, vasoconstrictor, pain killer, appetite suppressant, altitude sickness	Less addictive derivatives for anesthesia: benzocaine, lidocaine, Cepacol, Dermoplast, Lanacane	Perforation of nasal septum, renal failure, hyperthermia, cardiac arrest, seizures, dermatitis, tetany, septicemia, respiratory arrest, dehydration, sleep disorders, depression, impulsiveness, hostility, impaired memory	Fever, unresponsiveness, difficulty breathing, unconsciousness, stroke, death
2. Amphetamine (AMP)	Black beauties, Christmas trees, dexies, speed, double trouble, gaggler, beanies	Made in illegal laboratories	Smoked, injected, snorted	Appetite suppressant, central nervous system stimulant	Adderall, Citramine, DexAlone, Tanphetamin, Zamitam	Dependence, increased blood pressure, increased respiration, dilated pupils, sweating, tremors	Seizures, cardiac arrest
3. Methamphetamine (mAMP) Ecstasy XTC (MDMA)	Cat, crank, glass, speed, ice, love, Disco biscuits, Molly	Made in illegal laboratories	Oral, powder inhalant, crystals smoked	Nasal decongestant No medical use	Desoxyn	Dependence, psychosis, decreased appetite, restlessness, anxiety, heart failure, extreme fatigue, hunger, mental depression, dysrhythmias, lethargy, skin pallor, fits of rage	Seizures, cardiac arrest
4. Marijuana (THC) Hashish or Hash	Pot, weed, joint, reefer, roach, dope Hashish, hash oil, ganja	*Cannabis sativa*, hemp plant flowers and leaves	Smoked, eaten, injected	Pain relief (colitis), treatment of glaucoma, appetite stimulant, reduction of nausea from chemotherapy, euphoria, detachment, relaxation	Marinol, Dronabinol	Talkativeness, slowed time perception, inappropriate hilarity, paranoia, confusion, anxiety, short-term memory loss	Impaired lung structure, chromosomal mutation, micronucleic white blood cells, cancer, lack of motivation
5. Methadone (MTD)	Fizzies, chocolate chip cookies, jungle juice, juice wafer, biscuit	Laboratory manufactured	Oral, injection, powder	Treatment for narcotic addiction, pain	Methadose, Dolophine	Also addictive	**Danger of** respiratory and cardiac arrest and death if stopped suddenly
6. Opiates (OPI 2000) (also see MOP 300)	Heroin: smack, horse, chiva, junk, black tar, gunpowder, courage pills, bomb Opium: Big O, black stuff, clock, Dover's powder Fentanyl: Apache, Chia girl, King Ivory, Murder 8, tango	Poppy refined	Nasal, oral, intravenous injection, dermal patch	Potent pain killer, heroin, morphine, codeine, fentanyl	Demerol, Darvon, Vicodin, Dilaudid	Addiction in hospitals, constipation, dermatitis, malnutrition, hypoglycemia, dental caries, amenorrhea	**Danger of** acquired immunodeficiency syndrome (from sharing needles)

TABLE 9.3   Common Drugs of Abuse Detected on Multiple Drug Urine Screening Tests—cont'd

Drug (Test Code)*	Street Name Examples	Source	Route	Medical Use	Brand Names	Side Effects and Risks	Overdose
7. Oxycodone (OXY)	Oxy, OC, blues, killers, kickers, hillbilly heroin, Percocet: hillbilly heroin, percs, perks	Semisynthetic similar to codeine	Oral, injection	Moderate to heavy pain relief	OxyContin, Percodan, Percocet	Addiction in patients on long-term pain therapy	Death
8. Barbiturates (BAR)	Barbs, pinks, blockbusters, Christmas trees, goofballs, red devils, reds and blues, yellowjackets	Laboratory manufactured	Oral, intravenous injection	Depressant, sedative, hypnotic, anticonvulsant	Seconal, Amytal, Nembutal	Dullness, apathy, dependence	Respiratory arrest, coma, death
9. Benzodiazepines (BZO)	Roofies, downers, tranks, benzos	Laboratory manufactured	Oral, injection	Treatment for anxiety, seizures, sleeplessness, muscle relaxant	Valium, Xanax, Restoril, Versed	Carefree, detached, sleepy, disoriented, unconsciousness, amnesia, diminished reflexes	Coma; can be lethal when combined with alcohol
10. Buprenorphine (BUP)	Bupe, Subs	Laboratory manufactured	Under the tongue injection, skin patch, implant	Analgesic, treatment for opioid addiction	Buprenex, Suboxone, Subutex	Euphoria, respiratory depression, sedation	Causes severe respiratory depression when combined with benzodiazepines
11. Tricyclic antidepressants (TCAs)	Yellow	Laboratory manufactured	Oral, injection	Treatment for depression, attention-deficit hyperactivity disorder, migraines	Adapin, Norpramin, Anafranil, Pamelor, Tofranil, Elavil	Blurred vision, constipation and dry mouth, anxiety, restlessness, difficulty urinating, weight gain, drowsiness, muscle twitches, weakness, sweating, nausea, dizziness, cognitive and memory difficulties, increased heart rate, irregular heart rhythms	Panic attacks, hostile or angry feelings, impulsive actions, severe restlessness, very rapid speech
12. Lysergic acid diethylamide (LSD)	Acid, the Beast, California sunshine	Illicit laboratories, peyote (mescaline), psilocybin mexicana (mushroom), fungus on grains	Ingested orally	No medical use		Hallucinations, anxiety, depression, confusion, paranoia, panic attacks, impaired memory, inability to reason, flashbacks, increased blood pressure, high temperature, dilated pupils, increased heart rate	Psychosis, flashbacks
13. Phencyclidine (PCP)	Angel dust, peace pill, rocket fuel, wack, ozone, fry	Illegal laboratories	Oral, intravenous, sniffed, smoked	No medical use		Hallucinations, acute anxiety, dulled thinking, poor memory, depression, severe brain damage, hepatitis, respiratory arrest, panic reaction, confusion, blurred vision, high blood pressure	Violence, psychoses, self-injurious behavior, suicide

*Numbers 1 through 9 are the screened drugs for patients taking number 10, buprenorphine therapy (see Procedure 9.3).
MDMA, 3,4-Methylenedioxymethamphetamine; *THC*, tetrahydrocannabinol.

❖ ADVANCED CONCEPTS

Therapeutic Drug Monitoring

Therapeutic drug monitoring (TDM) is the process of measuring either the effects of a drug on a patient or the actual levels of a drug being administered to a patient. For example, we have already discussed monitoring the *effect* of insulin therapy by performing blood glucose levels, and we monitored the *effect* of Coumadin therapy by testing the patient's prothrombin time and international normalized ratio (INR). In this chapter, we will learn the importance of monitoring therapeutic drug levels in the patient's blood, urine, or both.

Most prescribed drugs have a therapeutic range that must be maintained for successful therapy. If a patient's drug level falls outside of the range, it may become ineffective if too low or toxic if too high. Table 9.4 lists therapeutic ranges and toxic levels for various drugs. Therapeutic ranges and the subsequent monitoring of the drug levels in the body give the physician guidelines for prescribing the medication and fine tuning the exact effective amount of medication to keep the patient within the range.

It is very important to collect the blood sample for TDM at a certain time—either before or after administering the drug. Otherwise, the test results will be useless and unreliable, or even worse, they may prompt the physician to initiate inappropriate treatment.

Common Therapeutic Drugs That are Tested for Toxicity

Amikacin	Paracetamol
Caffeine	Phenobarbital
Carbamazepine	Phenytoin
Cyclosporine	Primidone
Digoxin	Salicylic acid
Ethosuximide	Theophylline
Gentamicin	Tobramycin
Lithium	Valproic acid
Methotrexate	Vancomycin

Pharmacokinetics

For a better understanding of how drugs are used by the body, here is a brief look at the five stages of **pharmacokinetics** (the movement of drugs through the body from the time of introduction to elimination).

Liberation

Liberation is the release of the active ingredient in a drug from its dosage form. For the active ingredient to be liberated, it must first enter the body by way of a solution. For example, eye drops go into solution in the tears of the eye. Swallowed medication goes into solution in the gastric fluid. Liquid injections are inserted into the skin, muscle, or vein. The liberation phase extends from the time the drug was administered to the time it dissolves and is able to be absorbed.

Absorption and Distribution

Absorption is the movement of a drug from a body surface (e.g., the skin or mucous membrane) through the tissues and

TABLE 9.4   Drug Categories Showing Therapeutic Ranges and Toxic Levels

Drug	Therapeutic Range	Toxic Level
Antibiotics		
Amikacin	15–25 mcg/mL	>25 mcg/mL
Gentamicin	5–10 mcg/mL	>12 mcg/mL
Kanamycin	20–25 mcg/mL	>35 mcg/mL
Tobramycin	5–10 mcg/mL	12 mcg/mL
Anticonvulsants		
Carbamazepine (Tegretol)	5–12 mcg/mL	>12 mcg/mL
Ethosuximide (Zarontin)	40–100 mcg/mL	>100 mcg/mL
Phenobarbital (Luminal)	10–30 mcg/mL	>40 mcg/mL
Phenytoin (Dilantin)	10–20 mcg/mL	>30 mcg/mL
Primidone	5–12 mcg/mL	>15 mcg/mL
Antidepressants and Antipsychotics		
Amitriptyline (Elavil)	100–150 ng/mL	>500 ng/mL
Diazepam (Valium)	1–2 mg/L	>20 mg/L
Imipramine (Tofranil)	150–300 ng/mL	>500 ng/mL
Lithium (Lithonate)	0.8–1.2 mEq/L	>2 mEq/L
Antirheumatics		
Salicylate (aspirin)	Varies with use	>300 mcg/mL
Acetaminophen (Tylenol)	Varies with use	>250 mcg/mL
Barbiturates		
Amobarbital (Amytal)	2–10 mcg/mL	40–80 mcg/mL(lethal)
Pentobarbital (Nembutal)	10–30 mcg/mL	40 mcg/mL
Secobarbital (Seconal)	3 mcg/mL	10 mcg/mL
Cardiotonics		
Digoxin	0.8–2 mcg/mL	>2.4 mcg/mL
Disopyramide	2–5 mcg/mL	>5 mcg/mL
Lidocaine	1.5–5 mcg/mL	>5 mcg/mL
Procainamide (Pronestyl)	4–10 mcg/mL	>16mcg/mL
Quinidine	2–5 mcg/mL	>10 mcg/mL

Adapted from MedlinePlus. (2015). *Therapeutic drug levels.* Retrieved from https://medlineplus.gov/ency/article/003430.htm and DrugLib.com. Amytal (amobarbital sodium): drug interactions, contraindications, overdosage, etc. Retrieved from http://www.druglib.com/druginfo/amytal/interactions_overdosage_contraindications.

into the blood (also called *uptake*). The blood then carries the drug through the body (**distribution**) until it finds its target (e.g., antibiotics find the pathogen, anticonvulsants and antidepressants find the brain, cardiotonics find the heart and vessels).

Metabolism and Elimination

Next, the drug needs to be broken down (**metabolism**) into a water-soluble metabolite, which generally occurs in the liver, gut wall, kidney, or skin. After it is broken down, the drug metabolite is eliminated by way of bile from the liver or urine from the kidneys. Drug metabolites may also be excreted through the skin by way of sweat, the lungs by way of expired air, or the salivary or mammary glands.

Drug Half-Life and Specimen Collection

The amount of time necessary to eliminate 50% of a drug is referred to as its *half-life*. The half-life cycle varies for each individual depending on sex, age, body weight, and health status. For example, children and older adults are more prone to experiencing toxic levels of therapeutic drugs because of their body size or altered metabolic rates. These factors have an effect on whether a drug is prescribed, when to test for the drug, and what type of specimen is tested (e.g., urine, blood).

Drugs of abuse are generally tested using urine specimens for the qualitative result and urine or blood for the quantitative result. TDM generally uses blood specimens taken in a gold gel tube (serum separator tube) or a light green heparin tube with gel (plasma separator tube). NOTE: Do *not* use a lithium heparin tube when monitoring blood lithium levels. Be sure to refer to the laboratory manual when collecting toxicology specimens that are sent to the toxicology department of reference labs and hospitals. See the website listed at the end of the chapter for additional information on TDM testing and specimen collection.

Other Toxicology Tests

Other conditions in which a medical assistant may be asked to collect specimens for toxicology or perform drug screening tests are as follows:

Chronic lead poisoning may occur from the lead-based paint found in old homes. A tan or K2EDTA-topped tube is needed for a lead test specimen. Two tubes offered by BD have been FDA cleared for use in lead testing and are certified to have low lead content, thereby reducing the risk of false-positive lead test results. The BD microtainer K2EDTA tube (certified to contain <1 ng of lead) with BD Microgard is used for capillary collections from infants or children. The 3-mL BD K2EDTA Plus plastic tube with tan top can be used on older children or adults.

Always refer to the laboratory manual for any other directions regarding collection and processing of the specimen and for the following specimen collections:

- Acute iron poisoning in children who have taken adult iron tablets is a stat test.
- Chronic exposure to mercury and arsenic poisoning tests
- Forensic drug tests for court purposes
- Urine screening testing on pregnant mothers for drugs of abuse
- Urine and blood drug testing for on-the-job injuries to rule out an impaired employee

SUMMARY

We are constantly exposed to harmful and poisonous substances. Even prescription medications may be harmful if not used as directed. The physician needs to know whether a drug is at its therapeutic level or whether the drug level is becoming toxic. Toxicology is the study and monitoring of these drugs as well as the identification of drugs of abuse. The medical assistant must be aware of the proper timing and specifics of collecting toxicology specimens, as well as the legal processing of specimens that may contain illicit drugs (i.e., chain of custody protocol).

■ REVIEW QUESTIONS*

True or False

Indicate if the following statements are true or false:

1. Therapeutic drug monitoring is a way for the physician to measure the effects and levels of a drug being administered to a patient.
2. Pharmacokinetics is the study of drugs.

Fill in the Blanks

Complete the following statements:

3. _____ is the term meaning the release of the active ingredient of a drug from its dosage.
4. The movement of a drug from solution to the blood is called _____.
5. The transport of a drug throughout the body by way of the blood is called _____.
6. The term for the breakdown of a drug within the body is _____.
7. The two main organs that eliminate drugs are the _____ and the _____.
8. The time it takes to eliminate 50% of any drug is called its _____.
9. Poisonous metals may include _____, _____, _____, and _____.

10. The most widely used and abused legal drug in society is _____.
11. Methamphetamine is also known as _____ or _____.
12. Two examples of opiate-derived drugs are _____ and _____.

Multiple Choice

Circle the letter that represents the single best answer:

13. Drugs may be excreted through all of the following *except*
    a. skin.
    b. sweat.
    c. stool.
    d. tears.
    e. lungs.
14. Forensic laboratories prefer _____ for medical alcohol test.
    a. urine
    b. serum
    c. plasma
    d. whole blood
    e. breath

*Answers to these Review Questions are located in the Appendix on p. 279.

WEBSITES

DEA—Drug Enforcement Administration—Drug Fact Sheets: An excellent website for finding fact sheets on drugs of abuse, it provides an updated alphabetical index of the drugs and chemicals of concern:
www.justice.gov/dea/druginfo/factsheets.shtml

Drug abuse signs and symptoms (updated as of June 2013):
www.helpguide.org/mental/drug_substance_abuse_addiction_signs_effects_treatment.htm

Website for Screeners Dip Drug Test Kit:
www.lifelinemedical.net/ddd_dip_drug_test.html

Website with links to therapeutic drug monitoring testing and specimen collection information:
www.questdiagnostics.com/testcenter/testguide.action?dc=WP_DrugHalfLife

CHAPTER 10

Electrocardiography

OBJECTIVES

After completing this chapter, you should be able to do the following:

1. Define and match key terms and abbreviations related to electrocardiography (ECG) in this chapter.

Fundamental Electrocardiography Concepts

2. Identify the vessels and chambers of the heart related to pulmonary and systemic circulation.
3. Compare Einthoven's early ECG invention with the current equipment, supplies, and recordings produced by modern ECGs.
4. Identify the structures involved in the electrical conduction system of the heart and identify the electrical patterns on the ECG:
   - Identify the sinoatrial node, bundle of His, left and right bundle branches, and Purkinje network.
   - Identify the P, Q, R, S, T, and U waves and the baseline on the ECG tracing.
   - Compare the intervals and segments on an ECG tracing.
   - Compare a normal ECG tracing with one showing bradycardia.

Diagnostic Electrocardiography Testing

5. Prepare the patient and show awareness of the patients' concerns related to the ECG procedures.
6. Perform the 12-lead ECG diagnostic test according to the stated task, conditions, and standards listed in the Learning Outcome Evaluation in the student workbook.
7. Identify a successful ECG tracing and take appropriate steps to correct common artifacts found on the ECG tracing.
8. Succinctly and accurately report to the physician relevant information regarding the ECG test.

Advanced Electrocardiography Concepts

9. Perform or describe how to prepare the patient for cardiac monitoring using a Holter or Zio monitor.
10. Understand the terms related to various cardiac conditions as seen on the ECG tracing:
    - Premature atrial contractions and premature ventricular contractions
    - Atrial flutter, atrial tachycardia, and ventricular tachycardia
    - Fibrillation in atria and fibrillation in the ventricles

KEY TERMS

artifacts: tracings other than from the heart that will interfere with the interpretation of the ECG recordings

atria: the upper chambers of the heart; they receive blood from the body on the right side and from the lungs on the left side

atrioventricular (AV) node: node that transmits the electrical impulse to the Bundle of His

augmented limb leads: unipolar limb leads (aVR, aVL, aVF)

bradycardia: slow heart rate

cardiac cycle: a sequence of two phases: a contraction phase and a relaxation phase

clavicle: collarbone

diastole: the relaxation phase in the heart when there is no electrical activity within the cardiac muscle

ECG cycle: pattern of P, Q, R, S, T, and U waves on an ECG recording

electrodes: the 10 "sensors" placed on the limbs and chest that pick up the electrical activity of the heart

Holter monitoring: ambulatory ECG monitoring

intercostal: between the ribs

precordial leads: chest leads

pulmonary circulation: blood flowing to the lungs and back to the heart

Purkinje fibers: network that transmits electrical impulses to the ventricles, causing them to contract

septum: a muscular wall that divides the right and left sides of the heart

sinoatrial (SA) node: node that transmits an electrical impulse that starts the heartbeat

sinus bradycardia: slow heart rate

sinus rhythm: heart rhythm initiated by the sino-atrial (SA) node

sinus tachycardia: rapid heart rate

standard limb leads: Einthoven's first leads known as bipolar leads I, II, and III

sternum: breastbone

systemic circulation: blood flowing to the body and back to the heart

systole: the contraction phase of the heart when the cardiac muscle is being stimulated by electrical impulses

tachycardia: fast heart rate

ventricles: the lower chambers of the heart; they pump the blood out of the heart to the lungs and the body

ECG: electrocardiogram
PAC: premature atrial contractions

PVCs: premature ventricular contractions

❖ FUNDAMENTAL CONCEPTS

This chapter and Chapter 11 (Spirometry) are unique from the other laboratory testing chapters in that they do not use a specimen from the body to test. Instead they use various instruments applied to the body itself to evaluate cardiac and pulmonary function. Consequently, these cardiopulmonary tests are referred to as "diagnostic tests" rather than "laboratory tests." In this chapter, the heart is reviewed anatomically followed by discussions of the ways the electrocardiogram (ECG) is able to display various graphs and provide interpretations of the patient's heart.

Anatomy of the Heart

In Chapter 4, we studied the blood vessels in the cardiovascular system. This chapter focuses on the heart and how it is able to rhythmically and continuously pump the blood to the pulmonary circulation (lungs) and to the systemic circulation (upper and lower body) and return the blood to the heart after each circulation (Figure 10.1).

Chambers and Vessels of the Heart

Anatomically, the heart is divided into right and left sides by a muscular wall referred to as the septum. Both sides contain upper chambers, atria, that receive blood from the body (right atrium) and from the lungs (left atrium). The lower chambers on each side are ventricles that then pump the blood out of the heart. The right ventricle sends the blood to the lungs, and the left ventricle pumps the blood to the body (Figure 10.2).

The movement of the blood through the heart's chambers is the result of the muscles in both atria simultaneously contracting and pushing the blood into the ventricles. The atria then relax and fill up with the blood while the large muscles of the ventricles are stimulated to contract and push the blood into the pulmonary artery on the right, and the aorta on the left. These muscular contractions are initiated by electrical impulses from the nervous system that flow through the cardiac muscle from top to bottom, creating each heartbeat. See the Evolve animation to view the route of blood flow and the movement of the electrical current through the heart.

Cardiac Cycle and Electrical Conduction System in the Heart

The cardiac cycle is a sequence of two phases: (1) a contraction phase, or systole, when the cardiac muscle is being stimulated by electrical impulses; and a (2) relaxation phase, or diastole, when there is no electrical activity within the cardiac muscle. On average, each cycle lasts 0.8 second.

The specialized structures that regulate each cardiac cycle include the sinoatrial (SA) node, the atrioventricular (AV)

node, the bundle of His, the right and left bundle branches, and the Purkinje fibers (Figure 10.3).

During each cardiac cycle, the electrical impulses and muscular contractions flow as follows:

1. The SA node transmits an electrical impulse that starts the heartbeat and sets its rhythm, or pattern. The SA node is also known as the "pacemaker."
2. The electrical impulse from the SA node moves through the atria, causing them to contract first.
3. From the atria, the impulse travels to the AV node. Here, the impulse is slightly delayed to give the atria time to fully contract and fill the ventricles with blood.
4. Then the AV node transmits the electrical impulse to the bundle of His.
5. Next, the impulse splits and travels down the right and left bundle branches.

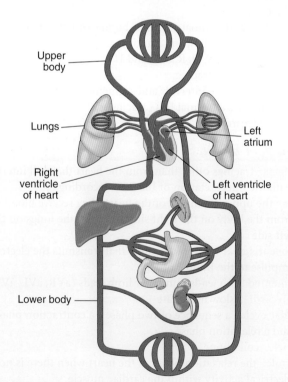

FIG. 10.1 Note how the right side of the patient's heart receives blood from the upper and lower body. The right ventricle then pumps the deoxygenated *(blue)* blood to the **pulmonary circulation** (lungs) and then back to the left side of the patient's heart. The oxygenated *(red)* blood in the heart's left ventricle is pumped to the **systemic circulation** (upper and lower body). (From Frazier M: *Human diseases and conditions,* ed 5, St. Louis, 2013, Saunders.)

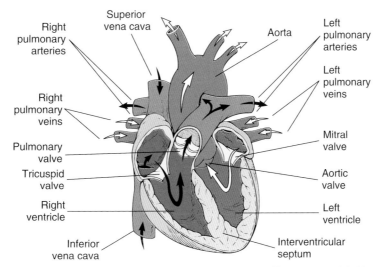

FIG. 10.2 Close-up view of blood circulation through the heart. (From Frazier M: *Human diseases and conditions,* ed 5, St. Louis, 2013, Saunders.)

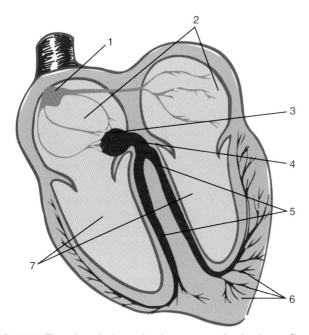

FIG. 10.3 The electrical conduction system in the heart flows as follows: *(1) The SA node* initiates the cycle, sending impulses that excite the atria. *(2) The atria* contract while *(3) the AV node* becomes stimulated and sends impulse to *(4) the bundle of His,* which sends the impulse down *(5) the right and left bundle branches,* which continue to branch into *(6) the Purkinje network* of fibers that excite *(7) the ventricles,* causing them to contract.

6. The impulse continues along the branches to the Purkinje fibers. This network of fibers transmits the impulse to the ventricles, causing them to contract.

Brief History of the Electrocardiogram

Willem Einthoven invented the first practical electrocardiogram (ECG or EKG) in 1903 and received the Nobel Prize in Medicine in 1924 for it. His research included placing his two arms into salt solutions and his right foot into a bucket to provide an electrical ground. He then measured the electrical activity that took place between his arms using a crude galvanometer that moved a stylus up and down on a moving background. The first picture of the heartbeats between the arms was labeled "Lead I."

He also measured the electrical activity between his right arm and left leg and saw that the picture of the electrical impulse that flowed through the heart from top to bottom created a more defined picture, and it was labeled "Lead II." A typical lead II recording is seen on the right side of Figure 10.4. Note the positive upward and negative downward deflections called "waves" that were produced with each heartbeat cycle during lead II. The waves were labeled P through T. The three color-coded areas (P, QRS, and T) relate to the following electrical activities in the heart:

- The *P wave* on the graph shows *atrial depolarization.* This wave occurs when the nervous impulse starts in the SA node, causing the atria to contract.
- The *QRS complex* of three waves shows *ventricular depolarization.* These waves occur as the impulse moves through the heart's AV node, bundle of His, and Purkinje fibers, causing the ventricles to contract.
- The *T wave* shows *repolarization.* This state occurs during a period of electrical recovery. Then the ventricles relax briefly before the cycle resumes.

NOTE: A small *U wave* may appear after the *T wave* for some patients. The cause is often unknown.

Einthoven also measured the left arm and left leg and created another picture of heartbeats that became known as "Lead III." Collectively, these three leads were referred to as the *bipolar limb leads* because they were measuring the electrical impulses that occurred between two limbs that were dipped into the two salt solutions. These first three "limb" leads are still referred to as *Einthoven's triangle* (Figure 10.5).

Modern Electrocardiography Monitors and Tracings

Einthoven's initial invention to detect the electrical activity in the heart has evolved into modern electrocardiograph instruments

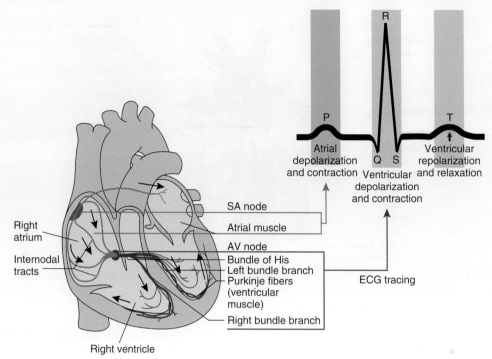

FIG. 10.4 Conduction system in the heart (labeled to the right of the heart) and its relationship to the three color-coded phases seen on the electrocardiogram (ECG). *AV*, Atrioventricular; *SA*, sinoatrial. (From Gould B: *Pathophysiology for the health professions*, ed 4, Philadelphia, 2011, Saunders.)

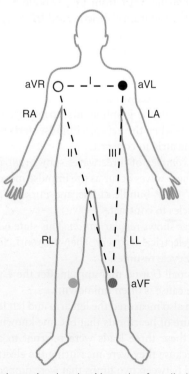

FIG. 10.5 Einthoven's triangle: Note the four limb electrodes: right arm (RA) *(white)*, left arm (LA) *(black)*, right leg (RL) *(green)*, and left leg (LL) *(red)*. The RL functions as a "ground," and the other three limbs form Einthoven's triangle, which is able to take six limb lead pictures of the heart: three bipolar leads (I, II, and III) and three augmented unipolar leads (aVR, aVL, and aVF).

and computers that are now able to record and analyze 12 leads in less than 15 seconds by recording 3 leads at the same time. See the ECG report in Figure 10.6. Each of the 12 leads, seen in the top 3 rows, shows a view of the heart from 12 different angles with the bottom graph showing a continuous lead II for rhythm analysis known as the *rhythm strip*. Together the leads give an overall picture of the electrical activity in the entire heart. By analyzing different leads, the physician is able to pinpoint the source of certain problems.

Electrodes

Einthoven's three salt solutions in buckets have been replaced by 10 disposable electrodes, or *sensors*, that are placed on the patient's limbs and chest. The disposable electrodes have an electrolyte gel and adhesive backing that are applied to the four limbs and six locations on the chest. They simultaneously detect the electrical impulses produced when the heart contracts (Figure 10.7).

From the electrodes, the impulses from the heart are then transmitted through their 10 designated "lead" wires that are connected to a patient cable that attaches to the electrocardiograph instrument as seen in Figure 10.8. The signal is amplified and sent to the galvanometer, which changes the electrical impulse into mechanical motion. The motion is then recorded on moving graph paper or to a computerized graph.

Limb Lead Wires

The lead wires that connect to the electrodes are labeled and color coded as follows:
- **RA** designates right arm—white
- **LA** designates left arm—black

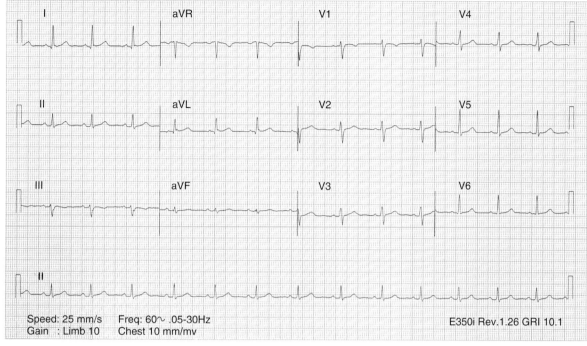

Name : Jane Doe
ID   : 34
Date : 04/06/73   Time : 11:37
Age : 20   Sex : Female
Hgt : 64 IN   Wgt : 130 LBS

Vent rate : 81   SINUS RHYTHM
                     WITHIN NORMAL LIMITS
- - Durations - -
P   : 84   SUMMARY: NORMAL
QRS : 92

I   aVR   V1   V4

II   aVL   V2   V5

III   aVF   V3   V6

II

Speed: 25 mm/s   Freq: 60∿ .05-30Hz
Gain : Limb 10   Chest 10 mm/mv

E350i Rev.1.26 GRI 10.1

FIG. 10.6 A three-channel electrocardiography report showing the six limb lead recordings on the left and the chest lead recordings on the right. Also notice the "rhythm strip" at the bottom showing lead II uninterrupted and the interpretation of the recording on the upper right. (From Bonewit-West K: *Clinical procedures for medical assistants,* ed 10, St. Louis, 2018, Elsevier.)

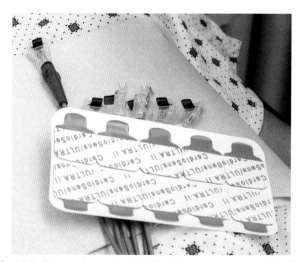

FIG. 10.7 Electrode card with 10 stick-on electrodes (4 will be placed on the limbs and 6 will be placed on the chest). Also, notice the blue-tipped alligator clips seen under the card that are attached to brown "lead" wires. The alligator clips will clamp on to the electrodes after they have been placed on the patient.

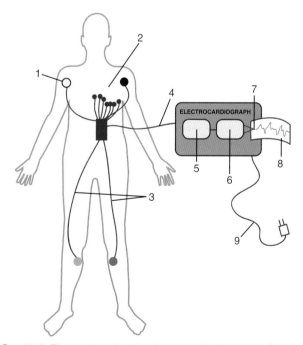

FIG. 10.8 Electrodes, lead wires, and electrocardiography (ECG) recorder. *1,* Right arm limb electrode; *2,* chest electrodes; *3,* lower limb lead wires; *4,* patient cable; *5,* amplifier; *6,* galvanometer; *7,* recording stylus; *8,* moving ECG paper; *9,* power cord.

- **RL** designates right leg—green
- **LL** designates left leg—red

Standard limb leads. The first three leads recorded on a routine ECG are called standard limb leads. They are Einthoven's first leads known as *bipolar leads* because they each monitor two limb electrodes. They show the following electrical activity between the electrodes:

- Lead I shows the voltage changes between the right arm and left arm.
- Lead II shows the voltage changes between the right arm and left leg.
- Lead III shows the voltage changes between the left arm and left leg.

Augmented limb leads. The next three limb leads are called augmented limb leads. They are known as *unipolar leads* because they each directly monitor only one limb electrode. Each lead shows the electrical activity between one limb electrode and a point midway between the other two limb electrodes in the triangle.

The electrical impulses recorded by these leads are small. As a result, the ECG machine must augment, or *increase,* their size in order for the tracing to be readable. These leads are labeled aV, denoting "augmented voltage."

- Lead aVR shows the voltage difference between the *right arm* and the midpoint of the left arm and left leg.
- Lead aVL shows the voltage difference between the *left arm* and the midpoint of the right arm and left leg.
- Lead aVF shows the voltage difference between the *left leg* and the midpoint of the right arm and left arm.

Refer to Figure 10.5, Einthoven's triangle, showing all six limb leads: I, II, III, aVR, aVL, and aVF.

Note the placement of the electrodes (sensors) on the lower limbs with the color-coded lead wires attached in Figure 10.9. The electrode placed on the right leg (green) is not used as part of the recording. Instead, it functions as an electrical ground and reference point.

Precordial Chest Lead Wires

In addition to the limb leads, there are six precordial leads, or *chest leads.* They are also unipolar leads that monitor the heart from one chest electrode at a time. Each precordial lead shows the electrical activity between a central point within the heart and a specific site on the front of the chest based on skeletal structures (i.e. clavicle).

Six electrodes are placed across the chest in a specific pattern based on the patient's skeletal structures. The precordial lead wires are each labeled with the letter V or C and a lead number 1 through 6. They monitor electrodes at the following sites:

- **V1:** fourth intercostal space on the right side of the sternum
- **V2:** fourth intercostal space on the left side of the sternum
- **V3:** midway between the V2 and V4 positions
- **V4:** fifth intercostal space on the left mid-clavicular line
- **V5:** horizontal to V4 at the left anterior axillary line
- **V6:** horizontal to V4 at the left midaxillary line

See Figure 10.10, which shows the four steps taken to locate the six chest leads using skeletal landmarks.

Standardization and Interpretation of the Electrocardiograph

Standardization. All electrocardiographs (instruments) must be standardized to produce a consistent electrocardiogram (picture) that records the electrical deflections produced by each person's heartbeats over time. All ECG tracing paper is divided into squares that form graph lines. The size and pattern of the squares are standard. As a result, physicians throughout the world are able to read and compare a patient's tracings in the same way (Figure 10.11).

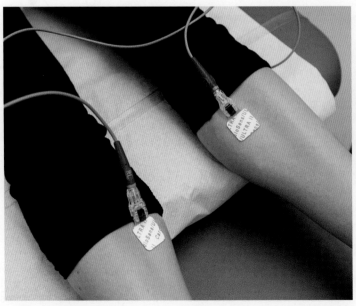

FIG. 10.9 Note the disposable electrodes with color-coded wires for the grounded right leg *(green-tipped wire)* and the lead wire for the left leg *(red-tipped wire).* (Photo by Zack Bent.)

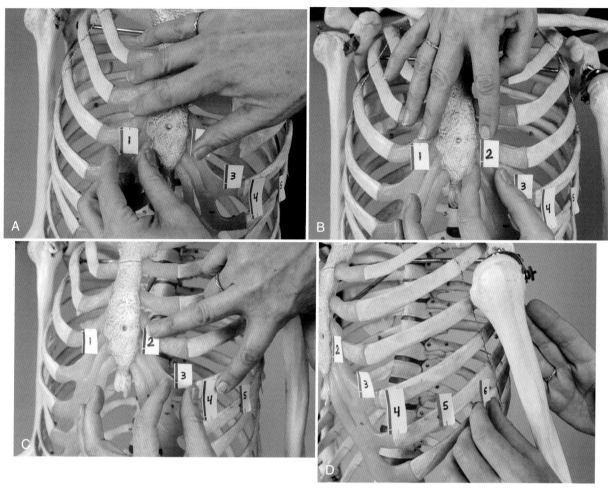

FIG. 10.10 A, *Step 1:* Locate V1 by palpating the top three intercostal spaces and then placing the electrode on the next fourth intercostal space on the right side of the patient's sternum. **B,** *Step 2:* Place V2 directly across from V1 over the fourth intercostal space on the left side of the patient's sternum. **C,** *Step 3:* Locate V4 by drawing an imaginary line from the mid-clavicle to the fifth intercostal space; then place V3 midway on an imaginary straight line between V2 and V4. **D,** *Step 4:* Place V5 in line with V4 at the anterior/lateral "corner" of the chest. And then place V6 in line with V5 at the midaxillary line on the left side of the chest.

Two sizes of squares are in the graph, small and large. Each small square is 1 mm by 1 mm. A large square is made up of 25 small squares. Therefore, each large square is 5 mm by 5 mm.
- The vertical lines on the graph measure voltage, or the strength of the electrical impulse. One small square represents 0.1 millivolt (mV), and two large squares (10 mm) represent 1 mV.
- The horizontal lines on the graph measure time. One small square represents 0.04 second, and five large squares (25 mm) represent 1 second.

The upward and downward deflections produced on the moving graph paper are standardized to a sensitivity showing 1 mV of electricity producing a 10-mm deflection on the graph paper as seen in Figure 10.11. NOTE: The standardized pulses were also seen at the beginning and end of each of the leads in Figure 10.6. The sensitivity may also be set at half when a large heartbeat needs to be diminished on the graph or at two times to magnify the recording of a small heartbeat.

The time it takes to produce each cardiac cycle is also standardized by setting the speed of the graph paper to move horizontally at a speed of 25 mm per second.

Interpretation of electrocardiogram. Physicians are now able to analyze the electrical patterns (vertical waves) and the specific timing (horizontal measurements) of each wave (P, Q, R, S, T, and the occasional U) (see Figure 10.11).

Cardiologists (and interpretive ECGs) also measure the following (as seen in Figure 10.11):
- The timing of the *QRS complex* related to ventricular stimulation and contraction
- The timing (or duration) of two *segments:* the *P-R segment,* showing the time when the impulse is delayed at the AV node before traveling down the bundle of His, and the *ST segment,* showing the time between ventricular depolarization and repolarization
- The timing (or duration) of two *intervals* related to atrial activity *(P-R interval)* and ventricular activity *(Q-T interval)*

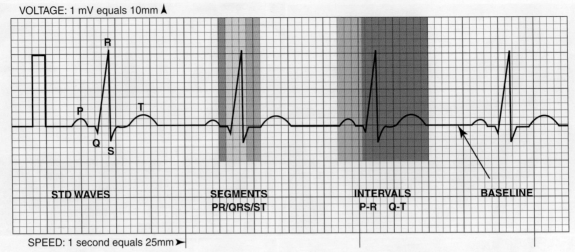

VOLTAGE: 1 mV equals 10mm ▲

STD WAVES   SEGMENTS   INTERVALS   BASELINE
                   PR/QRS/ST   P-R Q-T

SPEED: 1 second equals 25mm ➤

FIG. 10.11 Enlarged electrocardiography (ECG) graph paper showing the large boxes that have been divided into 5 × 5 1-mm small boxes. Notice the normal standardization pulse on the left: a 1-mV charge caused the stylus to jump up 10 mm (2 large squares) while the paper was moving, creating a 2-mm horizontal line that returned to the baseline. Notice how the waves (P, Q, R, S, and T) are identified and measured by the up and down movement of the stylus showing the voltage of each. The color-coded "segments" and "intervals" of each ECG cycle are also analyzed and measured based on the horizontal movement of the paper over time.

The *baseline* on the ECG is when the heart is at rest between beats, and no electrical activity is taking place. Cardiologists and computerized interpretive ECGs are able to calculate the rate and rhythm of the heartbeat per minute by observing the distance between the peaks of the R waves of each ECG cycle. See Figure 10.12, which displays an interpretation of sinus bradycardia (slow heart rate) with a ventricular rate of 58 beats/min, and compare the distance of the ECG cycles seen at the bottom of the ECG in Figure 10.6, which displays an interpretation of sinus rhythm (within normal limits) with a ventricular rate of 81 beats/min. If the cardiac cycles were very close together on the bottom "rhythm strip," the result would be sinus tachycardia.

❖ DIAGNOSTIC PROCEDURES: ELECTROCARDIOGRAPHY

In this chapter, the ECG is recording the results produced by the patient's heart rather than lab specimens. It is therefore necessary to prepare patients properly and to coach them with helpful instructions throughout the procedures to produce accurate reports. It is also important to identify and correct any artifacts (tracings other than from the heart that will interfere with the interpretation of the ECG or spirometer recordings) before submitting a final report to the physician.

Electrocardiography Patient Preparations, Instructions, and Identification of Artifacts
Patient Preparation
Call the patient into the room and sanitize your hands while confirming the patient's name with the same methods that are covered in Chapter 4: Ask each patient to spell his or her last name; provide his or her date of birth; and give one more

identifier, such as phone number or address, or show a driver's license.

Be aware of patients' anxiety level and assure them that the ECG test is "routine" and that when they are being connected to the lead wires, the procedure is not forcing any electricity into them. The wires are simply attaching to the sticky "sensors" (electrodes) that are placed on various places on their body to "take pictures" of the electrical activity generated by the heart and any other muscle in the body. Explain that it is important that they are very comfortable and relaxed so that the only muscular activity during the test should be from their hearts. Show them the gowns and have them disrobe from the waist up; then tell them you will return to their room when they are ready.

When you return, help them recline on their back with their head placed comfortably on the pillow and their arms rested on their sides in a comfortable position. NOTE: If a large person's body does not allow enough room for her or his arms on the table, have the person tuck their thumbs under her or his legs. This will reduce the muscular interference caused by using their arm muscles to keep the patient's arms on the table. Also make sure the patient's legs are relaxed by allowing their feet to turn outward.

When running the test, let the patient know when the ECG is recording and encourage him or her to be very still and relaxed with no talking or moving for the 15 seconds of recording.

Identifying and Correcting Electrocardiography Artifacts
When the patient's electrocardiogram tracing is printed on the 3-channel ECG paper, or "captured" on the computer screen, it is the medical assistant's responsibility to analyze the tracings on each of the 12 leads and identify any artifacts. See Figure 10.13, which shows a computer readout of all 12 leads.

Name : Jane Doe
ID : 27
Date : 08/28/03   Time : 04:17
Age : 48   Sex : Female
Hgt : 67 IN   Wgt : 150 LBS
Med1 :
Med2 :
Ccl1 :
Ccl2 :
Cmnt :

Vent rate : 58

- - Durations - -
P : 82
QRS : 92
- - Intervals - -
PR : 110
QT : 426
QTc : 423
- - Axes - -
P : -15
QRS : 34
T : 33

SINUS BRADYCARDIA
SUPRAVENTRICULAR EXTRASYSTOLES
    ST junctional depression
NON SPECIFIC ST CHANGES

SUMMARY: BORDERLINE NORMAL

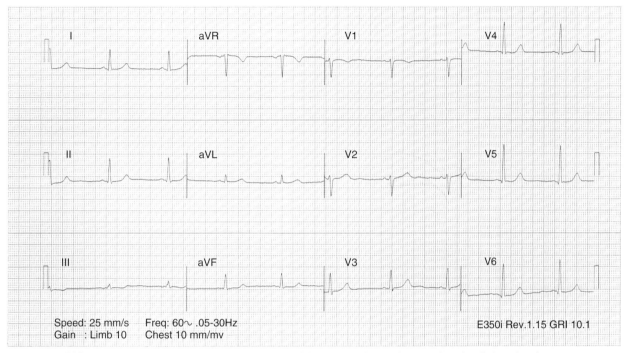

Speed: 25 mm/s   Freq: 60∿ .05-30Hz
Gain : Limb 10   Chest 10 mm/mv

E350i Rev.1.15 GRI 10.1

FIG. 10.12 Electrocardiography recording with interpretation at the top showing "sinus bradycardia." Notice how much farther apart the R spikes are compared with those in Figure 10.6. (From Bonewit-West K: *Clinical procedures for medical assistants*, ed 9, St. Louis, 2015, Saunders.)

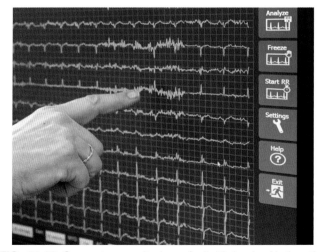

FIG. 10.13 Computer monitoring of all 12 leads. Notice the "artifacts" (erratic tracings attributable to patient movement) on three of the limb tracings. These artifacts would need to be corrected before printing the final report.

Notice the hand pointing at the erratic tracings on 3 of the 12 lead tracings. You may also notice that the erratic tracings appeared and then stabilized to the right of the artifacts, which means that the patient moved an arm during that part of the tracing. Obviously, you would not want to have that part of the tracing in the final report.

Figure 10.14 illustrates four examples of the most common artifacts found on ECG tracings (somatic tremors, wandering baseline, AC interference, and interrupted baseline). The four artifacts shown in the accompanying table explain the possible causes of each artifact.

If the medical assistant spots artifacts on any of the limb leads (I, II, III, aVR, aVL, or aVF), the problem needs to be located and corrected. Knowledge of Einthoven's triangle is helpful in locating the limb producing the artifact. For example, if there are muscle tremors or poor electrode contact on lead I and III but not on lead II, it can be deduced that the problem stems from the left arm because leads I and III both involve the left arm and lead II does not.

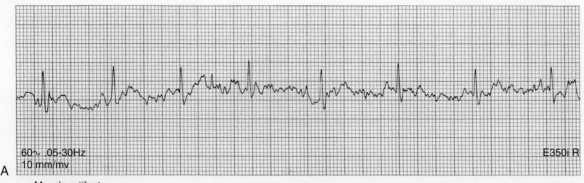

A

Muscle artifact

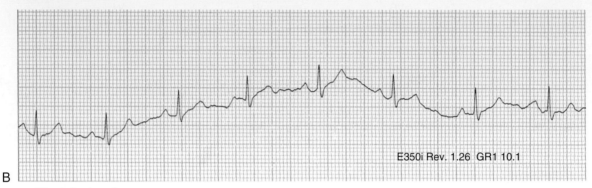

B

Wandering baseline

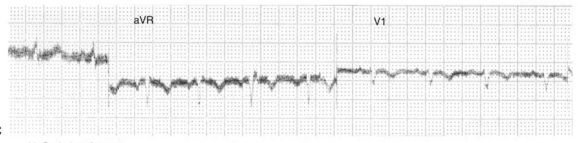

C

60-Cycle interference

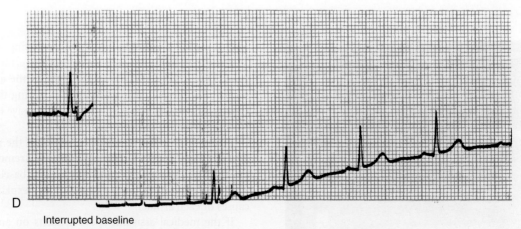

D

Interrupted baseline

FIG. 10.14 Electrocardiography artifacts (tracings caused by sources other than the patient's heart) that need to be corrected. Refer to the table on p. 253 showing the possible causes and ways to correct or eliminate each of these artifacts. (From Bonewit-West K: *Clinical procedures for medical assistants,* ed 10, St. Louis, 2018, Elsevier, with reference to Long BW: *Radiography essentials for limited practice,* ed 3, St. Louis, 2010, Saunders.)

ECG Artifacts	Ways to Correct
A. Muscle artifact: "somatic tremor"	1. Check to ensure the patient is comfortable and relaxed. 2. Provide a blanket if the patient is cold. 3. Provide the patient with a pillow. 4. Elevate the back of the exam table until the patient is comfortable. 5. Check if the patient's arms are slipping off the exam table. (Have the patient tuck her or his thumbs under her or his legs for better passive support.) 6. Explain that patient should not talk, chew, or move during the 15-second procedure. 7. If the patient has Parkinson disease with involuntary muscle tremors in the limbs, place the electrodes on the patient's trunk by the shoulders instead of the arms and the hips instead of the legs. Note the new locations on the recording and in the patient's medical record.
B. Wandering baseline	1. Check to see if the patient cable or the lead wires are dangling and unsupported. The lead wires should follow the contour of the body and not cross one another. 2. Have the patient hold his or her breath for 15 seconds if patient's rising and falling chest is causing the drifting baseline.
C. 60-cycle interference: "AC interference"	1. Check if the power cord is running under the exam table. If it is, find another plug or move the table. 2. Check if high-voltage wiring is running parallel in the walls or overhead (e.g., x-ray equipment uses high voltage). If this is true, turn the exam table at a 90-degree angle to the wiring.
D. Interrupted baseline	1. This is seen frequently when an electrode becomes dislodged (especially on the chest leads). Correct the problem by applying hypoallergenic tape to reinforce the electrodes. 2. The electrode is not making contact because of hair on the legs or chest. Shave the site and reapply a new electrode. 3. The cable showing the interrupted pattern may be damaged and in need of replacement.

If the problem is seen on one of the chest leads (V1, V2, V3, V4, V5, or V6), then go directly to the lead wire and its electrode location on the chest to correct it.

When all the artifacts have been corrected and a new acceptable final tracing is printed, the physician will then check the tracing and give his or her approval before having the lead wires and electrodes removed from the patient. It should be noted that most patients are anxious about the results, knowing that their heart is a very vital organ. So, be aware how you relate to patients during and after the procedure. Also remember that you are not authorized to tell the patient the results of the ECG and that the physician will be sharing the findings with the patient along with the whole picture of the patient's health status.

Prior to your ECG lab, you will want to complete the Fundamental Concepts and Diagnostic Procedures sections in your workbook, and view the ECG video on the Evolve website. Also, review Procedure 10.1 below.

PROCEDURE 10.1 Electrocardiography (Three Channel and Computerized with Interpretation)

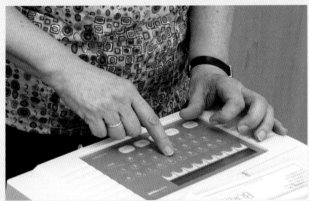

A, Place the three-channel electrocardiography instrument on the patient's left side and enter demographic data as prompted into the electrocardiograph: patient name, age, sex, height, weight, and medications.

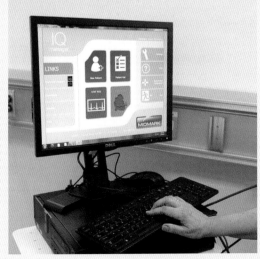

B, If using computerized electrocardiography, enter the patient's demographic data and digital vital signs into the patient's electronic record.

Continued

PROCEDURE 10.1   Electrocardiography (Three Channel and Computerized with Interpretation)—cont'd

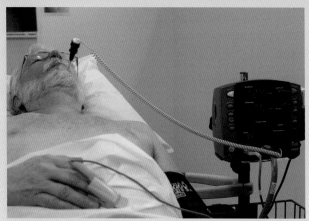

C, The computerized electrocardiography will also ask for the following vital signs: temperature from the digital thermometer, blood pressure from the digital blood pressure cuff, pulse rate, and percent saturated oxygen from the pulse oximeter.

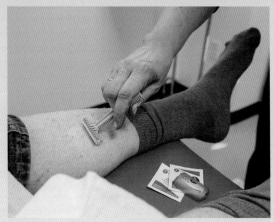

D, Prepare the lower limb electrode sites by shaving hair if necessary followed by rubbing with an alcohol swab. Allow the alcohol to completely dry while preparing the limb and chest electrode sites.

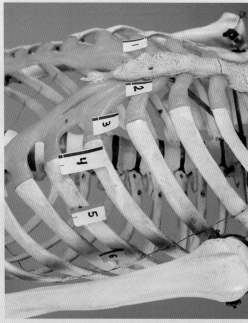

E, Visualize and palpate the skeletal landmarks on the patient's chest. The key landmarks are lead I at the fourth intercostal space to the right of the patient's sternum (with lead II directly across from it). Then lead IV on the fifth intercostal space is in line with the middle of the clavicle bone on the patient's left side. Lead III is placed midway between leads II and IV. Leads V and VI wrap around the chest in line with lead IV (on anterolateral line and the midaxillary line).

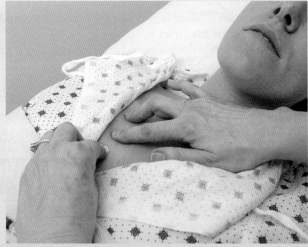

F, Palpate the first three intercostal spaces with your right hand and rub the alcohol swab on the next fourth intercostal space on the patient's right side of the sternum as seen in the illustration. Then rub alcohol directly across the sternum to the fourth intercostal space on the patient's left side of the sternum followed by a diagonal down to the fifth intercostal space at the midclavicular line. Continue rubbing the alcohol around the chest intersecting the anterior lateral line and the mid axillary line. Be aware of the patient's modesty when locating female chest sites.

PROCEDURE 10.1 Electrocardiography (Three Channel and Computerized with Interpretation)—cont'd

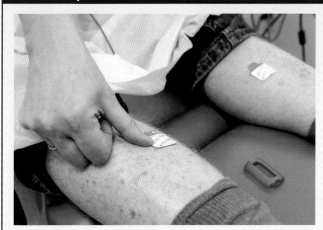

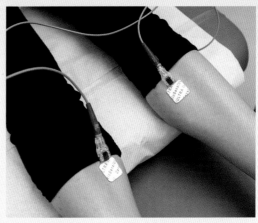

G, Return to the limbs and firmly press the sticky, tabbed electrodes with tabs up on the legs and tabs down on the arms.

H, Attach each of the alligator clips located on the four color-coded, limb lead wires starting with the **green RL** on the leg across from you. Then the **red LL** on the patient's left leg (closest to you) completes "Christmas." Find the **black LA** wire and clip it to the arm close to you (red LL is when funds are down, and black LA means you are up in funds). Then **white LA** goes to the opposite arm away from you (which is the opposite of black).

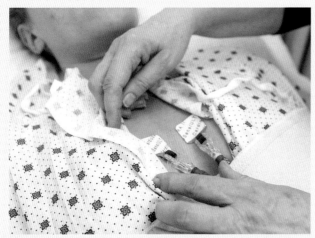

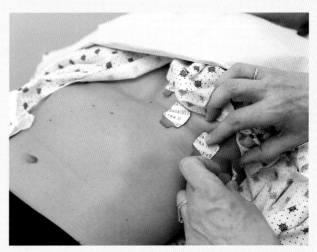

I, Return to the chest where the initial alcohol has dried. Re-palpate for the fourth intercostal space on the side away from you and press the electrode with the tabs down followed by placing the electrode for V2 directly across the sternum on your side. Clip on the V1 and V2 wires.

J, After locating the V4 site and applying the electrode at the fifth intercostal space in line with the middle of the clavicle, apply V3 electrode on the diagonal line between V2 and V4. Then place V5 electrode at the anterior lateral line and V6 electrode in line with the middle of the armpit (midaxillary line). These four leads and their respective lead wires may all be applied with the female's gown carefully lifted up just enough to expose the sites.

Continued

PROCEDURE 10.1   Electrocardiography (Three Channel and Computerized with Interpretation)—cont'd

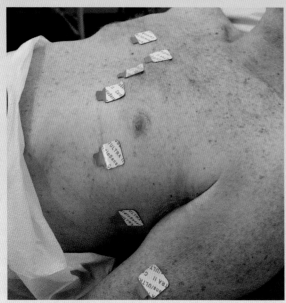

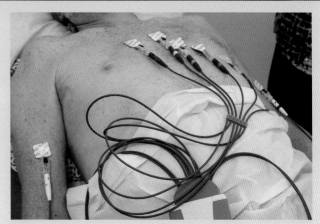

L, Clip the chest lead wires (V1 through V6) to the electrodes, taking care to note the proper numbered wire is attached to the proper site. The patient is now ready to have his or her electrocardiogram recorded.

K, On a male patient, all the chest electrodes may be placed on the bare chest followed by the lead wires. Note the following: V1 and V2 are parallel; V2, V3, and V4 are diagonal; and V4, V5, V6 are around the chest.

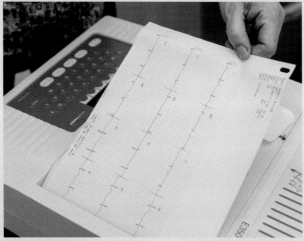

M, If running the three-channel electrocardiography, examine the printout for any artifacts. If artifacts are present, run another recording.

N, Alternatively, as the computerized electrocardiography is running, make sure all 12 leads are stable with no artifacts and then "freeze" the recording, followed by "analyze" and "print."

Electrocardiography Procedure
Equipment and Supplies

The two most common electrocardiography (ECG) analyzers are the three-channel type seen in Figure A and the computerized ECG (Figure B). Both are placed on the patient's left side of the exam table, and both share the following supplies (not pictured):

- Razor
- Alcohol
- 10 disposable electrodes
- Patient cable
- Power cord
- Graph paper or printer connected to computer

Preanalytical

1. Cleanse hands and prepare room with clean table paper, pillow, gown, and drape.
2. Greet the patient and confirm identity while entering demographic data (e.g., patient's name, number, age, address) (see Figures A and B).
3. Explain procedure and how to disrobe (from the waist up with the gown opening in the front). Provide the patient with privacy.
4. After returning, obtain the patient's vital signs (Figure C). Enter the vital signs into the computer.
5. Prepare the 10 sites in a routine order to avoid errors when stressed.
6. Prepare the lower limbs by dry shaving the inner calf muscles if necessary (Figure D) and then rub the areas with the alcohol swab to encourage circulation at the sites.

PROCEDURE 10.1   Electrocardiography (Three Channel and Computerized with Interpretation)—cont'd

7. While the lower limbs are drying, prepare the upper outer limbs with the alcohol swab followed by locating the general areas for the chest leads and rubbing the areas with the alcohol swab. See Figure E to help visualize the skeletal landmarks for V1 and V4 and their relationships with the other leads (as demonstrated in Figure 10.10 of the text). Figure F shows the three-finger method of locating V1 using three fingers for the first three intercostal spaces. Use the alcohol swab to cleanse the fourth intercostal area and then swab across the sternum for V2. Next, swab a diagonal line from V2 to V4. Finally, swab a line from V4 around the chest to the midaxillary area.

8. Return to the legs and arms and firmly press the electrode sensors with the tabs up on the legs (Figure G) and the tabs down on the arms. NOTE: It is important to let the alcohol dry completely before placing the electrodes on the prepared sites.

9. Connect the color-coded limb lead wires (Figure H) in the following order:
   - Start with the **green RL = right leg** for "go" and "ground" wire. (NOTE: You should always be working on the patient's left side, so this will always be on the leg farthest away.)
   - Next, the **red LL = left leg** is placed. NOTE: Green and red are always the "Christmas colors" on the legs.
   - After the LL comes the **black LA = left arm** on the same side closest to you. This wire is always coded black. (*Hint:* Red and black are the two colors used in accounting—red is in the hole (at the feet) and black is on top of finances (at the arm).
   - The only limb lead left is the **white RA = right arm**, which is the opposite of black. So, the arms are black and white!

10. The chest leads have been prepared with alcohol, but it is now necessary to relocate the actual sites and place the electrodes in the following order:
    - Palpate to locate the fourth intercostal space across the right side of the patient's sternum and then place the **V1 electrode** with the tab down followed by the **V2 electrode** directly across the sternum on the patient's left side (closest to you) (Figure I).
    - Next, locate the V4 lead location by following the fifth intercostal space to the mid-clavicular line and place the **V4 electrode** on the site followed by the **V3 electrode** midway between V2 and V4.

   - The last two leads follow a horizontal line based on V4's location around the ribs, with the **V5 electrode** being placed on the anterior-lateral line of the chest and the **V6 electrode** being placed at the midaxillary line of the chest (Figure J).
   - After all the electrodes are placed on the chest (Figure K), methodically connect the numbered **V lead wires** to each of their designated electrode locations (Figure L).

Analytical

11. The ECG is now ready to start recording. Before starting the recording, let the patient know that he or she needs to be very still and relaxed for about 15 seconds while the ECG is monitoring heartbeats. The patient should not talk or chew gum or do any muscular activity during the testing because the ECG instrument will pick up any patient movement.

12. When you are sure the patient understands the instructions and the patient is comfortable and still, start the recording.

Postanalytical

13. Observe the three-channel ECG printout (Figure M) or the computer results (Figure N) for the following:
    - Check the inserted 1-mV standard pulse for an upward rise of 10 mm (little squares) and a sideways line of 2 mm and then back down to the baseline.
    - Check each lead in the tracing for unwanted artifacts and correct them if possible (e.g., AC interference, muscle tremors, wandering or interrupted baseline). If artifacts are seen, re-record another tracing if necessary.
    - Allow the physician to see the final product before disconnecting the patient from the ECG.

14. Remove and dispose the electrodes and help the patient to a sitting position. Instruct the patient to get dressed and that the physician will be sharing the findings with him or her.

15. The ECG procedure is documented in the patient's chart or the electronic medical record, noting any variables due to artifacts or patient issues.

❖ ADVANCED CONCEPTS

Preparing the patient for ambulatory ECG monitoring using Holter monitoring and a Zio patch will be discussed followed by a brief overview of cardiac arrhythmias seen on ECG tracings. An atlas showing seven classic cardiac arrhythmias the physician will be interpreting is provided at the end of this section.

Ambulatory Electrocardiography Monitoring

The in-office ECG is a "snapshot" picture of the heart's electrical activity when the patient is at rest on the exam table. Often, the physician needs to see the heart's reaction to a variety of conditions the patient experiences outside of the office (e.g., after eating, after exercising, during the stress of work, while sleeping). There are now very sophisticated portable ECG monitors that the patient may wear home and be monitored for 1 to 14 days.

The first ambulatory ECG monitor was invented by Norman J. Holter and Dr. W. R. Glasscock in 1961, thus the name "Holter monitor." Since then, Holter monitors have become smaller and capable of monitoring and recording increasing amounts of valuable data.

The medical assistant is usually the person to set up and instruct the patient with the ambulatory ECG monitor. See the Evolve site for a video of one method and refer to Procedure 10.2 at the end of this section for the steps involved in the instruction and preparation of the patient for ambulatory ECG monitoring.

Zio Patch Wireless Electrocardiography Monitoring

The Zio patch is the most recent development in cardiac rhythm monitoring that provides continuous wireless monitoring. A single patch is applied to the chest and records the heart's activity for up to 14 days, after which the patch is returned by mail for interpretation. See the Zio patch figure at the end of

Procedure 10.2, which describes this new wireless method of ambulatory cardiac monitoring.

Cardiac Arrhythmias and the Electrocardiogram
Acute Myocardial Infarction

At the top of an interpretive ECG or the physician's interpretation, the term *sinus rhythm* means the normal pattern of waves and the rate of beats per minute are as expected. In contrast, when the neurologic pattern or rhythm is not as expected, it is referred to as *arrhythmia*. One possible cause of an arrhythmia is when a coronary artery on the heart becomes blocked. A portion of the heart muscle becomes damaged from lack of oxygen and it becomes a *myocardial infarct* or *heart attack*. The damaged cardiac muscle disrupts the flow of electricity and changes the ECG tracing. See the Evolve website for an animation of how myocardial infarcts in various locations affect ECG tracings.

Bradycardia and tachycardia were discussed earlier. They both have normal PQRST waves, but their beats (distance between the cardiac cycles) per minute occur slowly (far apart) in bradycardia and rapidly (close together) in tachycardia. Refer to the Atlas of Atrial Arrhythmias showing four additional arrhythmias that are caused by atrial dysfunction and the Atlas of Ventricular Arrhythmias showing three additional ventricular arrhythmias. It should be noted that ECG technicians are not qualified to interpret these examples. But an awareness of serious arrhythmias (e.g., ventricular fibrillation) should be brought to the physician's attention immediately.

Atlas of Atrial Arrhythmias

See Figures 10.15 to 10.18.

Atlas of Ventricular Arrhythmias

See Figures 10.19 to 10.21.

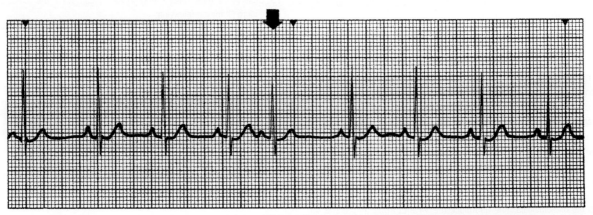

FIG. 10.15 Premature **atrial** contraction (PACs) seen between the fourth and fifth electrocardiography cycle causing a premature heartbeat. (From Huang SH, et al: *Coronary care nursing*, St. Louis, 1989, Saunders.)

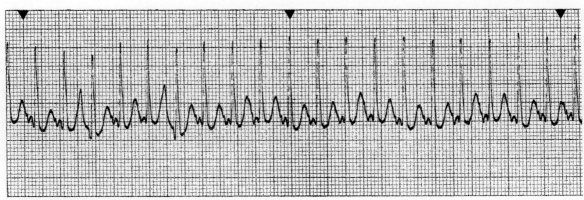

FIG. 10.16 Paroxysmal (sudden) **atrial** tachycardia (PAT) seen as rapid heartbeats initiated by atria. (From Huang SH, et al: *Coronary care nursing*, St. Louis, 1989, Saunders.)

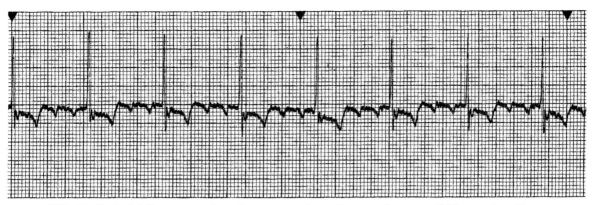

FIG. 10.17 Atrial flutter seen here has two to three P waves for every QRS complex. (From Johnson R, Swartz MH: *A simplified approach to electrocardiography*, St. Louis, 1986, Saunders.)

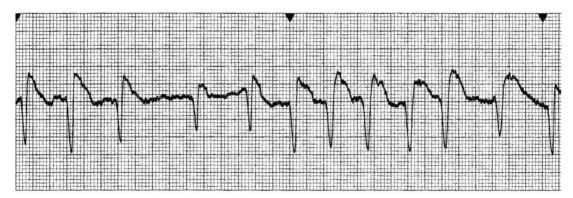

FIG. 10.18 Atrial fibrillation (A-fib) seen in this chest lead shows no P waves between the QRS complexes because the atria are not contracting in a coordinated way. (From Huang SH, et al: *Coronary care nursing*, St. Louis, 1989, Saunders.)

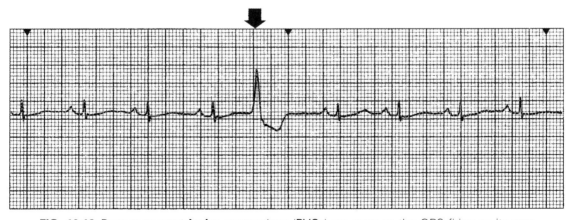

FIG. 10.19 Premature **ventricular** contractions (PVCs) are seen as the QRS firing on its own without any P wave preceding (see the fifth electrocardiography cycle). It is usually followed by a recovery pause and then regular beats. (From Huang SH, et al: *Coronary care nursing*, St. Louis, 1989, Saunders.)

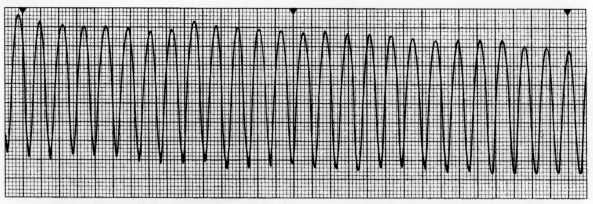

FIG. 10.20 Ventricular tachycardia (V-tach) is seen as rapid QRS complexes with no P waves because the ventricles are rapidly firing on their own. (From Huang SH, et al: *Coronary care nursing,* St. Louis, 1989, Saunders.)

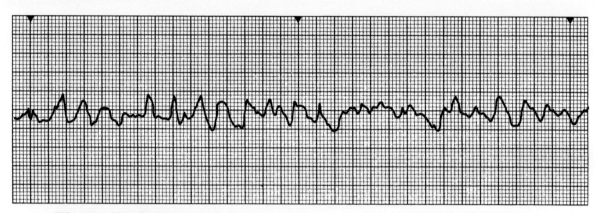

FIG. 10.21 Ventricular fibrillation (V-fib) is seen as an uncoordinated irregular line of jagged spikes. There are no recognizable P waves, QRS complexes, or T waves because the ventricles are twitching irregularly. Consequently, there is no circulation of the blood. This is a medical emergency requiring cardiopulmonary resuscitation and a defibrillator to return the heart to a coordinated effective rhythm. (From Huang SH, et al: *Coronary care nursing,* St. Louis, 1989, Saunders.)

PROCEDURE 10.2 Holter Monitoring

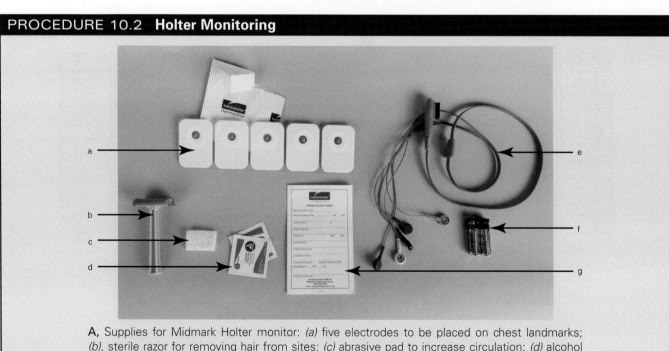

A, Supplies for Midmark Holter monitor: *(a)* five electrodes to be placed on chest landmarks; *(b),* sterile razor for removing hair from sites; *(c)* abrasive pad to increase circulation; *(d)* alcohol swabs for removing oil and sweat; *(e)* patient cable with four lead wires and a green ground wire; *(f)* new batteries for the monitor; *(g)* patient log for recording cardiac "events."

PROCEDURE 10.2 Holter Monitoring—cont'd

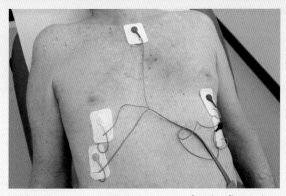

B, Midmark Holter monitor's recommended placement for the five color-coded lead and ground wires that snap onto the white electrodes. Note the looping of the wires to prevent tension during the 24 hours of monitoring.

Instrument and Supplies

A variety of Holter monitoring systems are in use. Most systems provide patient packets with all the supplies for patient preparation. See Figure A showing the following supplies for the Midmark monitor:

a. Five white electrodes to be placed on chest landmarks
b. Sterile razor for removing hair from sites
c. Abrasive pad to increase circulation at the sites
d. Alcohol swabs for removing oil and sweat
e. Patient cable with four lead wires and a green ground wire
f. New batteries for the monitor
g. Patient log for recording cardiac "events"

Preanalytical

1. Greet the patient and confirm her or his identity while sanitizing your hands.
2. Explain the procedure and how to disrobe (from the waist up with the gown opening in the front). Provide the patient with privacy.
3. After returning to patient's room, prepare the electrode sites by:
   • Dry shaving hair (if necessary)
   • Applying alcohol to remove lotions, oils, and dirt
   • Rubbing the abrasive pad over the sites to increase circulation
   • NOTE: There are different configurations of where to place the electrodes and the color-coded wires as seen in Figure B. Be sure to follow the manufacturer's diagram of the site locations or the physician's preference.
4. While the sites are drying from the alcohol, snap the color-coded wires to their electrodes.
5. Then, one at a time, peel off the backing of each sticky electrode with its colored lead wire and firmly press it on to its designated prepared site. Remember, each Holter system will provide its own diagram showing where each colored lead wire belongs. The latest Holter system, seen at the bottom of this procedure (Figure C), is wireless and only needs one kidney-shaped "patch" that is placed on the upper left side of the patient's chest.
6. The wires coming from each electrode must then be looped and taped down with surgical tape, or looped and held down by the lower sticky tab at the bottom of the electrode as seen in Figure B. This alleviates any tension on wires and prevents them from being accidentally pulled off during the monitoring.
7. Insert the digital flashcard or tape into the recorder.
8. Place the new batteries (provided in the supply kit) into the monitor and connect the lead cable to the monitor.

Analytical

9. Turn on the monitor and follow the manufacturer's directions for data input and quality control. Note the start time on the monitor and write it on patient's log.

10. Show the patient his or her log book and explain how the monitor works and is stored in its pouch. Emphasize that the monitor and wires should not get wet.
11. Then instruct the patient to do the following in the log book (diary):
    • Record the activities you do and exactly what time you do them using the clock on the Holter monitor screen. Activities include:
      • When you exert yourself
      • When you are at rest
      • When you eat
      • When you take medications
      • When you have bowel movements
    • Record any symptoms you have while you are wearing the monitor, such as:
      • Chest pain
      • Shortness of breath
      • Lightheadedness
      • Skipped heartbeats
    • The physician will be comparing the data from the Holter monitor recorder with your diary, which will help diagnose your condition.
12. Explain how long the patient needs to wear the monitor. (It may vary from 12 hours to 14 days based on the physician's order.)
13. Document in the patient record that all the above steps were performed and that the patient was informed when to return for a follow-up visit.

Postanalytical

14. When the monitoring period is over, the patient returns with the Holter monitor and his or her diary. Perform the following steps:
    • Check to ensure entries were made in the log (diary).
    • Turn off and disconnect the monitor per manufacturer's instructions.
    • Disconnect the cable from the monitor.
    • Remove the monitor from the pouch.
    • Carefully remove the electrodes from patient and from the lead wires and discard.
    • Clean the patient's chest of any residual gel from the electrodes.
    • Remove and discard the batteries from the monitor.
    • Remove the flashcard or tape from the monitor and submit it along with the patient's diary for interpretation.
    • Clean the Holter monitor and patient cable with its lead wires for next patient.
15. Document completed procedure.

Continued

PROCEDURE 10.2 Holter Monitoring—cont'd

Alternative Wireless Ambulatory Electrocardiography Monitoring System by Zio

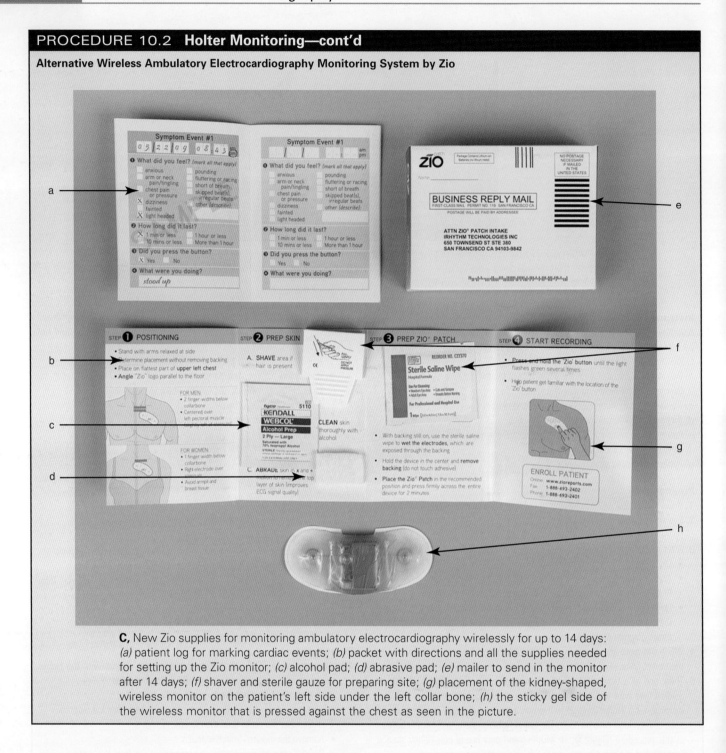

C, New Zio supplies for monitoring ambulatory electrocardiography wirelessly for up to 14 days: *(a)* patient log for marking cardiac events; *(b)* packet with directions and all the supplies needed for setting up the Zio monitor; *(c)* alcohol pad; *(d)* abrasive pad; *(e)* mailer to send in the monitor after 14 days; *(f)* shaver and sterile gauze for preparing site; *(g)* placement of the kidney-shaped, wireless monitor on the patient's left side under the left collar bone; *(h)* the sticky gel side of the wireless monitor that is pressed against the chest as seen in the picture.

Becoming proficient at electrocardiography tests. Now that you have learned about the significance of performing accurate cardiac diagnostic tests, take the time to complete the following:

1. Answer the text electrocardiography questions at the end of this chapter and do all of the exercises in Chapter 10 in the workbook using your student handout on the Evolve website.

2. View the animations and videos on the Evolve website to see the anatomy and physiology of the heart.

3. Perform the Chapter 10 online exercises, which are designed to reinforce your terminology, theory, and testing techniques for measuring heart function.

4. Study Procedures 10.1 and 10.2 before performing your lab procedures on ECGs and Holter monitoring.

▌REVIEW QUESTIONS*

1. Which chamber of the heart contracts to send oxygenated blood through the aortic valve and out to the body's cells?
   a. Left atrium
   b. Left ventricle
   c. Right atrium
   d. Right ventricle

2. Which of these tissues is known as the body's "natural pacemaker"?
   a. SA node
   b. AV node
   c. Bundle of His
   d. Purkinje fibers

3. Which component of the ECG cycle shows ventricular depolarization?
   a. P
   b. QRS
   c. T
   d. U

4. After the first precordial electrode is placed, what is the correct order for the next three electrodes?
   a. V2, then V3, then V4
   b. V3, then V2, then V4
   c. V2, then V4, then V3
   d. There is no recommended order.

5. Match the leads with their codes and circle the leads that form Einthoven's triangle.
   a. Augmented unipolar limb leads   (1) V1 through V6
   b. Precordial chest leads   (2) aVL, aVF, and aVR
   c. Standard limb leads   (3) I, II, III

6. Which of these items are placed on the patient's limbs and chest in an ECG to detect impulses?
   a. Amplifier
   b. Electrodes
   c. Galvanometer
   d. Stylus

7. Which limb electrode is used as a reference point and is not part of the ECG recording?
   a. Right arm (RA)
   c. Right leg (RL)
   b. Left arm (LA)
   d. Left leg (LL)

8. If ECG artifacts are seen on leads I and II, what is the likely source of interference?
   a. Left arm electrode
   b. Left leg electrode
   c. Right arm electrode
   d. Right leg electrode

9. What should the assistant do after seeing an urgent problem on an ECG tracing?
   a. Share the information with the patient right away.
   b. Notify the physician immediately.
   c. Look in the patient's chart for an explanation.

10. How many leads does a Holter monitor have?
    a. 2
    b. 3
    c. Up to 5
    d. Up to 12

11. What is the purpose of the patient diary in Holter monitoring?
    a. Reminds the patient about heart-healthy behaviors
    b. Supplies a link to patient activity at the time of any abnormal results
    c. Provides a place to document the results of the test
    d. Informs the patient of what items to avoid during the test

*Answers to these Review Questions are located in the Appendix on p. 279.

WEBSITE

http://cardiacmonitoring.com/holter-monitoring/holter-monitoring-companies/irhythm-technologies/zio-patch/

11 | CHAPTER

Spirometry

OBJECTIVES

After completing this chapter, you should be able to do the following:

1. Define and match key terms and abbreviations in this chapter.

Fundamental Spirometry Concepts

2. Explain the principle of spirometry and identify the airway structures in the lung related to chronic obstructive pulmonary disease.
3. Explain the following results seen on a spirometer report:
   - FVC, FEV$_1$, and PEF
   - The volume/time chart, the flow/volume chart, and the predictive indicators

Diagnostic Spirometry Testing

4. Prepare the patient and show awareness of the patients' concerns related to spirometry procedures.

5. Perform the forced vital capacity diagnostic test using a spirometer according to the stated task, conditions, and standards listed in the Learning Outcome Evaluation in the student workbook.
6. Identify a successful spirometer maneuver and take appropriate steps to correct common artifacts found on the spirometer recording.
7. Succinctly and accurately report to the physician relevant information regarding the spirometer test.

Advanced Spirometry Concepts

8. Explain why and how peak flow monitoring is performed and recorded.
9. Perform or describe ordered dosages administered with a nebulizer and the procedure followed for oxygen breathing treatment with a nasal cannula.

KEY TERMS

artifacts: tracings other than from the lungs that will interfere with the interpretation of the spirometer recordings

peak flow rate: a test that measures how fast a person can exhale

spirometer: instrument that measures the volume and flow of air that is breathed

spirometry: measurement of the volume and flow of air that is breathed

ABBREVIATIONS

COPD: chronic obstructive pulmonary disease

FEF$_{25\%-75\%}$: the breakdown of flow at 25%, 50%, and 75% of the maneuver

FET: forced expiratory time—the horizontal length of the line showing how long the patient exhaled in seconds (ideally the line should continue to 6 seconds)

FEV$_1$: forced expiratory volume in the first second; expressed in liters

FVC: forced vital capacity—the total volume of air exhaled in 6 seconds

PEF: peak expiratory flow

PFM: peak flow meter (a portable, handheld device used in ambulatory monitoring)

❖ FUNDAMENTAL SPIROMETRY CONCEPTS

In this section, the lungs will be reviewed anatomically followed by a discussion of the ways a spirometer is able to display various graphs and interpretations of the patient's lung health status.

Anatomy of the Lungs

Lung function tests are able to measure how much and how fast air is inhaled and exhaled from the lungs. They are generally used in primary care to identify breathing obstructions and restrictions in the respiratory system airways. A review of the structures in the respiratory tract and common obstructive diseases related to each are listed below and are seen in Figure 11.1. Note the upper respiratory tract at the top and the lower respiratory tract with its bronchial tubes (primary, secondary, and tertiary, and terminal) branching out like a tree until it terminates in alveoli (seen enlarged at the bottom), where gas exchange occurs.

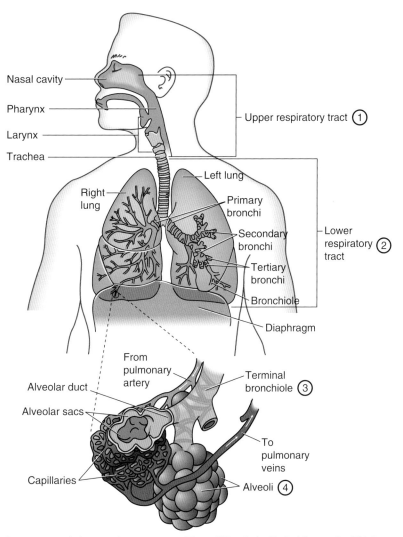

FIG. 11.1 Structures of the respiratory tract. (From Warekois R, Robinson R: *Phlebotomy: worktext and procedures manual*, ed 3, St. Louis, 2012, Saunders.)

Respiratory Structures

1. Upper respiratory tract (nasal cavity, pharynx, larynx)
2. Lower respiratory tract (trachea, primary bronchi, secondary bronchi, tertiary bronchi)
3. Terminal bronchioles (muscles capable of dilation or constriction)
4. Alveoli (air sacs where oxygen and carbon dioxide exchange takes place)

Common Obstructive Diseases

URI—upper respiratory tract infections such as colds, flu, allergies

Bronchitis—acute infection may follow URI; chronic form typically caused by smoking, toxic fumes, or other irritants

Asthma—bronchioles are inflamed (swollen) and thick mucus forms, causing difficulty during inspiration and expiration

Emphysema—walls of alveoli break down; most commonly caused by smoking

Modern Spirometry Testing and Tracings

Spirometry testing in the ambulatory setting is usually performed to screen a patient for known or suspected pulmonary dysfunction (e.g., chronic obstructive pulmonary disease [**COPD**]) or if a patient's respiratory system is at risk from inhaling toxins such as toxic gases or smoke.

A spirometer is an instrument that measures the volume and flow of air that is breathed. In ambulatory settings, the most common screening test is the **FVC** (forced vital capacity). In this diagnostic test, the patient is asked to fully inflate the lungs followed by exhaling the air from the lungs into the spirometer's disposable mouthpiece as fast and as forcibly as possible.

The FVC test requires the patient to complete the following three-step "forced expiratory maneuver":

Step 1—While holding the disposable mouthpiece that is attached to the spirometer, the patient uses full inspiration to fill the lungs and then holds his or her breath while sealing the lips around the disposable mouthpiece.

Step 2—The patient then exhales fast and hard to exhale most of the air within the first second of exhalation.

Step 3—The patient continues to exhale any remaining air for as close to 6 seconds as possible.

When the maneuver is performed correctly, the spirometer produces two graphs along with an analysis and interpretation of the results as seen in Figure 11.2.

Spirometry Report

Name:		Age:	37 years	Race:	Caucasian
ID:		Height:	73 inches	Weight:	Unspecified
Sex:	Male	Indication:			
Smoker:	No	Medications:			
COPD risk	Low	Lung age:	< 37 years		

Requested by:		Performed by:	MG
Test date:	03/15/13 14:35:28	Sensor S/N:	543679
Test date post:		Sensor calibrated:	01/30/12 14:10:58
Press/Temp:	760 mmHg/79 degrees F	Spiro control ver:	8.5.0
Bronchodilator:		Normals/interp:	Crapo/ATS (1991)

Measurement	Units	Predicted	Pre-Bronchodilator Trial					
			1		2		3	
			Actual	% pred.	Actual	% pred.	Actual	% pred.
FVC	L	5.68	5.95	105 %	5.83	103 %	5.80	102 %
FEV1	L	4.58	4.32	94 %	4.49*	98 %	4.44	97 %
FEV1/FVC	%	81 %	73 %	90 %	77 %	95 %	77 %	95 %
FEF25%	L/S	9.40	7.90	84 %	8.40	89 %	8.52	91 %
FEF50%	L/S	5.79	3.70	64 %	4.29	74 %	4.20	73 %
FEF75%	L/S	2.41	1.55	64 %	1.81	75 %	1.82	75 %
FEF25-75%	L/S	4.51	3.24	72 %	3.80	84 %	3.70	82 %
PEF	L/S	10.14	8.87	87 %	9.93	98 %	10.02	99 %
Exp. time	SEC.		5.93		3.60		3.38	
V ext.	L		0.14		0.09		0.09	

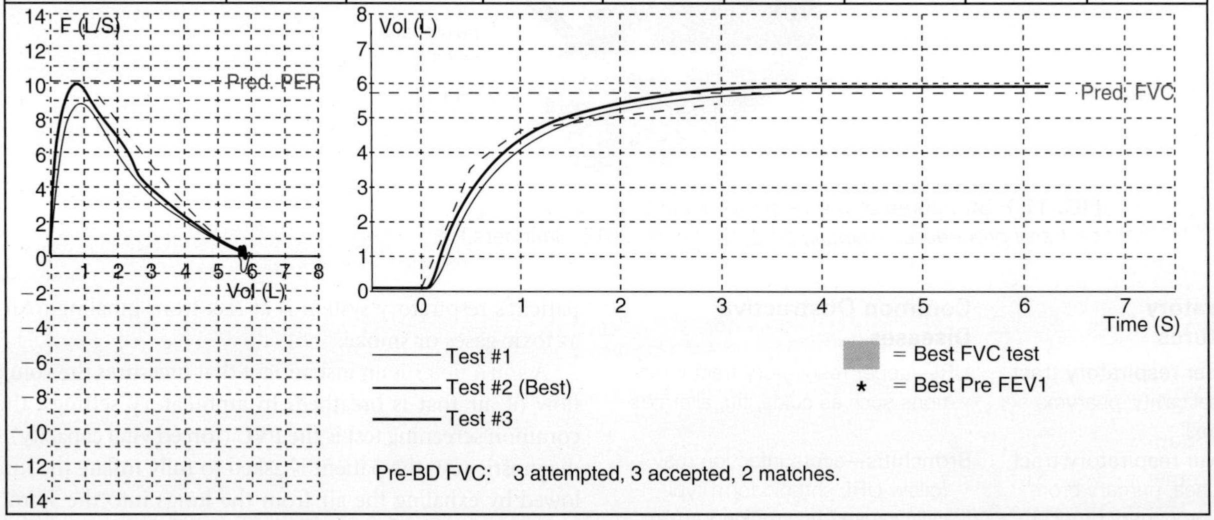
F (L/S)
Pred. PER
Vol (L)
Vol (L)
Pred. FVC
Time (S)
Test #1
Test #2 (Best)
Test #3
= Best FVC test
* = Best Pre FEV1
Pre-BD FVC: 3 attempted, 3 accepted, 2 matches.

Interpretation: Normal spirometry

Observations:

Unconfirmed report

Midmark Diagnostics Group Software Version: 8.5.0 Printed: 03/15/13 14:35:34 Page 1 of 1

FIG. 11.2 Spirometry report showing "normal spirometry." The volume/time graph (on the right) has a quick rise within the first second and then a steady upward rise plateauing for the next 6 seconds.

Volume/Time Chart

The graph in the lower right of the report (see Figure 11.2) provides the physician with the following information:

1. **FET**, or forced expiratory time, is the horizontal length of the curved line, which shows how long the patient exhaled in seconds (ideally the line should continue to 6 seconds).
2. **FVC**, or forced vital capacity, is the vertical height of the line, which shows how much air was exhaled in liters. (NOTE: The total volume will vary with patient based on size, age, gender, and race.)
3. FEV_1 is the forced expiratory volume in the first second and is expressed in liters.
4. **FEV_1/FVC ratio**—A healthy person is predicted to exhale 80% to 90% of their total volume (FVC) within the first second (FEV_1). This percentage is calculated by dividing the FEV_1 volume by the total FVC volume.

A good maneuver will show a volume/time chart with a quick rise within the first second and then a steady upward rise plateauing for up to 6 seconds. NOTE: A patient with an obstructive disorder will not be able to exhale rapidly in the first second and will consequently have a predicted percentage less than 80%.

Flow/Volume Chart—"Peak Flow Chart"

The graph in the lower left of the report (see Figure 11.2) provides the physician with the following information:

- **PEF**, or peak expiratory flow, is the highest point on the graph representing maximum flow during the maneuver.
- **$FEF_{25\%-75\%}$** is the breakdown of flow at 25%, 50%, and 75% of the maneuver.

A good maneuver should show a fast rise in the beginning of the graph with a gradual curve downward that ends on the baseline.

Predicted Values and Percentiles

A computerized, interpretive spirometer will also provide *predicted values* to compare the patient's results with a control group of others who share the same age, height, weight, gender, and race. This allows the physician to readily see when a patient lags behind predicted values (i.e., below 80% of predicted values), which may then necessitate more extensive pulmonary function tests.

Quality Control–Spirometer Calibration

The spirometer needs to be calibrated on each testing day using a large 3-L syringe as seen in Figure 11.3. A mouthpiece is applied to the syringe and the air is pushed into the spirometer in a rapid,

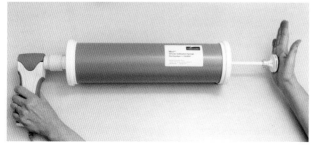

FIG. 11.3 Spirometer calibration syringe showing the right hand pushing 3 L of air through the mouthpiece held by the left hand. The spirometer result must register 3 L within ±3% to be in control.

steady motion. The spirometer then provides feedback if the calibration is successful (results will show a total exhaled volume within 3% of 3 L). If not, refer to the instruction manual for recommended ways to adjust the instrument. A typical adjustment is to enter the temperature and elevation settings (barometric pressure) for the testing area. Both of these variables affect the accuracy of the test. See the spirometer video on the Evolve website for a demonstration on calibrating the spirometer with the 3-L syringe.

❖ DIAGNOSTIC PROCEDURES: SPIROMETRY

In this chapter, the spirometer is recording the results produced by the patient's breathing rather than a lab specimen. It is therefore necessary to prepare patients properly and to coach them with helpful instructions throughout the procedures to produce accurate reports. It is also important to identify and correct any artifacts (tracings other than from the lungs that will interfere with the interpretation of the spirometer recordings) before submitting a final report to the physician.

Spirometer Patient Preparations, Instructions, and Identification of Artifacts

Similar to electrocardiogram testing, patients may be anxious to know the results of their spirometer test in hopes of "passing" the test. The success of their test requires an understanding of exactly what they need to do during the maneuver, and good coaching from the assistant or technician running the test.

Patient Preparation

When making the appointment for the spirometry test, the patient should be instructed to make the following preparations:

- Wear loose clothing.
- Avoid smoking and eating anything heavy 8 hours before the procedure.
- Do not use the bronchodilator 4 hours before the test based on the physician's recommendations.

On the day of the test, explain the procedure in a simple, clear manner, emphasizing that you will be performing a lung measurement test that does not hurt but will require effort and cooperation to produce two reproducible records for the physician to interpret. Explain and demonstrate the three steps of the maneuver using a mouthpiece that is not connected to the spirometer:

1. *Fully inflate* your lungs and then hold your breath while sealing your lips around the mouthpiece.
2. *Fully exhale* into the mouthpiece as fast and as hard as possible.
3. Give *full effort* to exhale the remaining air in your lungs for another 5 seconds without inhaling until the time has expired.

Show and explain the importance of standing upright during the maneuver and that the patient will have 1 minute to sit and rest between a minimum of three attempts.

Coaching the Maneuver

Watch the patient as he or she performs the maneuver, making sure you see all three steps: inspiration, rapid exhalation, and extended exhalation. Praise the patient for maneuvers performed well and communicate positive ways to improve the next maneuver. Do not give negative feedback. The following chart provides examples of positive versus negative comments.

Positive Corrective Feedback	**Negative Corrective Feedback**
"I need you to blow out really hard."	"You didn't blow hard enough."
"I need you to seal your lips firmly around the mouthpiece so all your breath is captured."	"You're not putting the mouthpiece far enough into your mouth."
"I need you to blow until I say stop."	"You didn't blow long enough."
"Keep your eyes on the screen."	"Don't look away."

Modern spirometers may also give coaching tips such as "blow harder" or "blow longer" based on the final curves produced on the recorded graphs on the spirometer. Computerized spirometers also provide the incentive to blow hard and continuously by displaying a tree with hidden monkeys behind the leaves that must be blown away, or a cake with candles, for example. Instruct the patient to stay focused on the progress seen on the screen and help the patient verbally by counting down "5-4-3-2-1" to keep the patient exhaling for the full 6 seconds without inhaling or coughing. NOTE: You should look at the patient, not the screen, to make sure the procedure is being performed correctly (e.g., mouth position, body position, signs of fatigue).

Most spirometers will also let you know when there was a successful maneuver by reporting "Good test!" See Figure 11.4, which illustrates a computerized spirometer confirmation of a successful maneuver along with the two graphs and predictors. The patient may need to attempt up to eight maneuvers, with 1 minute of rest in between each attempt, to produce the required two maneuvers with "Good test!" results. NOTE: If the patient has an obstructed airway, he or she may not be able to produce a "Good test" result. If this occurs, let the patient know there is still enough information to help with the diagnosis. Be sure to note any difficulties or issues during the maneuver on the patient's chart to help the physician with the final analysis.

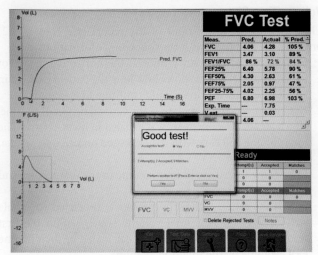

FIG. 11.4 Spirometer results on a computer showing a "Good test" maneuver. Note the upper time/volume curve shows a sharp rise within the first second and then a slight steady rise for the next 2 to 6 seconds. The lower volume/flow curve shows a fast rise in the beginning of the graph with a gradual curve downward that ends on the baseline.

Postbronchodilator Response

When adults demonstrate airway obstruction (COPD) with their FEV_1/FVC ratio less than 70% of predicted or when children with asthma show an FEV_1/FVC ratio less than 80%, the physician may order a postbronchodilator test. This consists of administering a prescribed bronchodilator dosage and then retesting the patient 20 minutes later to see if the patient's results are improved. Improved results after the bronchodilator may indicate the patient is a candidate for the medication.

You are now ready to perform a spirometer test. You will need to view the Spirometer video on the Evolve website before lab, and review the Behavioral 1.1 procedure in your workbook as well as Procedure 11.1 below.

PROCEDURE 11.1   Spirometry

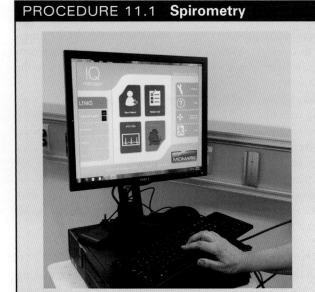

A, Enter patient demographic data and current height and weight plus the patient's gender, race, and age.

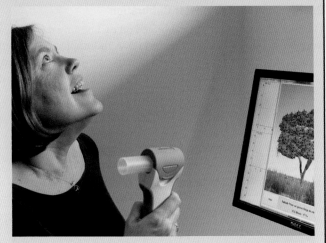

B, Fully inflate your lungs and then hold your breath while sealing your lips around the mouthpiece. Note the tree on the computer screen is filled with leaves.

PROCEDURE 11.1   Spirometry—cont'd

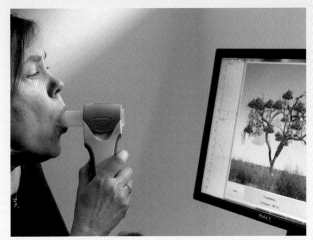

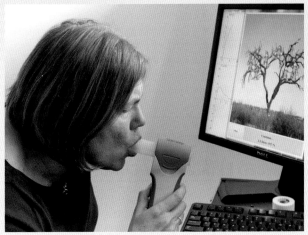

C, Fully exhale into the mouthpiece as fast and as hard as possible. Note that most of the leaves are gone, exposing the monkeys on the tree within the first second.

D, Give full effort to exhale the remaining air in your lungs for another 5 seconds if possible without inhaling until time has expired. Note that all the leaves are off the tree.

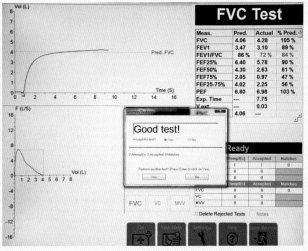

E, Spirometer results on computer showing "Good test" maneuver. NOTE: The upper left time/volume curve shows a sharp rise within the first second and then a slight steady rise for the next 2 to 6 seconds. In addition, the lower left volume/flow curve shows a fast rise in the beginning of the graph with a gradual curve downward that ends on the baseline.

Instrument and Supplies

Prepare the testing area with the following:
- Spirometer instrument or computer connected to a printer
- A disposable sterile mouthpiece connected to the plastic tubing on the spirometer. (Take care not to touch the area where the patient's mouth will be placed.)
- A nose clip (based on the physician's preference)
- A chair available for the patient to sit if he or she becomes fatigued during the maneuver

- Disposable gloves to be worn during and after the patient's test to avoid the transmission of possible respiratory viruses and other respiratory pathogens
- 3-L syringe for calibrating the spirometer

Preanalytical

1. Call the patient into the room and sanitize your hands while confirming the patient's name using three identifiers: have the patient spell his or her last name, give his or her date of birth, and provide one more identifier such as phone number or address, or show a driver's license.
2. Enter the following data into the spirometer or into the computer's spirometer patient record: name, ID number, age, height, weight, gender, and race. NOTE: All this information is critical for the spirometer to produce the appropriate "predicted" results that compare the patient's performance with others in his or her demographic pool (Figure A).
3. Confirm when the patient last took bronchodilator medication and if the patient has smoked and note it on the chart. Also, if appropriate, check to make sure the patient does not have loose dentures that will interfere with the breathing maneuver.
4. Explain and demonstrate the three steps of the maneuver using a mouthpiece that is not connected to the spirometer:
   - **Fully inflate** your lungs and then hold your breath while sealing your lips around the mouthpiece (Figure B).
   - **Fully exhale** into the mouthpiece as fast and as hard as possible (Figure C).
   - Give **full effort** to exhale the remaining air in your lungs for another 5 seconds without inhaling until the time has expired (Figure D).
5. Show and explain the importance of standing upright during the maneuver and that the patient will have 1 minute to rest and sit between a minimum of three attempts.

Analytical

6. Coach the patient as he or she performs the maneuver. Watch the patient, making sure he or she performs all three steps: inspiration, rapid exhalation, and extended exhalation. Praise what the patient did well and communicate positive ways to improve the next maneuver. Do not give negative feedback.

Continued

PROCEDURE 11.1 Spirometry—cont'd

7. Observe the two graph results and the spirometer feedback after each maneuver (Figure E) and have the patient rest for 1 minute.
  • The time/volume curve should show a sharp rise within the first second and then a slight steady rise for the next 2 to 6 seconds.
  • The volume/flow curve should show a fast rise in the beginning of the graph with a gradual curve downward that ends on the baseline.
8. Repeat at least three maneuvers until the patient is able to perform two reproducible results.

Postanalytical
9. Discard the patient's mouthpiece and your gloves in a biohazard container. Sanitize hands.
10. Chart the procedure and any difficulties or issues during the maneuver.
11. If the physician orders a postbronchodilator test, administer the prescribed bronchodilator dosage and then retest the patient 20 minutes later to see if the patient responds well and is a candidate for the medication.

❖ ADVANCED SPIROMETRY CONCEPTS

This section covers ambulatory pulmonary testing using peak flow rate meters. It then presents two pulmonary treatments commonly performed in offices when dealing with patients with asthma or COPD: nebulizer use and oxygen administration.

Peak Expiratory Flow Screening and Monitoring

The three common causes for COPD—bronchitis, asthma, and emphysema—were presented under Fundamental Concepts. Each has a distinct spirometry pattern seen during the initial in-office spirometry screening test and the postbronchodilator test as presented in the previous diagnostic section. PEF may also be measured with a peak flow meter (**PFM**), a portable, handheld device (Figure 11.5). These inexpensive devices only test the initial PEF segment of the FVC.

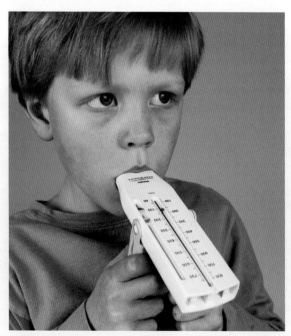

FIG. 11.5 Patient using a peak flow meter. The patient was instructed to (1) fully inflate the lungs and hold his breath while sealing his lips around the mouthpiece and (2) then fully exhale into the mouthpiece as fast and as hard as possible.

In this screening test, the patient performs the first two steps of the FVC maneuver:
1. *Fully inflate* the lungs and hold breath while sealing lips around the mouthpiece.
2. *Fully exhale* into the mouthpiece as fast and as hard as possible. NOTE: It is not necessary to continue exhaling for 6 seconds as in the FVC test.

The meter displays a result between 0 and 800 L/min of forced exhaled air. The result is compared with the predicted rate of individuals sharing the same gender, height, and age (see Table 11.1 at the end of Procedure 11.2). By dividing the predicted value from the table into the patient's value, a percent of predicted value may be obtained. A result less than 80% may be due to an airway obstruction and would require further evaluation.

Patients with COPD (especially asthma) may also be given the handheld PFM to monitor their lung health daily to predict and prevent an asthmatic attack. Figure 11.6 shows the anatomy, symptoms, and physical findings seen in a child experiencing an asthmatic attack and respiratory distress.

Daily peak flow monitoring, when used properly, may reveal the narrowing of the airways well in advance of an asthma attack. PFMs help determine the following:
• When the patient needs to seek emergency medical care
• The level of effectiveness of the patient's asthma management and treatment plan
• When to stop or add medication as directed by a physician
• What triggers an asthma attack (e.g., exercise-induced asthma)

Before receiving the portable PFM, the patient with asthma performs three peak expiratory flow maneuvers using the PFM. The highest of three readings, showing the patient's "best effort," is then used as the recorded value of the patient's specific peak expiratory flow rate (rather than using the predicted flow chart seen in Table 11.1 at the end of Procedure 11.2). The PFM is then classified into three zones of measurement according to the American Lung Association: green, yellow, and red.

Peak flow zones are based on the traffic light concept: red means danger, yellow means caution, and green means safe. The zones are different for each person. The goal of the peak flow zones is to recognize early symptoms of uncontrolled asthma.
• *Green*—This is the *go* zone. The green zone is from 80% to 100% of the patient's highest peak flow reading, or

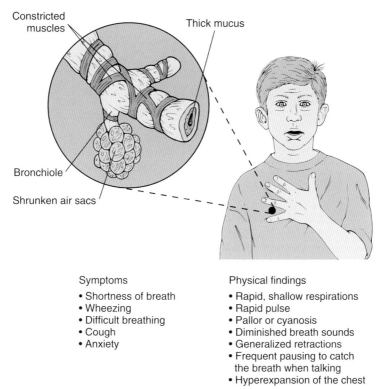

Constricted muscles

Thick mucus

Bronchiole

Shrunken air sacs

Symptoms
- Shortness of breath
- Wheezing
- Difficult breathing
- Cough
- Anxiety

Physical findings
- Rapid, shallow respirations
- Rapid pulse
- Pallor or cyanosis
- Diminished breath sounds
- Generalized retractions
- Frequent pausing to catch the breath when talking
- Hyperexpansion of the chest

FIG. 11.6 An asthma attack with respiratory distress. *Symptoms:* Shortness of breath, wheezing, difficult breathing, cough, anxiety. *Physical findings:* Rapid, shallow respirations, rapid pulse rate, pallor or cyanosis, diminished breath sounds, generalized retractions, frequent pausing to catch the breath when talking, hyperexpansion of the chest. (From Frazier M: *Human diseases and conditions,* ed 5, St. Louis, 2013, Saunders.)

personal best. Measurements in this zone signal that air is moving well through the airways and that the patient should continue to follow the asthma plan as directed by the physician.

- *Yellow*—This is the *caution* or *slow-down* zone. The yellow zone is from 50% to 80% of the patient's personal best. Measurements in this zone are a clue that the large airways are starting to narrow. The patient may begin to have mild symptoms, such as feeling short of breath, coughing, or feeling like the chest is tightening. The patient should notify the physician at this time.

- *Red*—This is the *stop* zone. The red zone is less than 50% of the patient's personal best. Readings in this zone indicate severe narrowing of the large airways has occurred. This is a medical emergency and requires immediate attention. The patient may experience coughing, shortness of breath, and wheezing when breathing. There may be problems walking and talking. The patient should take his or her rescue medication immediately and call the physician.

See Procedure 11.2: Peak Expiratory Flow Monitoring at the end of this section for ways to screen patients as well as instructing them in the daily monitoring of their peak expiratory flow.

Asthma Therapies: Inhalers, Nebulizers, and Oxygen

When the breathing of a patient with asthma reaches the yellow and red zones and the patient is experiencing respiratory distress, relief may be obtained in the following three ways:
- Inhale the prescribed bronchodilator medication using the correct inhaler.
- Breathe in a prescribed therapeutic dosage of medications via a nebulizer.
- Receive metered oxygen by nasal cannula.

The two basic types of drug therapies used in asthma treatment are as follows:
- *Antiinflammatory medications* (e.g., steroids) are the most important treatment for most people with asthma. These work by reducing the production of mucus and swelling in the airways. As a result, the airways are less likely to become constricted, and they will be less sensitive to asthma "triggers" such as allergens and emotional or exercise stressors.
- *Bronchodilators* relieve the respiratory distress symptoms of asthma by further relaxing the muscles that can tighten around the airways. Short-acting bronchodilators are referred to as rescue inhalers because they relieve the cough,

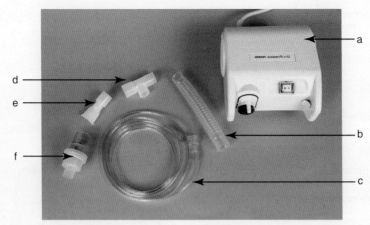

FIG. 11.7 Nebulizer and disposable supplies: *(a)* nebulizer; *(b)* reservoir tube; *(c)* supply tubing; *(d)* T tube; *(e)* mouthpiece; *(f)* medication jar.

wheeze, chest tightness, and shortness of breath caused by an asthmatic attack. They may also be used before exercise for people with exercise-induced asthma. These should *not* be used daily in the routine treatment of asthma. Long-acting bronchodilators, on the other hand, are used in combination with inhaled steroids for control of asthma symptoms.

The following two delivery systems are used by patients at home:

- *Metered-dosed inhalers* are the most common. They are an effective way to deliver asthma drugs to the lungs. They are available in different types of devices that require different techniques for use. Some inhalers deliver one medication and others contain two different medications. They are generally handheld devices and deliver a preset dosage of aerosol medication when activated and inhaled.
- *Nebulizers* are known as "breathing machines." The nebulizer forces air through the liquid medication, creating a mist that is then inhaled via a mouthpiece or mask. This method of asthma medication can be more easily inhaled into the lungs. Its use takes a few more minutes than an inhaler to take effect.

When a patient is in respiratory distress, the physician may order inhaled dosage medication via the nebulizer, and/or may order oxygen (as seen on the next page). It is therefore important to have a basic foundation of these two in-office treatments.

Nebulizer Procedure

1. Sanitize your hands.
2. Gather and assemble the sterile disposable supplies and nebulizer as seen in Figure 11.7.
3. Place the prescribed solution into the nebulizer jar after checking the label three times and connect firmly to the T tube.
4. Connect the mouthpiece to the T tube.
5. Connect the reservoir tube to the T tube.

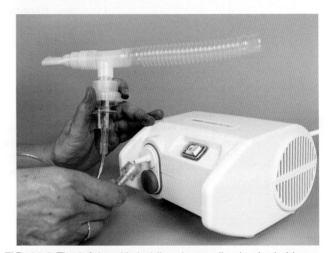

FIG. 11.8 The left hand is holding the medication jar (with green lid) that connects to the T tube where the mouthpiece and reservoir tube are also attached. The right hand is connecting the supply tubing to the nebulizer.

6. Attach the supply tubing between the medication jar and the nebulizer as seen in Figure 11.8.
7. Ask the patient to place the mouthpiece into the mouth and make a seal with the lips, without biting the mouthpiece. Instruct the patient to breathe normally during the treatment, occasionally taking a deep breath.
8. Turn the machine on using the on/off switch. Set the gas flow rate to 8 LPM (liters per minute) or according to the manufacturer's instructions. The medication in the jar will become a fine mist. Check for aerosol mist exiting out of the reservoir tube; if necessary, tap the device until it begins to nebulize.
9. Before, during, and after the breathing treatment, take and record the patient's pulse rate.
10. When the treatment is over and the medication is gone from the cup, turn the machine off and have the patient remove the mouthpiece.

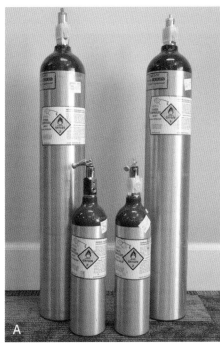

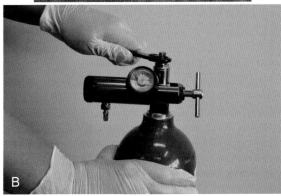

FIG. 11.9 A, Compressed oxygen cylinders. **B,** Oxygen cylinder with regulator and flow meter attached. (From Bonewit-West K: *Clinical procedures for medical assistants,* ed 10, St. Louis, 2018, Elsevier.)

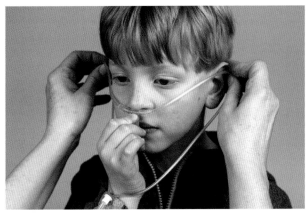

FIG. 11.10 While the patient is holding the two cannula tubes in his nose, bring the tubing from the front around each ear (creating a heart shape with the lower point at the chin). After the tubes are secure around the ears, tighten the lower tip under the chin with the white slider seen at the patient's wrist.

11. During treatment, periodically tap the nebulizer to minimize residual volume.
12. Disconnect the disposable treatment setup and dispose all parts into a biohazard container.
13. Sanitize your hands and document the procedure, including the patient's pulse rate before, during, and after the treatment.

Administering Oxygen by Nasal Cannula

Oxygen therapy is a treatment that provides extra oxygen to the patient with obstructed airways. When a patient arrives at your facility with severe respiratory distress, the patient may be in critical need of oxygen. It is important to be familiar with how oxygen may be administered to the patient from an oxygen tank, a metal cylinder as seen in Figure 11.9A.

The steps to take when preparing the oxygen tank are as follows:
1. Open the cylinder one full turn, counterclockwise. Check the pressure gauge (Figure 11.9B).
2. Attach the nasal cannula to the tubing and then to the flow meter.
3. Adjust the flow rate according to the physician's order (common standing order is 2 L/min). Check to see if there is air flowing out of the nasal cannula.
4. Place the tips of the cannula into the nares no more than 1 inch.
5. As the patient holds the cannula, adjust the tubing around the patient's ears and secure it under the chin using the slider (Figure 11.10).
6. Answer patient's questions while making sure the patient is comfortable.

Becoming Proficient at Spirometry Diagnostic Tests

Now that you have learned about peak flow monitoring and assisting in asthma therapies, take the time to complete the following:
1. Answer the text questions at the end of this chapter and do all of the exercises in Chapter 11 of the workbook using your student handouts on the Evolve website.
2. View the animations and videos on Evolve to see the anatomy and physiology of the lungs and to observe how to interact with patients when performing spirometry procedures.
3. Perform the Chapter 11 online exercises, which are designed to reinforce your terminology, theory, and testing techniques for measuring lung function.
4. Study Behavioral 11.1, and Procedure 11.2 Peak Expiratory Flow Monitoring below prior to your lab.

PROCEDURE 11.2 Peak Expiratory Flow Monitoring

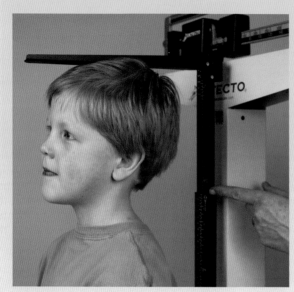

A, Before performing the peak flow screening test, accurately determine the child's height, age, and gender (all three are needed to compare the result against the predicted normal for the child's group).

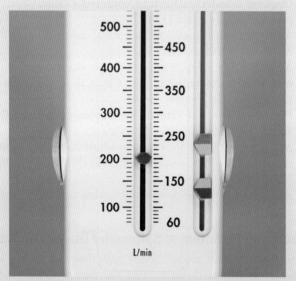

C, Peak flow result on the left registers 200 L/min. The preset green, yellow, and red indicators on the right indicate the patient is in the yellow zone.

Instrument and Supplies
- Height and weight scale
- Peak flow meter (PFM), new or sterilized
- PFM for demonstrating the maneuver
- Daily monitoring chart

Preanalytical
1. Call the patient into the room and sanitize your hands while confirming the patient's name using three identifiers: have the patient spell his or her last name, give his or her date of birth, and provide one more identifier such as phone number or address, or show a driver's license.

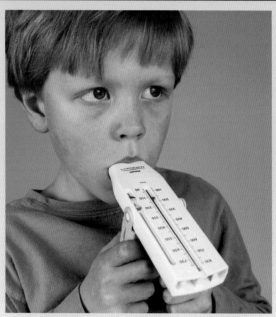

B, The patient is instructed to (1) fully inflate the lungs and hold her or his breath while sealing the lips around the mouthpiece and (2) fully exhale into the mouthpiece as fast and as hard as possible.

2. Confirm when the patient last took his or her bronchodilator medication and if the patient has ingested a heavy meal in the last 4 hours.
3. Measure the patient's height in inches and confirm the patient's age (to compare with the proper demographic group if it is a screening test) (Figure A).
4. Explain and demonstrate the two steps of the maneuver using a demo PFM.
   - **Fully inflate** your lungs and then hold your breath while sealing your lips around the mouthpiece.
   - **Fully exhale** into the mouthpiece as fast and as hard as possible (Figure B).
5. Show and explain the importance of standing upright during the maneuver and that the patient will have 1 minute to rest and sit between a minimum of three attempts to determine "personal best."

Analytical
6. Test and teach the patient through the following steps:
   a. Before each use, make sure the sliding pointer on the PFM is reset to the zero mark. See Figure C showing the red sliding pointer on the left after a maneuver.
   b. Stand up straight.
   c. Remove chewing gum or any food from your mouth.
   d. Take a deep breath and put the mouthpiece in your mouth. Seal your lips and teeth tightly around the mouthpiece.
   e. Blow out as hard and as fast as you can. Remember, a "fast blast" is better than a "slow blow."
   f. Note the number where the sliding pointer has stopped on the scale. See Figure C result.
   g. Reset the pointer to zero.
   h. Repeat this routine three times. You will know you have done the technique correctly when the three readings are close together.
   i. If you cough during a measurement, you should repeat it.
   j. Record the highest of the three readings on a graph or in a notebook. This is called your "best effort." Do not average the numbers together.
   k. Use the PFM once a day or as directed by your physician. Measure peak flows about the same time each day. A good time might be when you first wake up or at bedtime.

PROCEDURE 11.2 Peak Expiratory Flow Monitoring—cont'd

7. Coach the patient as he or she performs the maneuver. Make sure the patient performs both steps: inspiration and rapid exhalation. Praise good techniques to the patient and communicate positive ways to improve the next maneuver. Do not give negative feedback.

Postanalytical

8. If the patient is taking a screening test, locate his or her predicted value in Table 11.1 based on the patient's age, gender, and height. Divide the predicted value into the patient's result. If the result is less than 80%, the patient may need further evaluation.

9. If the patient has been prescribed daily peak flow monitoring, determine his or her "best effort" reading from three attempts. The personal best value will be used as a baseline for the patient's routine measurements. Show the patient the peak flow chart where he or she will be entering daily results. See Figure D above showing a completed patient chart.

10. Document the procedure.

Quality Control

Be aware of and correct the following issues that will prevent accurate readings:

- Coughing during the maneuver
- Forming a poor seal around the mouthpiece while performing the procedure
- Taking asthma medication before the PFM (especially the bronchodilator medication because it opens the airways and gives a false high reading)
- Using a dirty meter
- Blocking the mouthpiece with the tongue
- Using a different type or brand of PFM because the measurements may vary among brands and types of meters

Name __Doe, Johnny__   Week Beginning (date) __June 1, 20XX__

Peak Flow Zones: Green Zone ___> 240___ Yellow Zone___130 - 240___ Red Zone ___< 130___

Prescribed Medications (include dose and frequency)___Advair Diskus 100/50 1 inh qd in AM___

Peak Flow Recording Times: __8:00__ AM_____ PM

D, Peak flow chart showing daily monitoring results. Notice the readings that fell in the yellow zone on the days the patient was not using his inhaler.

TABLE 11.1 Peak Expiratory Flow Rates*

	GIRLS AND WOMEN: 6–20 YEARS OF AGE								
Height (inches)	42	46	50	54	57	60	64	68	72
Age 6	134	164	193	223	245	268	297	327	357
8	153	182	212	242	264	287	316	346	376
10	171	201	231	261	283	305	335	365	395
12	190	220	250	280	302	324	354	384	414
14	209	239	269	298	321	343	373	403	432
16	228	258	288	318	340	362	392	421	451
18	247	277	306	336	358	381	411	440	470
20	266	295	325	355	377	400	429	459	489

Continued

TABLE 11.1 Peak Expiratory Flow Rates*—cont'd

BOYS AND MEN: 6–25 YEARS OF AGE

Height (inches)	44	48	52	56	60	64	68	72	76
Age 6	99	146	194	241	289	336	384	431	479
8	119	166	214	261	309	356	404	451	499
10	139	186	234	281	329	376	424	471	519
12	159	206	254	301	349	396	444	491	539
14	178	226	274	321	369	416	464	511	559
16	198	246	293	341	389	436	484	531	579
18	218	266	313	361	408	456	503	551	599
20	238	286	333	381	428	476	523	571	618
22	258	306	353	401	448	496	543	591	638
24	278	326	373	421	468	516	563	611	658
25	288	336	383	431	478	526	573	621	668

WOMEN: 20–80 YEARS OF AGE

Height (inches)	58	60	62	64	66	68	70
Age 20	357	372	387	402	417	432	446
25	350	365	379	394	409	424	439
30	342	357	372	387	402	417	431
35	335	350	364	379	394	409	424
40	327	342	357	372	387	402	416
45	320	335	349	364	379	394	409
50	312	327	342	357	372	387	401
55	308	320	334	349	364	379	394
60	297	312	327	342	357	372	386
65	290	305	319	334	349	364	379
70	282	297	312	327	342	357	371
75	275	290	304	319	334	349	364
80	267	282	297	312	327	342	356

MEN: 25–80 YEARS OF AGE

Height (inches)	63	65	67	69	71	73	75	77
Age 25	492	520	549	578	606	635	664	692
30	481	510	538	567	596	624	653	682
35	471	499	528	557	585	614	643	671
40	460	489	517	546	575	603	632	661
45	450	478	507	536	564	593	622	650
50	439	468	496	525	554	582	611	640
55	429	457	486	515	543	572	601	629
60	418	447	475	504	533	561	590	619
65	408	436	465	494	522	551	580	608
70	397	426	454	483	512	540	569	598
75	387	405	444	473	501	530	559	587
80	376	405	433	462	491	519	5	

*Note that the values are the average normal values for healthy persons of a given age and height (Knudson, 1976). There will always be a range of normal values; not everyone can be expected to have exactly the same value. Men can have peak flow values as low as 100 L/min less than the average value shown and still fall within the normal range. Women can have peak flow values as low as 80 L/min less than the average value shown and still fall within the normal range.

From LSU Health Shreveport. Peak expiratory flow rates. http://www.sh.lsuhsc.edu/fammed/outpatientmanual/PeakFlowTables.htm. Accessed February 13, 2018.

REVIEW QUESTIONS*

1. Spirometry is used in primary care to
   a. determine the cause of lung diseases.
   b. screen and monitor pulmonary obstruction or restriction.
   c. determine exposure to pollutants.
   d. monitor how many cigarettes a patient has smoked.

2. Match the respiratory structure with its possible obstructive disorder:

   a. Terminal bronchioles   (1) emphysema
   b. Alveoli   (2) flu and colds
   c. Upper respiratory tract   (3) bronchitis
   d. Lower respiratory tract   (4) asthma

3. Spirometry is a pulmonary function test that measures
   a. airway inflammation.
   b. how much and how fast air is exhaled.
   c. how long you can hold your breath.
   d. how fast you can inhale and exhale.

4. A healthy person exhales what percentage of his or her total exhaled volume in the first second?
   a. 25% to 30%
   b. 75%
   c. 80% to 90%
   d. 100%

5. When looking at the volume/time curve, what indicates a good patient effort?
   a. A quick rise in the beginning
   b. A FET (forced volume expiratory time) of 6 seconds
   c. A Plateau of the curve at the end
   d. All the above

6. How often should the spirometer be checked with the calibrated syringe?
   a. Daily
   b. Weekly
   c. Monthly
   d. Not necessary if stable

*Answers to these Review Questions are located in the Appendix on p. 279.

WEBSITES

Information on Peak Flow monitoring:
www.hopkinsmedicine.org/healthlibrary/test_procedures/
   pulmonary/peak_flow_measurement_92,P07755/
Peak expiratory flow (PEF) charts for predicted normal:
www.sh.lsuhsc.edu/fammed/outpatientmanual/PeakFlow
   Tables.htm

Peak flow rate measurement on Medscape:
http://emedicine.medscape.com/article/1413347-overview#
   aw2aab6b4aa

A APPENDIX

Answers to Review Questions

CHAPTER 1

1. pathologist
2. venipunctures, blood draws
3. POLs (physician's office laboratories) and reference laboratories
4. Doctor of Medicine or Osteopathy
5. honesty, communication skills, efficiency, organizational skills, good eyesight, and dexterity
6. d, a, c, b
7. mL, dL, cm, mcm, cc
8. biohazards, chemical hazards, and physical hazards
9. fire, tornado, bomb, and electrical dangers
10. acids, caustics, flammables, inhalants
11. 10% solution of 1 part bleach and 9 parts water, or 70% alcohol
12. False
13. True

CHAPTER 2

1. All laboratories performing tests on specimens must register with CMS for permission to perform CoW, moderately complex, or highly complex tests based on the qualifications of the laboratory personnel and the difficulty of the tests performed to improve the accuracy and reliability of patient testing.
2. Laboratories performing moderately complex and complex tests must prove their proficiency by testing specimens from an outside accreditation agency twice a year and obtaining the correct results.
3. low
4. 10×
5. condenser
6. nosepiece
7. oil immersion
8. objective
9. c, a, b

CHAPTER 3

1. c
2. b
3. d
4. d
5. b
6. d
7. b
8. c
9. d
10. b
11. C
12. C
13. I—This would contaminate the urethral opening with bacteria from the rectal area.
14. I—Besides contaminating the urethral opening with bacteria from the rectal area, this step would also contaminate the opening with organisms from the other side.
15. C
16. C

CHAPTER 4

1. c
2. d
3. b
4. c
5. c
6. a
7. a
8. d
9. c
10. Light blue, red plastic (has clot activator—should not be drawn before the light blue), green, and lavender

CHAPTER 5

1. b
2. plasma, erythrocytes, granulocytes, anticoagulant, platelet, EDTA, megakaryocyte
3. g, h, b, e, c, d, f, a
4. prothrombin, fibrin
5. K
6. d, a, b, e, c
7. b, c, a
8. b, a, d, c, e
9. e, d, a, c, b

CHAPTER 6

1. whole blood from a fingerstick; serum from a red clot tube or gold SST of marbled red-gray rubber-topped SST tube
2. insulin
3. 90% to 95%

4. glucosuria
5. d
6. It provides a picture of average glucose levels over a 3-month period and helps determine whether the patient is keeping glucose levels under control.
7. from the diet (exogenous); from the liver (endogenous)
8. LDL adheres to the arteries, causing plaque, whereas HDL removes the plaque.
9. To check the instrument's optical performance and ensure quality results
10. poor specimen processing or technique; reagents stored at wrong temperature or expired; instrument dirty or faulty
11. less than 200 mg/dL; 200 to 240 mg/dL; greater than 240 mg/dL
12. f, d, c, e, a, b
13. To determine if bleeding is present within the colon or GI tract, which might indicate possible carcinoma:
    1. ColoScreen
    2. ColoCARE
    3. iFob—immunoassay fecal occult blood or FiT (Fecal immunoassay Test)
14. b, d, c, e, a

CHAPTER 7

1. b
2. c
3. d
4. a
5. b
6. a and c
7. d
8. b
9. d
10. B and Rh antigens
11. Blood; oral swab of the gums

CHAPTER 8

1. d
2. c
3. c
4. b
5. a
6. d
7. d

8. c
9. specimen—direct smear using swabbed specimen; colony growing on a solid medium; liquid medium with growth
10. d

CHAPTER 9

1. True
2. False (It is the mechanism of the drug's action in the body from introduction to elimination.)
3. Liberation
4. absorption
5. distribution
6. metabolism
7. kidney, liver
8. half-life
9. lead, arsenic, mercury, iron
10. alcohol
11. crank, speed
12. morphine, codeine, heroin
13. c
14. c

CHAPTER 10

1. b
2. a
3. b
4. c
5. a-2, b-1, c-3 (c-3 is Einthoven's triangle)
6. b
7. c
8. c
9. b
10. c
11. b

CHAPTER 11

1. b
2. a-4, b-1, c-2, d-3
3. b
4. c
5. d
6. a

Herb/Laboratory Test Interactions

Herb/Laboratory Test Interactions

Herb	Test Affected	Results
Aloe	Serum potassium	↓ Test values
Angelica	Plasma partial thromboplastin time (PTT)	←↑ In clients taking warfarin concurrently
	Prothrombin time (PT) and plasma ⊃⊃ International Normalized Ratio	↑ In clients taking warfarin concurrently
Astragalus	Semen specimen analysis	↑ Sperm motility in vitro
Cascara	Serum and 24-hour urine estrogens	↑ or ↓ Test values
Chaparral	Alanine aminotransferase (ALT)	
	Aspartate aminotransferase (AST)	
	Total bilirubin	
	Urine bilirubin	
Chaste tree	Serum prolactin	↓ Test values
Chromium	Blood glucose	↓ Test values
	High-density lipoprotein (HDL) levels	←↑ Test values
	Triglycerides	↓ Test values
Coffee	AST	↓ Test values in alcoholics
	Secretion provocation test	↑ Test values
	Serum 2-hour postprandial glucose	False ↑← if caffeine is ingested during test
	Specimen infertility screen	Possible ↓ in number of motile sperm with heavy coffee consumption
Comfrey	ALT	←↑ Test values
	AST	↑ Test values
	Total bilirubin	↑ Test values
Cranberry	Urine pH	↓ pH
Echinacea	ALT	←↑ Test values
	AST	←↑ Test values
	Lymphocyte counts	←↑ Lymphocyte counts
	Serum immunoglobulin E (IgE)	←↑ Test values
	Blood erythrocyte sedimentation rate (ESR)	↑ ESR
	Specimen semen analysis	High doses of herb interfere with sperm enzyme activity
Ephedra	AST	←↑ Test values
	ALT	←↑ Test values
	Total bilirubin	←↑ Test values
	Urine bilirubin	←↑ Test values
Fenugreek	Total cholesterol	↓ Total cholesterol
	Blood glucose	↓ Test values
	Low-density lipoprotein (LDL) cholesterol	↓ LDL cholesterol
Feverfew	Blood platelet aggregation	↓ Test values
	PT	↑ Values in clients taking warfarin concurrently
	PTT	↑ Values in clients taking warfarin concurrently
Figwort	Blood glucose	↓ Test values

Herb/Laboratory Test Interactions—cont'd

Herb	Test Affected	Results
Garlic	LDL cholesterol	↓ Test values with aged extract taken continuously
	Platelet aggregation	↓ Test values with aged extract taken continuously
	Triglycerides	↓ Test values with aged extract taken continuously
	Blood lipid profile	↓ Test values
	PT	↓ Test values
	Serum IgE	↓ Test values
Ginger	PTT	←↑ Values in clients taking warfarin concurrently
	PT	↑ Test values
Ginkgo	PT	↑← Test values
	Blood salicylate	←↑ Test values
	Platelet activity	↓ Platelet activity
	PTT	↑← Bleeding
	Acetylsalicylic acid tolerance test	←↑ Bleeding
Ginseng	Blood glucose	↓ Test values
	PTT	↓ Test values
	Serum and 24-hour urine estrogens	Additive effects to estrogen
	Serum digoxin	Falsely ↑← test value
Goldenseal	Bilirubin	←↑ Test values
	Blood osmolality	←↑ Test values
	Serum or urine plasma sodium	←↑ Test values
Guar gum	Blood cholesterol	↓ Test values
	Blood glucose levels	↓ Test values
Gymnema	Blood glucose	↓ Test values
	LDL cholesterol	↓ Test values
	Total cholesterol	↓ Test values
Hawthorn	Serum digoxin	Falsely ↑← test values
Lecithin	Blood lipid profile	↓ Total cholesterol test values
Licorice	Blood anion gap	↓ Test values
	Qualitative urine myoglobin	Possible positive test result
	Serum or urine plasma sodium	←↑ Test values (hypernatremia)
	Serum myoglobin	Possible positive test result
	Serum potassium	↓ Test values
	Serum prolactin (human prolactin)	↓ Test values
Mayapple	Red blood cells (RBCs)	↓ Test values
Mistletoe	ALT	←↑ Test values
	AST	↑ Test values
	Total bilirubin	↑ Test values
	Urine bilirubin	↑ Test values
	Lymphocyte counts	↑ Lymphocyte counts
	RBCs	↓ Test values
Mugwort	Serum bilirubin: total, direct (conjugated), and indirect (unconjugated)	Possible ↑← direct bilirubin
Pennyroyal	ALT	←↑ Test values
	AST	←↑ Test values
	Total bilirubin	←↑ Test values
	Urine bilirubin	←↑ Test values
	RBCs	↓ Test values
Plantain	Blood glucose	↓ Test values
	Cholesterol: total, LDL, HDL ratio tests	↓ Test values
	Serum digoxin	Falsely ↑← test values
Poppy	Urine heroin	False-positive test result
	Urine morphine	False-positive test result

Continued

Herb/Laboratory Test Interactions—cont'd

Herb	Test Affected	Results
Pycnogenol	Blood platelet aggregation	↓ Test values
Rauwolfia	Gastric analysis results	←↑ Test values
	Basal nocturnal acid output	←↑ Test values
	Serum or urine plasma sodium	←↑ Test values (hypernatremia)
	RBCs	↓ Test values
	Urine vanillylmandelic acid	↓ Test values
	Serum gastrin	↓ Test values
Saw palmetto	Bleeding time	↑← Bleeding time
	Specimen semen analysis	Metabolic changes in sperm
Schisandra	ALT	↓ Test values
	AST	↓ Test values
Senna	Serum and 24-hour urine estriol	↓ Test values
Siberian ginseng	Serum androstenedione	↑← Test values
	Blood glucose levels	↓ Test values
Skullcap	ALT	←↑ Test values
	AST	←↑ Test values
	Total and urine bilirubin	←↑ Test values
Soy	HDL cholesterol	←↑ Test values
	LDL cholesterol	↓ Test values
	Triglycerides	↓ Test values
	Total cholesterol	↓ Test values
Squill	RBCs	↓ Test values
St. John's wort	Growth hormone (somatotropin)	←↑ Test values
	Serum prolactin	↓ Test values
	Theophylline (aminophylline)	↓ Test values
	Serum iron	↓ Test values
	Serum digoxin	↓ Digoxin peak and trough concentrations
Valerian	ALT	←↑ Test values
	AST	←↑ Test values
	Total bilirubin	←↑ Test values
	Urine bilirubin	←↑ Test values

From Skidmore-Roth L: *Mosby's handbook of herbs and natural supplements,* ed 3, St. Louis, 2006, Mosby.

Common Laboratory and Diagnostic Tests

Values may vary according to laboratory reference values. These values are for reference only. Results of one test alone usually are not conclusive and should be considered with results of other diagnostic procedures, the symptoms and signs, and the physical examination to arrive at a diagnosis.

BLOOD ANALYSIS

Complete Blood Count

A complete blood count is the evaluation of cellular components of the blood. It includes red blood cell (RBC) count, RBC indices, white blood cell (WBC) count, WBC differential, hemoglobin (Hgb), hematocrit (HCT), and platelet count. Sometimes it is referred to as a *hemogram*. Often the differential must be ordered specifically as complete blood count (CBC) with differential.

Red Blood Cell Count

Count of erythrocytes in a specimen of whole blood.

Normal Levels

Adult male: 4.5.7 to 6.1 million/μl
Adult female: 4.0 to 5.5 million/μl
Infants and children: 3.8 to 5.5 million/μl
Newborns: 4.1 to 6.1 million/μl

An elevated RBC count is indicative of many disorders, including but not limited to erythremia, polycythemia, erythrocytosis, dehydration, burns, hypoxia, diarrhea, cardiovascular disease, poisoning, pulmonary disease, and smoking. A reduced RBC count also is indicative of many disorders, including but not limited to anemias, bone marrow suppression, hemorrhage, lead poisoning, liver diseases, thyroid disorders, cardiovascular disease, malnutrition, vitamin deficiency, and ingestion of certain drugs. When the RBC count is abnormal, cell morphology should be examined. As with most blood tests, results should be evaluated with other tests, along with symptoms and signs, to determine a diagnosis.

Hemoglobin Count

An Hgb count is the measurement of the oxygen-carrying pigment of the RBCs.

Normal Levels

Adult male: 13.0 to 18.0
Adult female: 12.0 to 16.0
Infants and children: 9.5 to 15.5
Newborns: 14 to 24

An elevated Hgb count is indicative of many disorders, including but not limited to congestive heart failure (CHF), chronic obstructive pulmonary disease (COPD), dehydration, burns, diarrhea, erythrocytosis, polycythemia, high altitudes, and thrombotic thrombocytopenia. A reduced Hgb count also is indicative of many disorders, including but not limited to iron-deficiency anemia, hemorrhage, hemolytic reaction to drugs or chemicals, liver diseases, systemic lupus erythematosus (SLE), and pregnancy.

Hematocrit Count

A HCT count is the measurement of the percentage of RBCs in a volume of whole blood.

Normal Levels

Adult male: 37% to 52%
Adult female: 36% to 48%
Infants and children: 28% to 65%
Newborns: 45% to 64%

An elevated HCT count is indicative of many disorders, including but not limited to dehydration, burns, diarrhea, eclampsia, pancreatitis, shock, and polycythemia. A reduced HCT count also is indicative of many disorders, including but not limited to anemia, bone marrow hyperplasia, CHF, fluid overload, burns, thyroid disorders, pancreatitis, pregnancy, pneumonia, malnutrition, and ingestion of certain drugs.

White Blood Cell Count

The WBC count is the count of WBCs in a whole blood specimen.

Normal Levels

Adult male: 4500 to 11,000/μl
Adult female: 4500 to 11,000/μl
Infants and children: 6000 to 17,500/μl
Newborns: 9000 to 35,000/μl

An elevated WBC count is indicative of many disorders, including but not limited to acquired hemolytic anemia, anorexia, abscess, appendicitis, bacterial infections, bronchitis, burns, biliary disorders, respiratory disorders, disorders of the gastrointestinal (GI) tract, renal disorders, blood disorders, lactic acidosis, lupus, poisoning, pregnancy, rheumatoid arthritis, sepsis, shock, tonsillitis, trauma, uremia, and ingestion of certain drugs. Similar to an abnormal RBC, a differential should be evaluated, and, as with most blood tests, results should be evaluated with other tests—along with symptoms and signs—to determine a diagnosis. A decreased WBC is indicative of many disorders, including but not limited to acquired immunodeficiency syndrome (AIDS), anemias, chemical toxicity, Hodgkin disease, influenza, legionnaires disease, radiation therapy, shock, septicemia, vitamin B_{12} deficiency, cirrhosis, hepatitis, hypothermia, leukopenia, tuberculosis, and ingestion of certain drugs.

Differential White Blood Cell (Leukocyte) Count

The differential WBC (leukocyte) count is an assessment by percentage of leukocyte distribution in a specimen of 100 WBCs.

Granulocyte Count

Normal Levels

Segmented neutrophils (SEGs; mature "fighter" cell) adult: 50% to 62%
Band neutrophils (immature "fighter" cells) adult: 3% to 6%
Eosinophil granulocytes (eosinophils) adult: 0% to 3%
Basophil granulocytes (basophils) adult: 0% to 1%
Monocytes adult: 3% to 7%
Lymphocytes adult: 24% to 44%

Increased neutrophils are indicative of many disorders, including but not limited to allergies, asthma, acute infections, appendicitis, burns, diabetic acidosis, cardiovascular disorders, disorders of the GI tract, leukemia, respiratory disorders, poisoning, pyelonephritis, septicemia, tonsillitis, and ingestion of certain drugs. A decrease in neutrophils is indicative of many disorders, including but not limited to endocrine disorders, anaphylactic shock, carcinoma, chemotherapy, anemias, pneumonia, influenza, septicemia, radiation therapy, and ingestion of certain drugs.

Increased eosinophils are indicative of many disorders, including but not limited to allergies, asthma, cancer, dermatitis, diverticulitis, eczema, Hodgkin disease, leukemia, parasitic infection, pernicious anemia, radiation therapy, sickle cell anemia, tuberculosis, and ingestion of certain drugs. Reduced eosinophils also are indicative of many disorders, including but not limited to aplastic anemia, CHF, eclampsia, infections, stress, and ingestion of certain drugs.

Increased basophils are indicative of many disorders, including but not limited to allergic reactions, Hodgkin disease, hypothyroidism, radiation therapy, sinusitis, urticaria, and ingestion of certain drugs. Decreased basophils also are indicative of many disorders, including but not limited to acute infections, anaphylactic shock, endocrine disorders, cancer, pregnancy, radiation therapy, stress, and ingestion of certain drugs.

Increased lymphocytes are indicative of many disorders, including but not limited to endocarditis, infectious mononucleosis, leukocytosis, lymphocytic leukemia, syphilis, toxoplasmosis chronic bacterial infection, viral infections, and ingestion of certain drugs. Decreased lymphocytes also are indicative of many disorders, including but not limited to aplastic anemia, Hodgkin disease, immunoglobulin deficiencies, leukemia, renal failure, SLE, uremia, sepsis, and ingestion of certain drugs.

Increased monocytes are indicative of many disorders, including but not limited to Epstein-Barr virus, Hodgkin disease, leukemia, rheumatoid arthritis, syphilis, SLE, tuberculosis, chronic inflammatory disease, and ingestion of certain drugs. Decreased monocytes are primarily indicative of aplastic anemia and hairy-cell leukemia.

Platelet (Thrombocyte) Count

The platelet (thrombocyte) count is the count of platelets in a whole blood specimen. Platelets help the blood clot.

Normal Adult Levels

150,000 to 400,000/μl

Increased platelet count (thrombocytosis) is indicative of many disorders, including but not limited to anemias, carcinoma, fractures, liver disorders, heart disease, hemorrhage, acute infection, inflammation, leukemia, pancreatitis, pregnancy, rheumatoid arthritis, surgery, and ingestion of certain drugs. A decreased platelet count (thrombocytopenia) is indicative of many disorders, including but not limited to anemias, bone marrow disorders, autoimmune disorders, severe burns, carcinoma, liver disorders, disseminated intravascular coagulation (DIC), hemolytic disease of the newborn, infections, radiation therapy, leukemia, celiac disease, vitamin K deficiency, and ingestion of certain drugs.

BLOOD CHEMISTRIES

Chemistries

Normal chemistry profile may contain blood serum levels for albumin, alkaline phosphatase, aspartate aminotransferase (AST), bilirubin, calcium, creatinine, lactate dehydrogenase (LDH), phosphorus, total protein, urea nitrogen, and uric acid.

Albumin

Albumin is the measurement of one of two major protein factions of blood.

Normal Adult Levels

3.5 to 5.0 g/dl

Increased levels of serum albumin are indicative of many disorders, including but not limited to dehydration, diarrhea, hepatitis, meningitis, carcinoma, myeloma, nephrosis, nephrotic syndrome, peptic ulcers, pneumonia, rheumatic fever, SLE, uremia, vomiting, and ingestion of certain drugs. Below normal levels of serum albumin are indicative of many disorders, including but not limited to ascites, alcoholism, burns, CHF, Crohn disease, cystic fibrosis, diabetes mellitus, edema, hypertension, kidney disorders, malnutrition, GI disorders, trauma, stress, and ingestion of certain drugs.

Alkaline Phosphatase

Alkaline phosphatase is the measurement of enzyme found in bone, liver, intestine, and placenta.

Normal Adult Levels

25 to 100 U/L

Elevated alkaline phosphatase levels are indicative of many disorders, including but not limited to alcoholism, liver disorders, diabetes mellitus, fractures, GI disorders, endocrine disorders, hepatitis, Hodgkin disease, leukemia, neoplasms, myocardial infarction (MI), bone disorders, disorders of the pancreas, kidney disorders, and ingestion of certain drugs. Below normal levels of alkaline phosphatase are indicative of many disorders, including but not limited to pernicious anemia, cretinism, hypothyroidism, malnutrition, nephritis, and ingestion of certain drugs.

Aspartate Aminotransferase (Serum Glutamic Oxaloacetic Transaminase)

AST (serum glutamic oxaloacetic transaminase [SGOT]) is the measurement of enzyme found primarily in heart, liver, and muscle.

Normal Adult Levels

Female: 10 to 36 U/L
Male: 14 to 20 U/L

Elevated AST levels are indicative of many disorders, including but not limited to acute MI, alcoholism, liver disorders, mononucleosis, insult and injury to tissue (including trauma), cerebral and pulmonary infarctions, and ingestion of certain drugs. Reduced AST levels are indicative of many disorders, including but not limited to diabetic ketoacidosis, liver disease, uremia, vitamin B_6 deficiency, and ingestion of certain drugs.

Bilirubin

Bilirubin is a byproduct of Hgb breakdown. Bilirubin is produced in the liver, spleen, and bone marrow.

Normal Adult Levels

Total: <1.5 mg/dl
Direct: 0.0 to 0.3 mg/dl
Indirect: 0.1 to 1.0 mg/dl

Total bilirubin is divided into direct bilirubin, primarily secreted by the intestinal tract, and indirect bilirubin, primarily circulating in the bloodstream. Obstructive or hepatic jaundice results in an increased amount of direct bilirubin entering the bloodstream rather than entering the GI tract and being filtered and eliminated by the kidneys. Conditions that cause an increase in direct bilirubin include, but are not limited to, biliary obstruction, pancreatic cancer (head of pancreas), cirrhosis, hepatitis, and ingestion of certain drugs. Hemolytic jaundice causes the indirect bilirubin to accumulate in the blood because of the increased breakdown of Hgb. Conditions that cause an increase in direct bilirubin levels include, but are not limited to, pernicious and sickle cell anemia, autoimmune hemolysis, cirrhosis, hepatitis, intracavity and soft tissue hemorrhage, MI, septicemia, hemolytic transfusion reaction, and ingestion of certain drugs.

Creatinine

Creatinine is a measurement of an indicator of renal function.

Normal Adult Levels

Female: 0.5 to 1.1 mg/dl
Male: 0.6 to 1.2 mg/dl

Serum creatinine is excreted continually by the renal system, and elevated levels are indicative of a slowing of glomerular filtration. Other conditions that may contribute to elevation of serum creatinine include, but are not limited to, CHF, diabetes mellitus, kidney disorders, hypovolemia, metal poisoning, endocrine disorders, subacute bacterial endocarditis, SLE, and ingestion of certain drugs. Decreased serum creatinine levels are indicative of diabetic ketoacidosis and muscular dystrophy.

Lactate Dehydrogenase

LDH is the measurement of body tissue intracellular enzyme released after tissue damage.

Normal Adult Levels

100-250 IU/L

Elevated LDH levels are indicative of many disorders, including but not limited to alcoholism, anoxia, burns, cardiomyopathy, cerebrovascular accident (CVA), cirrhosis, CHF and MI, neoplasms, anemias, leukemia, renal disorders, pancreatitis, mononucleosis, muscle and bone pain, respiratory disorders, shock, trauma, and ingestion of certain drugs. Decreased levels of LDH develop after radiation and after the ingestion of oxalates.

Total Protein

Total protein is a reflection of the total amounts of albumin and globulins in blood serum.

Normal Adult Levels

6.0 to 8.0 g/dl

Increased total protein is indicative of many disorders, including but not limited to Addison disease, dehydration, diarrhea, renal disease, vomiting, protozoal diseases, and ingestion of certain drugs. Decreased total protein is indicative of many disorders, including but not limited to autoimmune disease, burns, cholecystitis, cirrhosis, CHF, Crohn disease, diarrhea, hyperthyroidism, edema, leukemia, peptic ulcer, nephrosis, malnutrition, ulcerative colitis, and ingestion of certain drugs.

Urea Nitrogen/Blood Urea Nitrogen

Urea nitrogen/blood urea nitrogen (BUN) is an assessment of the urea content in the blood that gives an indication of the functioning of the renal glomeruli.

Normal Adult Levels

5 to 20 mg/dl

An elevated urea nitrogen level can be indicative of many disorders, including but not limited to kidney disease, dehydration, burns, urinary tract blockage, and a high protein diet. Decreased urea nitrogen level can be indicative of many disorders, including but not limited to malnutrition, overhydration, and liver damage.

Uric Acid

Uric acid is an end-product of the metabolism of purines.

Normal Adult Levels

Female: 2.4 to 6.0 mg/dl
Male: 3.4 to 7.0 mg/dl

Elevated uric acid levels are indicative of many disorders, including but not limited to gout, hyperuricemia, hemolytic and sickle cell anemias, hypothyroidism, acute infections, lead poisoning, leukemia, neoplasms, nephritis, kidney stones and polycystic kidney, renal failure, malnutrition, psoriasis, uremia, urinary obstruction, and ingestion of certain drugs. Reduced uric acid levels are indicative of many disorders, including but not limited to acromegaly, carcinomas, Hodgkin disease, pernicious anemia, and ingestion of certain drugs.

Thyroid Function Tests

An evaluation of all three thyroid levels is important in diagnosing thyroid disorders.

Thyroxine

The hormone thyroxine (T_4) is produced in the thyroid gland from iodide and thyroglobulin in response to stimulation by thyroid-stimulating hormone (TSH) produced by the pituitary gland. T_4 stimulates triiodothyronine (T_3) to be produced. It also stimulates the basal metabolism. In the process of negative feedback, circulating levels of T_4 influence the levels of TSH.

Normal Adult Levels

5.0 to 12.0 µg/dl

Increased levels of T_4 usually indicate the presence of hyperfunctioning thyroid disorders, including Graves disease, hyperthyroidism, thyrotoxicosis, and ingestion of certain drugs. Decreased levels of T_4 are indicative of hypothyroid disorders, including acromegaly, cretinism, and goiter, as well as hypothyroidism, liver disease, endocrine disorders, GI tract disorders, pituitary tumor, and ingestion of certain drugs.

Triiodothyronine

T_3 stimulates the basal metabolic rate for metabolism of carbohydrates and lipids, protein synthesis, vitamin metabolism, and bone calcium release.

Normal Adult Levels

80 to 230 ng/dl

An increase in T_3 levels is indicative of, but not limited to, Graves disease, hyperthyroidism, thyrotoxicosis, and ingestion of certain drugs. Decreased levels of T_3 are indicative of, but not limited to, iodine and thyroid deficiency disorders, including goiter and myxedema, renal failure, starvation, thyroidectomy, and ingestion of certain drugs.

Thyroid-Stimulating Hormone

TSH, produced in the anterior lobe of the pituitary gland, stimulates the production and release of T_3 and T_4 by the thyroid gland.

Normal Adult Levels

0.4 to 4.2 IU/L

An increase in TSH levels may be indicative of, but not limited to, Addison disease, goiter, hyperpituitarism, hypothyroidism, thyroiditis, and ingestion of certain drugs. A decrease in

TSH may be indicative of, but not limited to, Hashimoto thyroiditis, hyperthyroidism, and hypothyroidism.

Lipid Profile

A lipid profile consists of comparison of results of four serum lipids: total cholesterol, triglycerides, high-density lipoproteins (HDLs), and low-density lipoproteins (LDLs). One consideration is the ratio of HDL:LDL; the recommended ratio is 3.4:5.0.

Total Cholesterol

Total cholesterol is a widely-distributed sterol that facilitates the absorption and transport of fatty acids. Cholesterol helps build cells and produce hormones.

Normal Adult Levels

Desirable: <200 mg/dl
Borderline: 200 to 240 mg/dl
High risk: >240 mg/dl

Elevated serum cholesterol levels are indicative of many disorders, including but not limited to atherosclerosis, CHF, biliary disorders, kidney disorders, lipid disorders, and ingestion of certain drugs. Decreased levels of serum cholesterol are indicative of many disorders, including but not limited to anemias, carcinoma, cirrhosis, liver disease, hepatitis, endocrine disorders, GI tract disorders, and ingestion of certain drugs.

Triglycerides

Triglycerides, the principal lipids in blood, are simple fat compounds of three molecules of fatty acid: oleic, palmitic, or stearic. Triglycerides give energy to the muscle and store energy.

Normal Adult Levels

Normal: Below 150 mg/dl
Borderline: 150 to 199 mg/dl
High: 200 to 499 mg/dl
Very high: Above 500 mg/dl

Elevated triglyceride levels are indicative of many disorders, including but not limited to arteriosclerosis, MI, aortic aneurysm, hypercholesterolemia, hyperlipoproteinemia, alcoholism, diabetes mellitus, gout, renal disease, and malnutrition. Decreased triglyceride levels are indicative of many disorders, including but not limited to cirrhosis, malabsorption, hyperalimentation, and ingestion of certain drugs.

High-Density Lipoprotein Cholesterol

HDL transports cholesterol and other lipids to the liver for excretion. HDL is believed to reduce the risk of coronary artery disease. It is often referred to as the "good cholesterol."

Normal Adult Levels

Desirable: 60 mg/dl or higher
Acceptable: 40 to 59 mg/dl
Undesirable: Less than 50 mg/dl

Increased levels of HDL are indicative of, but not limited to, alcoholism, hepatic disorders, cirrhosis, and ingestion of certain drugs. Reduced levels of HDL are indicative of many disorders, including but not limited to arteriosclerosis, hypercholesterolemia, hyperlipoproteinemia, CHD, diabetes mellitus, liver disease, kidney disease, bacterial infections, and ingestion of certain drugs.

Low-Density Lipoprotein Cholesterol

LDL has high cholesterol content, and it delivers lipids to body tissues. It is often referred to as the "bad cholesterol."

Normal Adult Levels

Optimal: Less than 100 mg/dl
Near optimal: 100 to 129 mg/dl
Borderline: 130 to 159 mg/dl
High: 160 to 189 mg/dl
Very high: 190 and above

Elevated levels of LDL are indicative of many disorders, including but not limited to diabetes mellitus, anorexia nervosa, renal failure, hepatic disease, and ingestion of certain drugs. Decreased levels of LDL are indicative of, but not limited to, hyperlipoproteinemia, arteriosclerosis, pulmonary disease, stress, and the ingestion of certain drugs.

Electrolytes

Electrolytes are examined in the blood serum test for chloride, potassium, sodium, carbon dioxide. Other electrolytes that maybe be included or can be tested individually are calcium, magnesium, and phosphorus.

Chloride

Chloride is an anion found predominately in extracellular spaces. It helps keep the balance of fluid inside and outside the cells.

Normal Adult Levels

97 to 106 mEq/L

Increased blood serum levels of chloride may be the result of several disorders, including but not limited to metabolic disorders, dehydration, diabetes insipidus, hyperventilation, hyperparathyroidism, acidosis, respiratory alkalosis, CHF, Cushing disease, nephritis, renal failure, and ingestion of certain drugs. Reduced blood serum levels of chloride may be the result of several disorders, including but not limited to metabolic alkalosis, diabetes, severe vomiting, burns, overhydration, salt-losing diseases, some diuretic therapies, central nervous system (CNS) disorders, diaphoresis, fasting, fever, heat exhaustion, acute infections, gastric obstructions, uremia, and ingestion of certain drugs.

Potassium

Potassium is the major positive ion found inside of cells. Potassium is important in nerve conduction, muscle function, osmotic pressure, acid-base balance, and myocardial activity.

Normal Adult Levels

3.5 to 5.3 mEq/L

Increased blood serum levels of potassium may be the result of several disorders, including but not limited to renal failure, dehydration, burns, trauma, chemotherapy, metabolic acidosis, Addison disease, uncontrolled diabetes, dialysis, hemolysis, intestinal obstruction, sepsis, shock, pneumonia, uremia, and ingestion of certain drugs. Reduced blood serum levels of potassium may be the result of several disorders, including but not limited to alkalosis, anorexia, vomiting, diarrhea, malabsorption, starvation, diuresis, excessive sweating, draining wounds, severe burns, endocrine disorders, pancreatitis, cystic fibrosis, GI stress, and ingestion of certain drugs. Abnormally elevated or decreased potassium can cause life-threatening cardiac arrhythmias.

Sodium

Sodium is the major positive ion found outside the cell and the main base in the blood. Its functions include chemical maintenance of osmotic pressure, acid-base balance, and nerve transmission.

Normal Adult Levels

135 to 145 mEq/L

Increased blood serum levels of sodium may be the result of several disorders, including but not limited to dehydration, excessive fluid loss caused by vomiting, diarrhea, sweating, Cushing disease, kidney disease, diabetic ketoacidosis, diabetes insipidus, hyperaldosteronism, hypertension, hypovolemia, edema, and ingestion of certain drugs. Decreased blood serum levels of sodium may be the result of several disorders, including but not limited to CHF, cirrhosis, cystic fibrosis, hypothyroidism, poor nutrition, psychogenic polydipsia, syndrome of inappropriate antidiuretic hormone secretion (SIADH), severe burns, sweating, vomiting, diarrhea, and ingestion of certain drugs.

Carbon Dioxide

Carbon dioxide in normal blood plasma comes from bicarbonate.

Normal Adult Levels

20 to 30 mEq/L

Increased blood serum levels of carbon dioxide may be the result of several disorders, including but not limited to emphysema, aldosteronism, severe vomiting, dehydration, COPD, Cushing disease, bradycardia, cardiac disorders, renal disorders, and ingestion of certain drugs. Decreased blood serum levels of carbon dioxide may be the result of several disorders, including failure, alcoholic ketosis, dehydration, high fever, head trauma, malabsorption syndrome, uremia, and ingestion of certain drugs.

Calcium

Calcium studies include measurement of calcium levels in blood.

Normal Adult Levels

8.2 to 10.2 mg/dl

Ionized Calcium

Ionized calcium is the amount of calcium that is not attached to protein in the blood.

Normal Adult Levels

4.4 to 5.3 mg/dl

Calcium is the most abundant mineral found in the human body. Calcium acts in bone formation, impulse conduction, myocardial and skeletal muscle contractions, and the blood-clotting process. Elevated serum calcium levels are indicative of many disorders, including but not limited to endocrine disorders, hepatic disease, respiratory acidosis, leukemia, neoplasms, blood disorders, respiratory disorders, and ingestion of certain drugs. Reduced serum calcium levels are indicative of many disorders, including but not limited to alkalosis, bacteremia, burns, chronic renal disease and other renal disorders, endocrine disorders, osteomalacia, rickets, vitamin D deficiency, and ingestion of certain drugs.

Magnesium

Magnesium studies include measurement of magnesium levels in the blood.

Normal Adult Levels

1.5 to 2.4 mg/dl

Magnesium is an important mineral found in the bones and inside the cells. It is needed for proper nerve function, muscle maintenance and bone strength. Elevated levels of magnesium are indicative of many disorders, including but not limited to chronic renal failure, dehydration, Addison disease, and diabetic ketoacidosis. Decreased levels of magnesium are indicative of many disorders, including but not limited to pancreatitis, alcoholism, cirrhosis of liver, chronic diarrhea, and malabsorption disorders.

Phosphorus

Phosphorus studies include measurement of phosphorus in blood.

Normal Adult Levels

2.4 to 4.1 mg/dl

Phosphorus is the second most abundant mineral found in the human body. It is needed to help build bone and teeth, for muscles to contract, and for nerve function. Elevated levels of phosphorus may be indicative of, but not limited to, renal disease, diabetic ketoacidosis, liver disease, and hypoparathyroidism. Decreased levels of phosphorus may be indicative of, but not limited to alcoholism, malnutrition, hypercalcemia, and hyperparathyroidism.

CLOTTING AND COAGULATION STUDIES

Partial Thromboplastin Time

Partial thromboplastin time (PTT) is an evaluation of the functioning of the coagulation sequence. PTT is a screening process used for coagulation disorders and to monitor the effectiveness of heparin therapy.

Normal values or standardized times must be checked with the laboratory, because various processes may be used.

Increased standardized times may be indicative of many disorders, including but not limited to cardiac surgery, DIC, abruptio placentae, factor defects, hemodialysis, obstructive jaundice, vitamin K deficiency, presence of circulating anticoagulants, and ingestion of certain drugs. Decreased standardized times are indicative of acute early hemorrhage and extensive cancer.

Prothrombin Time

Prothrombin time (PT) is a measurement of the time taken for clot formation after the addition of reagent tissue thromboplastin and calcium to citrated plasma. In the clotting process, prothrombin converts to thrombin. Adequate vitamin K is necessary for adequate prothrombin production. This test helps in the evaluation of the clotting mechanism and in monitoring oral anticoagulant therapy.

Normal Adult Levels

10.0 to 13.0 seconds; may vary according to laboratory.

International normalized ratio (INR) is the standardized result used with treatment of anticoagulation therapy.

Critical Value

1.0 to 1.4 seconds

An increase in PT may be indicative of several disorders, including but not limited to vitamin K deficiency, liver disorders, anticoagulant therapy, prothrombin deficiency, salicylate intoxication, DIC, SLE, clotting disorders, biliary obstruction, CHF, pancreatitis, snakebite, vomiting, toxic shock syndrome, and ingestion of certain drugs. A reduced PT may be indicative of certain disorders, including but not limited to deep vein thrombosis, MI, peripheral vascular disease, spinal cord injury, pulmonary embolism, and ingestion of certain drugs.

Bleeding Times

Bleeding time is a screening test for coagulation disorders, a measurement of the time required for the platelet clot to form. It is often measured by the Ivy method. The Ivy method is done by placing a blood pressure cuff on the arm, inflating it to 40 mm Hg, and using a lancet or scalpel to make an incision on the underside of the forearm. The incision is to be shallow at 1 mm depth and about 10 mm long. Filter paper is used to "wick" the blood from the cut every 30 seconds until bleeding has ceased.

Normal time at most laboratories is less than 9 minutes.

Increased bleeding times are indicative of several disorders, including but not limited to thrombocytopenia, DIC, aplastic anemia, platelet dysfunction, vascular disease, leukemias, liver disorders, aspirin ingestion, and ingestion of certain drugs. Decreased bleeding time is clinically insignificant.

Erythrocyte Sedimentation Rate

Erythrocyte sedimentation rate (ESR) is the rate at which RBCs (erythrocytes) fall out of well-mixed whole blood to the bottom of the test tube. An alteration in blood proteins occurs during inflammatory and necrotic processes, causing an aggregation of red cells, thereby making them heavier and thus causing them to fall rapidly when placed in a special vertical test tube. A higher ESR is the result of faster settling of the cells. Although not diagnostic of any particular disease process, an elevated ESR gives an indication of an ongoing disease process.

Normal Values by Westergren Method

Adult male: 0 to 15 mm/hr
Adult female: 0 to 20 mm/hr
Children: 0 to 10 mm/hr

Normal Values by Wintrobe Method

Adult male: 0.41 to 0.51 mm/hr
Adult female: 0.36 to 0.45 mm/hr

Increased ESRs may be indicative of many disease processes, including but not necessarily limited to collagen diseases, infectious processes, inflammatory disorders, cancer, heavy metal poisoning, toxemia, pelvic inflammatory disease (PID), anemia, pain, pregnancy, pulmonary embolism, renal disorders, arthritis, subacute bacterial endocarditis, and ingestion of certain drugs. Decreased levels may be found in CHF and ingestion of certain drugs.

GLUCOSE MONITORING

Glucose Tolerance Test

Glucose tolerance test (GTT) is a test that evaluates patients who have symptoms of diabetes mellitus or diabetic complications, as well as screening for gestational diabetes. The test measures blood glucose levels at the following intervals: fasting, 30 minutes, 1 hour, 2 hours, and 3 hours after ingestion of a dose of glucose. Urine samples also are taken at these intervals.

Normal Adult Levels

Fasting: 70 to 110 mg/dl
30 minutes: 110 to 170 mg/dl
1 hour: 120 to 170 mg/dl
2 hours: 70 to 120 mg/dl
3 hours: 70 to 120 mg/dl

All urine samples should test negative for glucose.

Increased glucose values or decreased glucose tolerance are indicative of certain disorders, including but not limited to diabetes mellitus, excessive glucose ingestion, certain endocrine disorders, hepatic damage, CNS lesions, pancreatitis, pheochromocytoma, and ingestion of certain drugs. Decreased glucose values or increased glucose tolerance may be indicative of certain disorders, including but not limited to Addison disease, hypoglycemia, malabsorption, pancreatic disease, liver disease, hypoparathyroidism, hypopituitarism, and ingestion of certain drugs.

Fasting Blood Glucose Levels

Fasting blood glucose (FBG) levels are measured by the amount of glucose found in the blood after 8 hours of fasting.

Normal Adult Levels

Serum: 70 to 99 mg/dl

Increased levels of blood glucose are indicative of several disorders, including but not limited to diabetes mellitus, excessive glucose ingestion, certain endocrine disorders, hepatic damage, post gastrectomy, CNS lesions, pancreatitis, pheochromocytoma, and ingestion of certain drugs. Decreased glucose values may be indicative of certain disorders, including but not limited to Addison disease, hypoglycemia, malabsorption, pancreatic disease, liver disease, hypoparathyroidism, hypopituitarism, and ingestion of certain drugs.

Two-Hour Postprandial

Two-hour postprandial levels the measurement of blood glucose levels 2 hours after fasting for 10 to 12 hours and then consuming a normal meal.

Normal Adult Levels

70 to 145 mg/dl

Increased postprandial levels of blood glucose are indicative of several disorders, including but not limited to diabetes mellitus, excessive glucose ingestion, certain endocrine disorders, hepatic damage, post gastrectomy, CNS lesions, pancreatitis, pheochromocytoma, and ingestion of certain drugs. Decreased postprandial glucose values may be indicative of certain disorders, including but not limited to Addison disease, hypoglycemia, malabsorption, pancreatic disease, liver disease, hypoparathyroidism, hypopituitarism, and ingestion of certain drugs.

Glycosylated Hemoglobin/Glycohemoglobin

Glycohemoglobin (HgbA1c) is a measurement of the blood glucose bound to Hgb and gives an overall view of the past 120 days of glucose saturation.

Normal Adult Levels

Normal: Less than 5.7%
Prediabetic: 5.7% to 6.4%
Diabetic: 6.5% and higher

Increased glycohemoglobin levels are indicative of several disorders, including but not limited to poorly-controlled diabetes mellitus, iron deficiency anemia, splenectomy, alcohol or lead toxicity, and hyperglycemia. Decreased levels of glycohemoglobin may be indicative of certain diseases, including but not limited to hemolytic anemia, chronic blood loss, chronic renal failure, and pregnancy.

TOXICOLOGY STUDIES AND DRUG SCREENS

Toxicology studies are conducted on blood, primarily serum, and on urine. Blood levels of various medications are checked by toxicology levels to determine whether the medications are at a therapeutic level or approaching or at a toxic level. Blood alcohol levels are the preferred method of screening for blood alcohol content to provide the desired qualitative information. Urine drug screens are used to detect the presence of various drug substances, primarily drugs of common abuse and/or illegal origin, as well as blood alcohol. Drugs detected by urine screening include depressants, hallucinogens, sedatives, and stimulants.

BLOOD SCREENING TESTS

Drug Levels

Common blood serum testing for therapeutic drugs includes, but is not limited to, digoxin, digitoxin, theophylline, lidocaine, lithium, and various drugs for therapeutic or toxic levels.

Digoxin

Digoxin is a cardiac glycoside used to treat CHF and cardiac arrhythmias. Blood level studies produce information about the therapeutic or toxic levels.

Normal Therapeutic Levels

0.8 to 2 ng/ml

Levels above 2.5 ng/ml indicate a toxicity of the drug. Medical intervention is necessary to return to therapeutic levels. Levels below 0.8 ng/ml indicate that more digoxin is necessary to achieve the expected therapy.

Digitoxin

Digitoxin is a cardiac glycoside used to treat CHF and cardiac arrhythmias. Blood level studies provide information about the therapeutic or toxic levels.

Normal Therapeutic Levels

20 to 35 ng/ml

Levels above 35 ng/ml indicate a toxicity of the drug. Medical intervention is necessary to return to therapeutic levels. Levels below 20 ng/ml indicate that more digitoxin is necessary to achieve the expected therapy.

Theophylline

Theophylline, a bronchodilator, is used to treat asthma and obstructive respiratory disorders. Blood level studies give information about the therapeutic or toxic levels.

Normal Therapeutic Levels

10 to 20 µg/ml

Levels above 20 µ/ml indicate a toxicity of the drug. Medical intervention is necessary to return to therapeutic levels. Levels below 8 µg/ml indicate that more theophylline is necessary to achieve the expected therapy.

Lidocaine

Lidocaine is used to treat ventricular arrhythmias. Blood level studies give information about the therapeutic or toxic levels.

Normal Therapeutic Levels

1.5 to 6 µg/ml

Levels above 6 µg/ml indicate a toxicity of the drug. Medical intervention is necessary to return to therapeutic levels. Levels

below 1.5 µg/ml indicate that more lidocaine is necessary to achieve the expected therapy.

Lithium

Lithium is used to treat bipolar disorders.

Normal Therapeutic Levels

0.6 to 1.4 mEq/L

Levels above 1.5 mEq/L indicate a toxicity of the drug. Medical intervention is necessary to return to therapeutic levels. Levels below 0.6 mEq/L indicate that more lithium is necessary to achieve the expected therapy.

Prograf (Tacrolimus)/FK-506

Prograf (Tacrolimus)/FK-506 is an immunosuppressive medication used in patients that have had organ transplants. It is used prophylactically for organ rejection.

Normal Therapeutic Levels

5 to 20 µg/L

Therapeutic levels vary with other factors, such as organ of transplant, length of time with transplant, race, and other medication therapies.

Phenytoin (Dilantin)

Phenytoin (Dilantin) is an anticonvulsant medication used to control seizures.

Normal Therapeutic Levels

10-20 mcg/ml

Levels 30 mcg/ml and above indicate a toxicity of the drug. Medical intervention is necessary to return to therapeutic levels. Levels below 20 mcg/ml indicate more phenytoin is needed to achieve expected therapy.

Alcohol Levels

Normal Levels

0%

States have established blood levels or content of alcohol that are considered "legally drunk or intoxicated." Refer to state guidelines for these levels.

CARDIAC ENZYMES/CARDIAC ISOENZYMES

Cardiac enzymes and isoenzymes are released by the myocardium as a result of an MI. Monitoring the levels of these enzymes helps evaluate the extent of the insult to the myocardium and the progress of the healing process.

C-Reactive Protein

The tissues of the body release C-reactive protein, a protein that can be detected, helping to evaluate the general amount of inflammation in the body. In addition, a high sensitivity

C-reactive protein measures the risk for potential heart problems. Baseline studies are recommended as a reference for future measurement of arterial condition.

Normal Adult Levels

High risk: 0 to 1.0 mg/dl
Low risk: Less than 1.0 mg/dl
Average risk: 1.0 to 3.0 mg/dl
High risk: Greater than 3.0 mg/dl

An elevation may be indicative of MI, rheumatic fever, rheumatoid arthritis, tuberculosis, cancer, pneumococcal pneumonia, SLE, or use of oral contraceptives. This protein is normally elevated in the last half of pregnancy. An inflammation in the body's tissues also must be considered as a source of the elevation.

Creatine Kinase

Creatine kinase (CK), an enzyme found in certain body tissues, becomes elevated with damage to cardiac and skeletal muscles.

Normal Adult Levels

Female: 26 to 140 U/L
Male: 38 to 174 U/L
Values may vary according to the laboratory.

In an MI, levels begin to rise in 4 to 6 hours, peak at 12 to 24 hours, and return to baseline 3 to 5 days after the onset of the MI. The increased levels should be part of the total evaluation to confirm an MI.

Creatine Kinase Isoenzymes

Isoenzymes increase during an MI and are more specific in the diagnosis of an MI.

Normal Values

MM-CK (muscle): 97% to 100%
MB-CK (heart): 0% to 4%
BB-CK (brain): 0%

MB-CK begins to rise within 2 to 6 hours after the myocardial insult; it usually peaks at 15 to 24 hours and then returns to normal within 72 hours.

Lactate Dehydrogenase

LDH, an enzyme found in tissue of the kidney, heart, skeletal muscle, brain, liver, and lung, is released from the cell, increasing serum levels and indicating cellular necrosis.

Normal Values

100 to 250 IU/L
Values may vary according to the laboratory.

Levels of LDH begin to rise at 12 hours post insult, reach a peak at 24 hours, and return to normal later than CK.

Lactate Dehydrogenase Isoenzymes

LDH isoenzymes are found in many body tissues and are released when tissue necrosis occurs. There are five different LDH isoenzymes, and elevation of LDH1 and LDH2 usually point to cardiac involvement and subsequent necrosis of myocardial tissue.

Normal Values: Percentage of Total

LDH1: 17% to 32%
LDH2: 25% to 40%
LDH3: 19% to 27%
LDH4: 5% to 13%
LDH5: 4% to 20%

LDH1 and LDH2 usually are increased in myocardial insult and necrosis. LDH1 will peak first, and then in 48 hours the ratio between LDH1 and LDH2 reverses.

Aspartate Aminotransferase (Serum Glutamic Oxaloacetic Transaminase)

AST (SGOT) is a measurement of enzyme found primarily in heart, liver, and muscle.

Normal Adult Levels

Female: 8 to 20 U/L
Male: 8 to 26 U/L

Elevated AST levels are indicative of many disorders, including but not limited to acute MI, alcoholism, liver disorders, insult and injury to tissue (including trauma and cerebral and pulmonary infarctions), and ingestion of certain drugs. Decreased AST levels are indicative of many disorders, including but not limited to diabetic ketoacidosis, liver disease, uremia, and ingestion of certain drugs.

Alanine Aminotransferase (Serum Glutamic Pyruvate Transaminase)

Alanine aminotransferase (ALT; serum glutamic pyruvate transaminase [SGPT]) evaluates liver insult and is a measurement of an enzyme product found in the liver, certain body fluids, and in the liver, heart, kidneys, pancreas, and musculoskeletal tissue.

Normal Adult Levels

Female: 7 to 35 U/L
Male: 10 to 40 U/L

Elevated ALT levels are indicative of certain disorders, including but not limited to liver insult and liver disease, CHF, muscle injury, MI, pancreatitis, pulmonary embolism, severe burns, trauma, shock, and ingestion of certain drugs. Decreased levels of ALT are not found.

URINE STUDIES

Urinalysis/Clean Catch Urinalysis

A urinalysis/clean catch urinalysis is a physical, chemical, and microscopic analysis of a urine specimen. A clean catch is the method of collection used. Measurements include pH and specific gravity of the urine and presence of ketones, protein, sugars, bilirubin, and urobilinogen. Color and odor are noted, as is the presence of abnormal blood cells, casts, bacteria, other cells, and crystals.

Routine Urinalysis
Normal Characteristics
Color and clarity: Pale to darker yellow and clear
Odor: Aromatic
Chemical nature: pH is generally slightly acidic, 6.5
Specific gravity: 1.003 to 1.030; reflects amount of waste, minerals, and solids in urine

Normal Constituent Compounds
Protein: None or small amount
Glucose: None
Ketone bodies: None
Bile and bilirubin: None
Casts: None or small amount of hyaline casts
Nitrogenous wastes: Ammonia, creatinine, urea, and uric acid
Crystals: None to trace
Fat droplets: None

Refer to Table 11-1 for abnormal findings and related pathology.

Culture and Sensitivity of Urine
Culture
Sample of urine specimen is placed in/on culture medium to see whether microbial growth occurs. If growth occurs, the pathogenic microbe is identified.

Sensitivity
A portion of the specimen is placed on a sensitivity disk (that has been impregnated with specific antibiotics) to determine the antibiotic to which the pathogen is resistant or to which it will be responsive.

Normal Result
No growth

Growth indicates pathogens residing in urinary tract. Sensitivity identifies antimicrobials to which pathogens are sensitive.

CARDIOLOGY TESTS

Electrocardiogram (12 Lead)
A recording of electrical activity of the myocardium used to diagnose ischemia, arrhythmias, conduction difficulties, and activity of cardiac medications.

Normal Result
No dysrhythmias/arrhythmias

A 12-lead electrocardiogram (ECG) consists of three limb leads—I, II, III; three augmented limb leads—aV_R, aV_L, aV_F; and six precordial chest leads—V_1, V_2, V_3, V_4, V_5, and V_6. The conduction of the impulse through the myocardium is traced by three specific areas of the systolic and diastolic complex. The P wave represents atrial depolarization, the conduction of the stimulus from the sinoatrial (SA) node through the atrium to the atrioventricular (AV) node. The QRS complex represents ventricular depolarization, that is, the conduction

of the stimulus from the upper portion of the ventricle and below the AV node through the bundle of His, through the right and left bundle branches, and through the Purkinje fibers, followed by its relay throughout the ventricular myocardium. The T wave represents the repolarization of the ventricular myocardium. The 12-lead ECG is used to detect conduction abnormalities, dysrhythmias, myocardial ischemia, and myocardial damage; to monitor recovery from an MI; and to assist in evaluation of the effectiveness of cardiac medications. Lead II normally is used to evaluate cardiac rhythm. Refer to Table 10-1 for an explanation of cardiac arrhythmias/dysrhythmias.

Echocardiogram
An echocardiogram is an ultrasound (acoustic imaging) examination of the cardiac structure to define the size, shape, thickness, position, and movements of the cardiac structures, including valves, walls, and chambers.

Normal Result
Shows no abnormalities

This noninvasive procedure assists in diagnosing cardiac diseases and disorders, including structural abnormalities, congenital defects, myocardial damage, and blood flow through all structures of the heart.

Cardiac Stress Echocardiogram
A cardiac stress echocardiogram uses ultrasound imaging at rest and then during stress to evaluate the heart's walls, valves, and pumping action. The stress part of this examination can be done two different ways—either (1) by walking on a treadmill or use of a stationary bike or (2) chemically. The chemical agent that can be used to simulate exercise in the body is dobutamine, which is given intravenously. This test is performed in a safe environment and a physician or cardiologist is present, along with a specially trained staff.

Normal Result
Negative
Low risk of cardiac disease
Normal appearance of heart chambers and valves
No significant changes on ECG

Holter Monitor
A Holter monitor is a miniature electrocardiograph that records the electrical activity of the heart for an extended period of time, usually 24 to 48 hours. The patient records all activities during the time period to allow the examiner to correlate activity with cardiac abnormalities.

Cardiac Event Recorders
Cardiac event recorders are battery-powered, portable devices that record electrical activity of the heart while the patient goes about their everyday activities. The monitors record the heart's rate and rhythm. Some monitors are attached to the chest using electrodes, whereas some are placed on the wrist. There are two

types of monitors: (1) the loop memory recorder and (2) the symptom event monitor. The *loop memory recorder* records the ECG for a short period of time. One must push a button when symptoms (such as, faint, dizziness or feeling of irregular heartbeat) occur, and the monitor records the period before and after the event. The *symptom event monitor* is similar to the loop memory recorder in that one must place or activate the recorder during a symptom or event. But unlike the loop recorder, it is unable to record an ECG prior to the event. Both recorders have the capability to be transmitted over the phone to your physician's office. They may be worn for several days to several weeks depending on what your physician determines necessary.

Normal Result

No dysrhythmias
Refer to ECG

Multigated Blood Pool Study Scan

A multigated blood pool study (MUGA) scan is a nuclear medicine scan that assesses the function of the left ventricle, evaluates cardiac output, and identifies abnormalities of the myocardial walls.

Normal Result

50% to 70% ejection fraction
Symmetrical contraction of the left ventricle

A radioactive isotope "tracer" is injected, which attaches to RBCs to show all four chambers and the great vessels simultaneously. A series of images are taken during both systole and diastole, and then either is shown as a movie (or superimposed) to relate ventricular function and to allow the ejection fraction to be calculated. This test may be performed either under stress or without the stress factor.

Cardiac Stress Test (Cardiac Perfusion Scan)

A cardiac stress test (cardiac perfusion scan) is used to detect and evaluate coronary artery disease. This test measures blood flow to the heart during stress and rest. The stress part of this examination can be done two different ways—either (1) by walking on a treadmill or (2) chemically. Chemical agents that can be used to simulate exercise in the body are dobutamine, dipyridamole (Persantine), adenosine, or regadenoson (Lexiscan). Myoview, Cardiolite, and thallium are all radioactive agents used, and this test may be referred to accordingly. This test is performed in a safe environment, and a physician or cardiologist is present, along with a specially trained staff.

Normal Result

Good blood flow during both resting and exercise portion
   of test
No coronary blockage

Exercise Tolerance Test

An exercise tolerance test is an assessment of cardiac function during moderate exercise on a treadmill or stationary bicycle

after a 12-lead ECG. No chemical agent is used to stress the heart during exercise.

Normal Result

Negative

The stress test measures the effects of exercise on myocardial output and oxygen consumption by the concurrent evaluation of the monitored ECG and oxygen consumption. This test is performed in a safe environment to identify individuals who are prone to myocardial ischemia during activity.

Hepatobiliary (Gallbladder) Scan with Ejection Fraction

A hepatobiliary (HIDA; or gallbladder) scan with ejection fraction is a nuclear imaging scan used to evaluate the gallbladder and the ducts leading into and out of the gallbladder.

Normal Result

Negative scan
Ejection fraction: 30% to 50%

Pulse Oximeter

A pulse oximeter is an instrument (spectrophotometer) that provides a noninvasive measurement of the oxygen saturation of the arterial blood.

Normal Result

Arterial blood oxygen saturation: 95% or greater

Cardiac Catheterization

Cardiac catheterization is the fluoroscopic visualization of the right or left side of the heart by passing a catheter into the right or left chambers and injecting dye. In angiograms, the catheter is passed into the coronary vessels, where the dye is injected and fluoroscopic images are recorded.

Normal Result

Varies with the area being assessed
Indicates normal anatomy and physiology, normal chamber
   volumes and pressures, normal wall and valve motion,
   and normal patent coronary arteries

Normal Value for Cardiac Output

5 to 8 L/min

IMAGING STUDIES

Radiographs

Radiographs show a visualization of internal organs and structures by electromagnetic radiation. Radiographs of bone; the abdomen; the chest; paranasal sinuses; kidneys, ureters, and bladder (KUB); and mammograms do not require contrast medium. Contrast medium is used to distinguish soft tissue and some organs (such as, the gallbladder, esophagus, stomach, and small and large intestines). Normal results vary with the area being studied by the imaging process. The imaging is interpreted by the radiologist with a report and then dictated and transcribed for the ordering physician. The ordering physician often visually inspects the films or images to evaluate the area himself or herself.

Magnetic Resonance Imaging/Magnetic Resonance Angiogram Scan

A magnetic resonance imaging (MRI)/magnetic resonance angiogram (MRA) scan uses a magnetic field instead of radiation to visualize internal tissues. It is possible to view tissue and organs in three dimensions with MRI. An MRA scan is used to examine major blood vessels in the body and to study the condition of blood vessels to detect tumors, to differentiate healthy and diseased tissues, and to detect sites of infection. It helps determine blood flow to tissues and organs. The patient is not exposed to ionizing radiation during MRI. A contrast material (gadolinium) may be required for some examinations. Gadolinium does not contain iodine and is given intravenously. It is important to screen patients before the scan to see if they have any metal implants or pacemaker, if they work with metal shavings, or if they are claustrophobic.

Normal results vary with the area being studied during the MRI scan. The MRI scan is interpreted by the radiologist with a report, and then dictated and transcribed for the ordering physician. The ordering physician may ask to see the films so that he or she may evaluate the area of concern.

Computerized Tomography Scan

A computerized tomography (CT) scan is a radiographic technique using a scanner system that can provide images of the internal structure of tissue and organs both geographically and characteristically. Depending on the area to be scanned and the reason indicated for the scan, oral and/or intravenous (IV) contrast may be required. Iodinated contrast can result in nephrotoxicity and renal failure, and therefore, it is important to screen patients before they receive IV contrast. Any patient receiving IV contrast should be screened for the following risks:

- History of kidney disease; including tumor, surgery to kidneys, or transplant
- Myeloma
- Diabetes
- Potentially nephrotoxic medications (e.g., metformin, chemotherapy, and/or long-term use of nonsteroidal antiinflammatory drugs [NSAIDs])
- 70 years of age and older

If there are any of these risk factors, a serum creatinine level is needed to assess the glomerular filtration rate (GFR). If GFR is below 45 mn/min/1.73 m^2, intervention may be required before receiving contrast to protect the kidneys.

Normal results vary with the area being studied during the CT scan. The scan is interpreted by the radiologist with a report, and then dictated and transcribed for the ordering physician. The ordering physician often visually inspects the films or images of the CT scan to evaluate the area.

Fluoroscopy

A real-time imaging process, fluoroscopy provides continuous visualization of the area being imaged. Films are made of the process for more extensive examination. Fluoroscopy is used in procedures and to study the functioning of tissues and organs.

Normal results vary with the area being studied during fluoroscopy. The procedure is interpreted by the radiologist with a report, and then dictated and transcribed for the ordering physician. The ordering physician often performs a procedure using fluoroscopy as a diagnostic tool and also as a guide for the procedure.

Sonogram, Ultrasound, and Echogram

Sonograms, ultrasounds, and echograms all use an imaging system that projects a beam of sound waves into target tissues or organs and receives the waves as they bounce back off the target structure. An outline of the structure is produced and recorded on film for examination. Tissues, organs, and systems that may be studied by ultrasound include, but are not limited to, abdominal aorta, brain, breast, gallbladder, pelvis for gynecologic and obstetric diagnostic examination, heart, kidneys, liver, lymph nodes, pancreas, prostate, spleen, thyroid, urinary bladder, and upper GI tract.

Normal Result

Varies with the area being examined

The ultrasound scan is interpreted by the radiologist with a report, and then dictated and transcribed for the ordering physician. The ordering physician may request to visually inspect the films or images of the ultrasound to evaluate the area himself or herself.

Myelogram

A myelogram is an imaging examination of the spinal cord and spinal nerve roots. Contrast medium (dye) or air is injected into the subarachnoid space and recorded on radiographic film. Fluoroscopy generally is used in this procedure.

Normal Result

Reveals no lesions or abnormalities

It is used to diagnose ruptured or bulging disks, spinal cord lesions and tumors, spinal cord and spinal nerve trauma and edema, and other conditions involving the spinal cord and spinal nerves.

Positron Emission Tomography Scan

A molecular imaging study indicates how the organs and tissues are actually functioning. It measures blood flow, oxygen use, and sugar metabolism. It is used to diagnose a variety of diseases, including many types of cancers, heart disease, and certain brain abnormalities and CNS disorders. It is also helpful in assessing the effectiveness of cancer therapy.

A radioactive material called a *radiotracer* is injected intravenously or sometimes inhaled as a gas. The energy that the tracer gives off is then detected and recorded by the gamma camera and positron emission tomography (PET) scanner, and with the aid of a computer, three-dimensional images are created.

Results are interpreted by a nuclear radiologist who has received specialized training in nuclear medicine and are available in 2 to 3 days. Standardized uptake value (SUV) is the amount of chemical activity in a certain spot and assists the radiologist in their interpretation. Generally speaking, cancer has an SUV greater than 2.5. However, there are many other factors and variables that are taken into consideration by the physician.

STOOL ANALYSIS

Hemoccult/Guaiac Test

The hemoccult/guaiac test looks for hidden (occult) blood in a stool sample. It is a qualitative detection of RBCs in the stool.

Normal Result

Negative

Presence of blood in the stool specimen is indicative of trauma, lesion, or other insult to the GI mucosa, producing blood.

Ova, Larva, and Parasite Tests

Ova, larva, and parasite tests are microscopic examinations of stool to detect the presence of parasites at various stages of development.

Normal Result

None detected

A positive examination result indicates parasitic infection of the GI tract.

ENDOSCOPY TESTS

Endoscopy

Endoscopy is the visual inspection of internal organs or cavities of the body through the use of a fiberoptic instrument with the appropriate scope. In addition, pathology may be removed and insult to the tissue may be repaired during the diagnostic procedure.

Esophagogastroduodenoscopy/Upper Endoscopy

Esophagogastroduodenoscopy (EGD)/upper endoscopy is a visualization of the esophagus, stomach, and duodenum in a single procedure using an endoscope. Biopsies and endoscopic therapies, such as esophageal dilation, may be performed.

Normal Result

Appearance of esophagus, stomach, and duodenum within normal limits

Abnormal findings may include, but are not limited to, hiatal hernia, Barrett esophagus, gastroesophageal reflux disease (GERD), esophagitis, and ulcers.

Esophagoscopy

Esophagoscopy is a visualization of the esophagus using an esophagoscope.

Normal Result

Appearance of the esophagus mucosa normal

Foreign bodies may be visualized and removed. Inflammation may be noted and biopsies can be taken.

Gastroscopy

Gastroscopy is a visualization of the stomach by a gastroscope.

Normal Result

Appearance of upper GI tract within normal limits

Hemorrhagic areas or erosion of a vessel may be revealed. Additional abnormal findings may include neoplasm, gastric ulcers, hiatal hernia, gastritis, and esophagitis.

Colonoscopy

Colonoscopy is a visualization of the colon with a colonoscope.

Normal Result

Appearance of large intestinal mucosa normal

Inflammation, areas of ulceration, bleeding areas, strictures, polyps, colitis, diverticula, benign or malignant tumors, or foreign bodies may be observed in abnormal findings.

Sigmoidoscopy

Sigmoidoscopy is a visualization of the sigmoid portion of the colon and the rectum with a sigmoidoscope.

Normal Result

Normal appearance of mucosa of sigmoid colon

Inflammatory bowel disease, polyps, benign and cancerous tumors, and foreign bodies may be some of the abnormal findings during a sigmoidoscope examination.

Proctoscopy

Proctoscopy is a visualization of the rectum with a proctoscope.

Normal Result

Normal appearance to rectal mucosa and to anal canal

Rectal prolapse, hemorrhoids, rectal strictures, fissures, abscesses, and fistulas are some of the abnormal findings during a proctoscopic examination of the rectum.

Cystoscopy

Cystoscopy is a visualization of the structures of the urinary tract with a cystoscope.

Normal Result

Urethra, urethral orifices, urinary bladder interior, and male prostatic urethra appear normal

Cancer of the bladder, benign prostatic hyperplasia (BPH), bladder calculi, prostatitis, ureteral strictures, urinary fistulas, vesicle neck stenosis, ureterocele, polyps, and abnormal bladder capacity are some of the abnormal findings during a cystoscopic examination of the urinary bladder.

Ureteroscopy

Ureteroscopy is a visualization of the ureters and pelvis of the kidney.

Normal Result

Normal appearance of the ureters and pelvis of the kidney and its structures

Renal or ureteral stones, inflammation or bleeding of the urethral mucosa, and lesions or abnormal structures of the renal pelvis are some of the abnormal findings in a ureteroscopic examination.

Bronchoscopy

Bronchoscopy is visualization of the trachea and bronchi with a bronchoscope.

Normal Result

Nasopharynx, larynx, trachea, and bronchi are normal in appearance

Abnormalities revealed in a bronchoscopic examination include, but are not limited to, bronchitis, carcinoma and other tumors, inflammatory processes, tuberculosis, abnormal structure and disorders of the larynx and trachea, foreign bodies, and various pulmonary infections.

Arthroscopy

Arthroscopy is visualization or inspection of the inner aspect of a joint with an endoscope called an *arthroscope*. Biopsy specimens may be obtained.

Normal Result

Normal appearance of the inner aspect of the joint

Abnormal findings in the knee may include tears of meniscus, bone or cartilage fragments, and damage to other structures within the joint. Surgical repair may be attempted. Refer to Chapter 7 for additional information on arthroscopy.

ARTERIAL BLOOD GASES

Arterial Blood Gas Analysis

Arterial blood gas (ABG) analysis is a measurement of dissolved oxygen and carbon dioxide in arterial blood. It is also a measurement of pH and oxygen saturation of the arterial blood. ABGs are used to assess oxygenation and ventilation, along with acid-base balance. In addition, they produce information about the effectiveness of therapy and the status of critical patients and are used in conjunction with pulmonary function studies.

Normal values are listed; however, these studies are complex and require interpretation by a physician, along with other diagnostic studies and consideration of symptoms and signs to produce a diagnosis or an evaluation.

Normal Adult Values

Acidity (pH): 7.35 to 7.45
Carbon dioxide tension (PaCO$_2$): 35 to 45 mm Hg
Arterial oxygen tension (PaO$_2$): 75 to 100 mm Hg
Amount of bicarbonate (HCO$_3$) in the blood: 22 to 30 mEq/L
Oxygen (O$_2$) saturation: 95% to 100%

Increased pH is indicative of several disorders, including but not limited to alkali ingestion, diarrhea, vomiting, hyperventilation, high-altitude sickness, metabolic acidosis, fever, and ingestion of certain drugs. Decreased pH is indicative of several disorders, including but not limited to asthma, COPD, cardiac

disease, MI, renal disorders, pulmonary disorders, respiratory acidosis, sepsis, shock, and malignant hyperthermia.

Increased PaCO$_2$ is indicative of several disorders, including but not limited to late-stage asthma, brain death, CHF, respiratory disorders, hypoventilation, renal disorders, poisoning, pneumothorax, respiratory acidosis, near drowning, and ingestion of certain drugs. Decreased PaCO$_2$ is indicative of several disorders, including but not limited to early-stage asthma, hyperventilation, dysrhythmias, respiratory alkalosis, metabolic acidosis, and ingestion of certain drugs.

Increased PaO$_2$ is indicative of, but not limited to, hyperventilation and hyperbaric oxygen exposure. Decreased PaO$_2$ is indicative of several disorders, including but not limited to acute respiratory distress syndrome (ARDS), asthma, cardiac disorders, head injury, anoxia, hypoventilation, respiratory disorders, pneumothorax, respiratory failure, shock, smoke inhalation, and CVA.

Increased O$_2$ saturation is indicative of hyperbaric oxygenation. Decreased O$_2$ saturation is indicative of several disorders, including but not limited to anoxia, cardiac anomalies and disorders, carbon monoxide poisoning, adult respiratory distress syndrome (ARDS), CVA, hypoventilation, respiratory disorders, pneumothorax, shock, smoke inhalation, and near drowning.

PULMONARY FUNCTION STUDIES

Pulmonary function studies are complex and include evaluation of results from several tests. Most tests are performed by respiratory therapists and can be done with or without bronchodilators. Results usually are reported to a pulmonologist for evaluation and correlation with symptoms and signs. Normal values are reported here; however, the significance of these values is incomplete without the review and opinion of the pulmonologist, which is often assisted by the respiratory therapist.

Pulse Oximeter

A pulse oximeter is an instrument (spectrophotometer) that produces a noninvasive measurement of the oxygen saturation of the arterial blood.

Normal Result

Arterial blood oxygen saturation 95% or greater

Peak Flow

Peak flow is a measurement of inspiratory effort.

Normal Result

Approximately 300 L/min
Based on sex, height, and age

Spirometry

Spirometry is a measurement of lung capacity, volume, and flow rates used in the evaluation of asthma, bronchitis, COPD, and emphysema.

Methacholine Challenge

Methacholine challenge is a measurement of lung volumes before and after inhalation of methacholine chloride, which is used for diagnosis of asthma.

Normal Result

Negative

Sputum Studies

Sputum studies are analyses and cultures of sputum (material expelled from the respiratory tract) to detect the presence of pathogens. Common studies ordered on sputum include cytology testing, gram stain, and culture and sensitivity.

Normal Result

Negative

Positive results might include respiratory disorders, such as fungal infections, mycobacteria, tuberculosis, or carcinoma.

Pulmonary Function

Normal findings are reported in percentages of observed values and by expected values calculated to include allowances for age, sex, weight, and height. Abnormal results are considered to be less than 80% of calculated values. Consult a respiratory therapist or pulmonologist for interpretation of values.

Normal Values

Tidal volume: 500 ml
Expiratory reserve volume: 1500 ml
Residual volume: 1500 ml
Inspiratory reserve volume: 2000 ml

MISCELLANEOUS TESTS

Culture and Sensitivity Studies

For culture and sensitivity studies, specimens are obtained from various tissues and fluids of the body, placed on or in a medium to grow, and then studied for microbes present. The specimens are also placed on a disk impregnated with various antibiotics to determine which antibiotic will be effective in destroying or curbing the reproduction of the microbe.

Tissues and fluids include blood, sputum, cerebrospinal fluid (CSF), urine, exudates from lesions, nasal secretions, stool, wound drainage, and any excised tissue.

Normal Result

No growth

The growth of any microbes requires microscopic identification. The antibiotic-impregnated disk requires inspection and identification of antibiotics showing effectiveness against the microbes.

Bone Marrow Studies

For bone marrow studies, aspiration of bone marrow is obtained by needle from the sternum, posterior superior iliac spine, or the anterior iliac crest for diagnosis of neoplasms, metastasis, and blood disorders. Bone marrow studies produce a basis for evaluation of hematologic disorders and infectious diseases.

Immune and Immunoglobulin Studies

Immune and immunoglobulin studies examine the functioning and malfunctioning of the immune system.

Normal Adult Levels

Immunoglobulin A (IgA): 60 to 400 mg/dl
Immunoglobulin G (IgG): 700 to 1600 mg/dl
Immunoglobulin M (IgM): 40 to 230 mg/dl
Immunoglobulin D (IgD): 0.13 to 15.27 mg/dl
Immunoglobulin E (IgE): 3 to 42 IU/ml

Increased levels of immunoglobulins are indicative of many disorders and need to be evaluated by a physician. Some disorders include arthritis, cancer, chronic infections, sinusitis, asthma, food and drug allergies, liver disease, SLE, and ingestion of certain drugs. Decreased levels of immunoglobulins are indicative of many disorders, including but not limited to AIDS, bacterial infection, advanced cancer, hypogammaglobulinemia, and ingestion of certain drugs.

Biopsies

Biopsies are the excision of tissue from the living body, followed by microscopic examination, for purpose of exact diagnosis.

Normal Result

No abnormal cells seen

Abnormal findings depend on cell structure discovered during microscopic examination.

Lumbar Puncture

Lumbar puncture is a surgical procedure to withdraw spinal fluid for analysis. It is a measurement and analysis of the chemical components of the CSF used in diagnosis of CNS diseases and disorders.

Normal Adult Results

Appearance: Clear, colorless
Specific gravity: 1.006 to 1.009
Pressure: 90 to 180 mm H_2O
AST: 05 to 35 U
Bicarbonate: 22.9 mEq/L
WBC count: 0.0 to 0.8 mm^3
Glucose: 40 to 80 mg/dl
Total protein: 15 to 45 mg/dl
Lactic acid: 10 to 24 mg/dl
Venereal Disease Research Laboratory (VDRL): Negative
    titer for syphilis
Bacteria or viruses: None present

Pressure depends on height and whether patient is positioned in a sitting or horizontal position.

Abnormal findings are indicative of disorders or insults to the CNS.

Electroencephalogram

An electroencephalogram (EEG) is a recording of the electrical activity of the brain. A neurologist interprets the brain wave activity to determine presence of a neurologic disorder or any other medical condition.

Normal Result

Shows symmetric patterns of electrical brain activity

Abnormal findings include information indicative of CNS or brain insults, hematomas, CVAs, epilepsy, brain tumors, and seizure activity. Lack of any activity is an indication of brain death.

Electromyelography

Electromyelography (EMG) is an electrodiagnostic assessment and recording of the electrical activity of skeletal muscle at rest and contraction. It is a nerve conduction study used to assess the speed and strength in which the nerves can send the electrical signals. EMG tests and nerve conduction tests are often done in combination with each other.

Normal Result

Nerve conduction normal
Muscle action potential normal

Abnormal findings help to identify the site and cause of muscle disorders and neuronal lesions, particularly of involvement of the anterior horn of the spinal cord.

Gastric Analysis

Gastric analysis is used in the diagnosis of pernicious anemia and peptic ulcers. The contents of the stomach are analyzed for acidity, appearance, and volume.

Normal Adult Levels

Bile: 0 or minimal
Mucus: Evenly mixed
Blood: 0 or scant
Fasting acidity: 2.5 mEq/L
Quantity: 62 ml/hr
pH: 1.5 to 3.5

Increased levels of gastric acid are indicative of certain disorders, including but not limited to status post small-intestinal resection, gastric or duodenal ulcer, hyperplasia, and hyperfunction of gastric cells. Reduced gastric acid levels are indicative of several disorders, including but not limited to pernicious anemia, status post vagotomy, renal failure, rheumatoid arthritis, gastric cancer, and atrophic gastritis.

Human Chorionic Gonadotropin

Human chorionic gonadotropin (hCG) is used in diagnosis of pregnancy, abortion, ectopic pregnancy, and uterine pathology.

Normal Result

Negative

A positive result is indicative of pregnancy, either intrauterine or ectopic.

SCREENING

Tuberculosis Screening (Mantoux)

An intradermal injection of tuberculin is given, usually on the inner aspect of the lower arm. Results are read in 48 and 72 hours.

Normal Result

Negative

Positive Result

Red, raised, hardened area at injection site, which measures 10 mm induration or greater

Positive reaction requires further investigation, usually including a chest radiograph.

Cancer or Tumor Markers as Screening Tools

Certain substances are produced by some tumors or cancer, including enzymes, antigens, and hormones. These substances may be present in the blood in higher-than-normal levels and may be an indication of the presence of a tumor. Cancer or tumor markers cannot be used alone to diagnose the presence of cancer or a tumor. Some benign tumors may stimulate the production of these markers. In addition, elevated cancer markers are not always present, especially in the early stages of the disease process. Some physicians track the progress of tumor growth, as well as using them to measure the effectiveness of treatment and for possible recurrence of the tumor. There are several markers, and many are specific in nature. The most widely used screening tool of this nature is the prostate-specific antigen (PSA). Other markers include CA 125, carcinoembryonic antigen, alpha-fetoprotein (AFP), CA 19-9, CA 15-3, and the Pap smear.

Prostate-Specific Antigen

A serum blood test used to determine the level of the PSA. This is a screening test that should be followed by a digital rectal examination (DRE) of the prostate gland to identify any abnormalities. Additional diagnostic studies often are indicated.

PSA blood tests are reported as nanograms per milliliter.

PSA is considered a marker in the screening for prostatic cancer. Zero to 4 ng/ml usually is considered to be in the normal range; 4 to 10 ng/ml is considered borderline; values greater than 10 ng/ml are considered high. Increasing age makes slightly higher values acceptable:

- 40 to 49 years: 0 to 2.5 ng/ml
- 50 to 59 years: 0 to 3.5 ng/ml
- 60 to 69 years: 0 to 4.5 ng/ml
- 70 to 79 years: 0 to 6.5 ng/ml

Any increase of 20% or more in the PSA value in 1 year is suspicious and requires further investigation. Above-acceptable levels may be indicative of cancer. Additional investigation, including biopsy, is recommended.

The PSA screening should be completed before the DRE. A constant increase in the PSA leads to suspicion of prostate cancer. PSA levels that fluctuate up and down usually are not indicative of cancer but of an inflammatory process in the prostate or of BPH. PSA is a screening tool and must be combined with a DRE for a more accurate screen. Men older than 50 years of age are encouraged to have prostate screening on an annual basis; men older than 70 years of age may or may not be subjected to screening because of the high incidence of prostatic cancer in this group and the treatment protocol of watchful waiting without significant intervention.

CA 125

CA 125 may reflect an increase in production of a marker that may be indicative of cancer of the ovaries.

Normal Levels

<35 U/ml (conventional units)

An elevation above normal may be indicative of cancer of the ovaries, pelvic organs (including the uterus and cervix), pancreas, liver, breasts, colon, lung, and digestive tract.

CA 19-9

CA 19-9 may reflect an increase in marker levels in the presence of colorectal cancer.

Normal Levels

<37 U/ml (conventional units)

An elevation may be indicative of the presence of colorectal, pancreatic, stomach, and bile duct cancer.

CA 15-3

CA 15-3 may reflect an increase in marker levels in the presence of breast cancer.

Normal Levels

<35 U/ml (conventional units)

An elevation may be indicative of the presence of breast cancer, benign conditions of breast and ovarian disease, PID, endometriosis, pregnancy, lactation, and hepatitis.

Carcinoembryonic Antigen

Carcinoembryonic antigen may be elevated in some people without any form of cancer. This test is used to monitor the spread or metastasis of colorectal cancer and other cancers.

Reference value varies with the health of the individual as well as the smoking history and the presence of existing intestinal or other disease processes. A baseline should be established and monitored for effectiveness of treatment or exacerbation of the condition.

Alpha-Fetoprotein

Under normal circumstances, AFP is produced by the developing fetus with maternal levels decreasing after birth. However, certain conditions involving the fetus may cause an abnormal elevation of this protein as pregnancy progresses, suggesting a possible neural tube deficit or other anomaly in the developing fetus. A maternal AFP level that does not return to normal after parturition is an indication of possible liver or germ cell cancer that demands additional testing.

To compare or confirm normal values for amniotic fluid levels as well as blood serum AFP levels, check with reference laboratory for their normal levels.

Elevations in maternal serum levels and amniotic fluid may be indicative of neural tube deficits, including in the nonpregnant female and the male population.

Papanicolaou (Pap) Smear

A Papanicolaou (Pap) smear is a cytologic examination of cells that have been scraped or aspirated from the cervix and cervical os. A screening test is recommended every 2 to 3 years, and a pelvic exam is recommended yearly.

Results of Pap smears are now reported in two different formats. The two methods of reporting results to the physician are: (1) a system based on classes and (2) the Bethesda system, which is a system using descriptive diagnostic terms.

Class System

The system based on classes used to report Pap smear results to the physician is:

- Class I: Negative with no abnormal or unusual cells seen.
- Class II: Negative smear—but with some reservation based on the presence of inflammatory cells or evidence of infection. Additional causes may be regeneration of cervical cells or changes related to trauma, infections, or childbirth. A repeat Pap smear and treatment of the underlying cause may be indicated.
- Class III: Presence of some abnormal cells that may be considered premalignant. Changes may vary from mild dysplasia to severe dysplasia. Further evaluation is indicated, possibly including colposcopy.
- Class IV: Indicative of a high degree of suspicion for malignancy. Prompt and complete evaluation is indicated.
- Class V: Indication of high probability of more extensive malignancy. Prompt and complete evaluation to determine the extent of disease is indicated.

Bethesda System

When using the Bethesda system, the physician may relate the results as normal or abnormal because surface cervical cells may appear abnormal but are not always malignant.

The descriptive diagnostic terms are as follows:

- Dysplasia: Although not cancer, dysplasia may develop into very early cancer of the cervix. The cells in dysplasia undergo a series of changes in their appearance, appear abnormal in microscopic examination, and have not invaded nearby healthy tissue. The cells are described as mild, moderate, or severe according to their appearance under the microscope.
- Squamous intraepithelial lesion (SIL): Describes the appearance of abnormal changes on the surface of the cervix. SIL cells are classified further as low grade, having early changes in size, shape, and number, or high grade, containing a large number of precancerous cells with an appearance very different from normal cells.
- Cervical intraepithelial neoplasia (CIN): A description of a new abnormal growth of surface layers of cells. Additional

information is provided by using CIN and the numbers 1, 2, and 3 to describe how much of the cervix contains abnormal cells.

- Carcinoma *in situ*: Refers to a preinvasive cancer that has not invaded deeper tissues and contains only surface cells.
- Atypical glandular cells of undetermined significance (AGC-US): Describe slightly abnormal glandular cells of the cervix.
- Atypical squamous cells of undetermined significance (ASC-US): Describe slightly abnormal squamous cells of the cervix, possibly caused by a vaginal infection or by human papillomavirus (HPV).
- Inflammation: Inflammation is present in the cervical cells, and WBCs also are seen.
- Hyperkeratosis: Hyperkeratosis describes dried skin cells on the cervix, often resulting from cervical cap or diaphragm usage or a cervical infection.

Abnormal results range from insignificant to precancerous to invasive cancer of the cervix. Repeat Pap smears in 6 months are often all that is indicated for mild dysplasia and class II Pap smears. Colposcopy and further investigation may be indicated in other abnormal findings. The physician discusses abnormal findings with the patient, and a course of treatment or follow-up is determined.

Mammogram

A mammogram is a radiographic examination of the soft tissues of the breast. This is a screening test performed on an annual basis for women older than 40 years of age to detect the presence of breast disease. This screening should be accompanied by a manual examination of the breast tissue by a physician. Monthly breast self-examinations are recommended.

Normal Result

Negative for disease

Identification of abnormal conditions may indicate further investigation. Various benign disorders, including fibrocystic disease of the breast, calcifications, and asymmetric densities may be responsible for a positive interpretation and require additional mammogram views with ultrasound. It may also be recommended that in 6 months, a repeat mammogram and/or ultrasound be done to follow up on any abnormality. An ultrasound-guided breast biopsy or stereotactic breast biopsy may be indicated to confirm presence of a malignant neoplasm.